WL
141
C738
1981

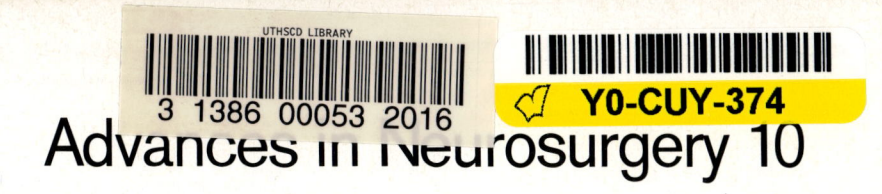

Advances in Neurosurgery 10

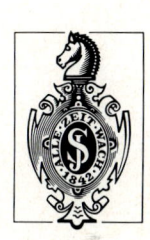

Computerized Tomography
Brain Metabolism
Spinal Injuries

Edited by
W. Driesen   M. Brock   M. Klinger

With 186 Figures and 75 Tables

Springer-Verlag
Berlin Heidelberg New York 1982

Proceedings of the 32nd Annual Meeting of the
Deutsche Gesellschaft für Neurochirurgie
Tübingen, April 22–25, 1981

ISBN 3-540-11115-8 Springer-Verlag Berlin Heidelberg New York
ISBN 0-387-11115-8 Springer-Verlag New York Heidelberg Berlin

Library of Congress Cataloging in Publication Data
Deutsche Gesellschaft für Neurochirurgie. Tagung (32nd: 1981: Tübingen, Germany)
Computerized tomography, brain metabolism, spinal injuries. (Advances in neurosurgery; 10)
"Proceedings of the 32nd Annual Meeting of the Deutsche Gesellschaft für Neurochirurgie,
Tübingen, April 22–25, 1981" – T.p. verso. Includes bibliographies and index.
1. Nervous system-Surgery-Congresses. 2. Tomography-Congresses. 3. Brain-Congresses.
4. Spine-Wounds and injuries-Complications and sequelae-Congresses. I. Driesen, W.
(Wilhelm), 1921-. II. Brock, M. (Mario), 1938-. III. Klinger, M. (Margareta), 1943-. IV. Title.
V. Series [DNLM: 1. Brain-Metabolism-Congresses. 2. Brain-Radiography-Congresses.
3. Neurosurgery-Congresses. 4. Spinal injuries-Congresses. 5. Tomography, X-ray
computed-Congresses. WI AD684 v.10 / WL 141 D486 1981c]   RD593.D47   1981   617'.48
82-3223   ISBN 0-387-11115-8 (U.S.)   AACR2

This work is subject to copyright. All rights are reserved, whether the whole or part of the
material is concerned, specifically those of translation, reprinting, re-use of illustrations,
broadcasting, reproduction by photocopying machine or similar means, and storage in
data banks. Under § 54 of the German Copyright Law, where copies are made for other
than private use, a fee is payable to 'Verwertungsgesellschaft Wort', Munich.

© by Springer-Verlag Berlin Heidelberg 1982
Printed in Germany

The use of registered names, trademarks, etc. in this publication does not imply, even in
the absence of a specific statement, that such names are exempt from the relevant protective laws and regulations and therefore free for general use.

Offsetprinting and Binding: Beltz Offsetdruck, Hemsbach/Bergstr.
2122/3140-543210

Preface

W. DRIESEN

This volume contains the original text of 60 papers delivered at the 32nd Annual Meeting of the German Society for Neurosurgery, held in Tübingen, 22nd to 25th April, 1981. They represent a selection from 91 papers submitted, a third of which had to be excluded on critical analysis. This was deemed necessary on account of costs, and in order to keep the volume of a size and standard usually achieved within the last few years.

Three main subjects were considered:
1. changes in methods of investigation and treatment of neurosurgical conditions, brought about by the use of computerised axial tomography (C.A.T. scanning);
2. papers dealing with fundamental research concerned with normal and abnormal cerebral metabolism;
3. trauma to the vertebral column and spinal cord, and its sequelae; and,
4. free communications.

The organisers of this meeting tried, in contradistinction to previous custom, to shift the emphasis away from highlighting major communications, and so to remain true to their intention to allow experts in their fields to introduce their subjects and pin-point problems, to which subsequent speakers could then address themselves in detail in their own papers. In my view, this did occur in a meaningful way, although not to perfection; a goal always difficult to attain.

As so often happens, a great pioneer in neurological surgery, OTFRID FOERSTER, was remembered and honoured. The OTFRID FOERSTER Medal was presented to H. KUHLENDAHL, Director Emeritus of the Neurosurgical Clinic in Düsseldorf, for his services to Neurosurgery and its development in Germany and Europe. Professor KUHLENDAHL then gave the OTFRID FOERSTER Memorial Lecture, in which he emphasised particularly how his life's work was dominated by study of the functional anatomy and clinical pathophysiology of the nervous system.

Later in life, OTFRID FOERSTER was concerned to put into practice what he had learned, and to develop neurological surgery. OTFRID FOERSTER taught himself the techniques of modern neurosurgery. KUHLENDAHL drew attention to FOERSTER's theories about the biomechanics of the central nervous system. Encapsulated within the hollow skull and vertebral column, the C.N.S. presents a model for research concerning biomechanical factors affecting internal organs. Trauma and disease processes may deform or destroy the brain, the spinal cord and the peripheral nerves. These neural structures may tolerate such insults up to a point without functional loss, but beyond that point such loss occurs, and neurological deficit will be detected by the trained observer. (H. KUHLENDAHL is of the opinion that currently too much neurosurgery is undertaken, and some of it attempts to be too subtle; this is due to the fact that even modern methods of investigation cannot, as yet, take account of all the biomechanical and neuropathological processes. The writer concurs with this opinion of FOERSTER and KUHLENDAHL, namely: Neurosurgery is the logical extension of Neurology, only employing different techniques).

For our first main subject: "Changes in methods of investigation and treatment due to the use of C.A.T. scanning", we had papers from experts in their fields. It is not the ease alone that is remarkable with which the C.A.T. scan can detect intracranial disease processes from their inception, and sometimes reveal their pathology, but also that diagnosis can be achieved at a single session, and, in addition, its great advantage accrues from the fact that it can be repeated with little risk and inconvenience to the patient to check the results of surgery, whether it has been successful or not, and if not, whether mistakes or complications require further intervention. Neurosurgeons are facing, in the C.A.T. scan, a task-master reminding them of their commitment to great care and attention to technical detail, and to humility in the evaluation of their results.

The second main theme, concerning cerebral metabolism, was found to present a broad field. New discoveries are the basis of further research, both in neurology and neurosurgery. The subject is wide open, and interest spans from oxidative cerebral metabolism and sphingolipids, catecholamines, cortisol and prolactins, to metabolic processes involving cell volume and oxygen exchange of in vitro cultures of glial and neural cells.

From our third main theme, no new fundamental concepts were disclosed regarding spinal cord and vertebral column trauma. Improvements in the techniques for stabilisation of the injured vertebral column were noted and found to be efficient. Several authors reported new methods of internal fixation of the vertebral column in its various sections from the neck to the pelvis. Successes are recorded which would have been impossible without the use of "plates", the component materials of which are accepted by the body. We are still a long way from seeing recovery following destructive lesions of the spinal cord, owing to lack of fundamental biological knowledge.

Fourthly, the free communications were notable for the new light they threw on problems of regional cerebral blood flow following microvascular anastomosis, using diaphanoscopy, Doppler, measurement of temperature of the cerebral cortex, inhalation methods employing Xenon 133. A paper from our clinic was of interest, inasmuch as it demonstrated that following micro-vascular anastomoses, thrombi could develop at the suture line, and, as we know, can be detected as emboli in the area of distribution of the vessel in question. Other papers emphasized the possibility of immediate discovery of air embolism in the sitting position. We all hope that, after further perusal of the papers and their linguistic corrections, this Volume 10 of Advances in Neurosurgery will, through the good offices of the Springer Verlag, be published soon, in the usual high quality and standard we have come to expect from our publishers.

We should like to express our sincere thanks to all concerned.

Contents

H. Kuhlendahl: Patho-Biomechanik - die neue nosogenetische Dimension am Zentralnervensystem Otfrid-Foerster-Gedenkvorlesung, Tübingen 24.4.1981 XV

Computerized Tomography

W. Kluge and C. Sprung: Has Computed Tomography Led to Earlier Diagnosis of Brain Tumors? 3

H.-U. Thal, A. Wanis, U. Pasch, and M. Weizsäcker: Conflicting Neuropathological and Computertomographic Findings in Cases of Suspected Brain Tumors or Retrobulbar Tumors 7

W. Haßler, J. Gilsbach, W. Birg, H.-R. Eggert, and W. Seeger: Computer Tomographic Findings of Brain Tumors Projected on X-Rays and Scalp 11

F. Mundinger and W. Birg: Stereotactic Brain Surgery with the Aid of Computed Tomography (CT-Stereotaxy) 17

H.C. Nahser, H.-E. Nau, L. Gerhard, W. Grote, and V. Reinhardt: Necessity for Biopsy After the Introduction of Computerized Tomography 25

W. Huk and M. Klinger: The Value of Computerized Tomography in the Preoperative Diagnosis of Brain Tumors 33

H. Arnold and D. Kühne: Metrizamide CT for Diagnosis of Intracranial Cystic Lesions 36

J. Menzel and U. Schmidt-Gayk: The Effect of Computed Tomography on Diagnosis, Operative Techniques and Prognosis of Tumors of the Middle Cranial Fossa (Petrous Apex) 42

R. Schönmayr, A. Laun, A.L. Agnoli, and O. Busse: Spontaneous Brain Stem Lesions. CT-Findings and Clinical Data in Respect to Morbidity 47

J. Gilsbach, H.R. Eggert, Ch. Ostertag, and W. Seeger: CT Localization and Operative Approaches in Posterior Fossa Lesions 52

H.R. Eggert, J. Gilsbach, and W. Seeger: Operative Approaches to the Rostral Brain Stem According to the CT-Findings 57

W. Entzian: On the Extended Indication for Operation of Deep Seated Brain Tumors 64

H. Klinge, U. Muhtaroglu, and M. Rautenberg: CT in Diagnosis and Treatment of 20 cases with Brain Abscesses and Subdural Empyemas 73

F. Brandt, H.C. Nahser, H.-E. Clar, and H.M. Mehdorn: Diagnosis and Two-Dimensional Localization of Intracranial Metastases with Computerized Tomography 80

Th. Grumme, W. Lanksch, and D. Kolodziejczyk: The Influence of Computerized Tomography on Treatment of Spontaneous Intracerebral Hematoma 84

E. Heiß, F. Albert, and H. Weiland: The Prognosis of Traumatic Intracranial Hematomas Before and After the Introduction of Computerized Tomography 90
J.R. Moringlane, M. Samii, and K.D. Lerch: Postoperative CT-Follow-Up of Chronic Subdural Hematoma 95
H.M. Mehdorn, W. Grote, H.C. Weichert, A. Buch, and S. Bergner: Cranial Computed Tomography: Its Influence on Results of Treating Traumatic Intracranial Extradural Hematomas 101
U. Dietrich, N. Nicola, and H.K. Seibert: Value of Computerized Tomography in Setting the Indication for Surgical Treatment of Extradural Hematomas with a Delayed Course 108
H. Kretschmer, P. Tzonos, and R. Gustorf: Surgery in Traumatic Intracerebral Bleeding Based on Computerized Tomographical Findings 112
S. Tiyaworabun, U. Pasch, N. Nicola, M. Schirmer, and H.K. Seibert: Detection of the Angiographically Cryptic Cerebrovascular Malformations by Computerized Tomography 117
W. Mauersberger and E. Lins: The Use of Computer Tomography in the Diagnosis and Postoperative Observation of Cerebral Aneurysms 132
H. Wassmann, R. Bollbach, and E. Lins: Computerized Tomography in the Operative Treatment of Cerebrovascular Disease 139
Th. Herter and H. Altenburg: The Diagnostic Value of Computerized Tomography in Follow-Up Studies After CSF Drainage 147
C. Sprung and B. Schulz: Correlation of Postoperative Clinical Course and Ventricular Size Determined by Computed Tomography in Normal Pressure Hydrocephalus 156
H.-J. Schmitz, M. Brock, and G.B. Bradac: B-Waves and Periventricular Lucency (PVL) in Intermittently Normotensive Hydrocephalus 164
S. Tiyaworabun, H.H. Kramer, R. Kiekens, and H.K. Seibert: Slit Ventricle Syndrome - Computerized Tomography Aid in the Evuluation and Management 173
H.K. Seibert, D.P. Lim, W.J. Bock, and C. Lumenta: Radiological Diagnosis Before and After Introduction of Computerized Tomography 183

Brain Metabolism

S. Hoyer: Normal and Abnormal Oxidative Brain Metabolism 189
G. Klingelhöffer and E. Halves: Neuroendocrinological Aspects in Cases of Brain Death After Severe Brain Injury 200
D. Heuser, P.J. Morris, and D.G. McDowall: Criteria for the Choice of Drugs Suitable for Controlled Hypotension in Neuroanaesthesia 203
R. Preger and G. Schwarzmann: Sphingolipids in the Progress of Head Injury - A Preliminary Report 208
H.W. Bothe, Th. Wallenfang, A. Khalifa, and K. Schürmann: The Relationship Between Brain Edema, Energy Metabolism, Glucose Content and rCBF Investigated by Artificial Brain Abscess in Cats 214
D. Ratge, A. Hadjidimos, K.H. Holbach, and H. Wisser: Circadian Rhythms of Catecholamines, Cortisol and Prolactin in Patients with Apallic Syndrome 222
R. Schubert, K. Zimmer, and J. Grote: Tissue Oxygen Supply Conditions in the Brain Cortex During Arterial Hypocapnia ... 229

W. Heller, B. Domres, W. Hacker, and U. Oehler: The Behavior of Sodium, Potassium, Magnesium and Zinc in the Brain with Special Attention to Cerebral Edema Following Experimentally Induced Burns 236
D.P. Lim, D. Reinhardt, and W.J. Bock: Determination of Dexamethasone with Radioimmunassay in Case of Head Injury ... 244
M. Brandt, H. Wagner, K.H. Krähling, and H.-J. König: Investigations of the Effects of Dexamethasone on Surgical Stress in Neurosurgical Patients, on the Basis of Radioimmunological Hormone Determinations (LH, FSH, GH, ACTH, Cortisol, Testosterone) 248
O. Kempski, U. Gross, and A. Baethmann: An in Vitro Model of Cytotoxic Brain Edema: Cell Volume and Metabolism of Cultivated Glial- and Nerve-Cells 254
D. Stolke and H. Dietz: Barbiturate Influence on Subcellular Organelles in Experimental Cold Lesion 259
K.E. Richard and T. Hashimoto: Dead Space Ventilation and Intracranial Volume Capacity 266

Spinal Injuries

W. Driesen: Injuries of the Spinal Cord and Their Prognosis 275
B. Hübner, K. Leyendecker, and A. Pihera: Indications for the Operative Treatment of Spinal Injuries and Technical Problems in Stabilizing the Spine 277
K. Leyendecker, B. Hübner, and A. Pihera: Preliminary Results with Surgery in Trauma to the Thoracic and Lumbar Spine, Using the Harrington Method 281
W. Elies and H. Kretschmer: Transoral Fusion of the First and Second Cervical Vertebra 287
B.N. Rana and O. Orio-Glaunec: Spinal Epidural Hematoma 293
J. Lemke, F. Koschorek, U. Larkamp, and H.-P. Jensen: 30 Cases of Traumatic Central Cervical Spinal Cord Injury 299
A. Karimi-Nejad: Early and the Still Possible Late Surgical Treatment of Cervical Spine Injuries 305
B. Rama, H. Koch, and O. Spoerri: Subluxations, Fracture Dislocations and Compression Fractures of Cervical Vertebral Column. Results of Surgical and Conservative Treatment 312
V. Reinhardt, K. Roosen, H.-E. Nau, and L. Gerhard: Pathomorphological and Clinical Basis of the Prognosis in Cervical Injuries 315
K. Roosen and W. Grote: Surcigal Treatment of Cervical Spine Injuries - Prognostic Aspects on Operative Procedures and Timing 322

Free Topics

J. Bockhorn, A. Brawanski, and M.R. Gaab: Regional Cerebral Blood Flow and Extra-Intracranial Bypass Surgery 333
H. Wismann and R. Meyermann: Early Morphological Changes in Microvascular Anastomoses 340
E. Wintermantel: Diaphanoscopy of Blood Vessels, Visualization of Emboli Originating from Blood Clots Formed Close to Suture Lines 344
D. Voth, M. Schwarz, N. Hüwel, and E. Mahlmann: Shunt Therapy in Medulloblastoma? 348

K. von Wild, L. Glusa, A. Sepehrnia, and M. Samii: Effect of
6-Methylprednisolone on the Brain Function in Patients with
Solitary Circumscribed Supratentorial Tumors 357
M.R. Gaab, I. Haubitz, A. Brawanski, J. Faulstich, and
H.E. Heissler: Pressure/Volume (P/V)-Test and Pulse Wave
(PA)-Analysis of ICP 367
F. Münch, K. van Deyk, D. Rinker, E. Epple, and H. Junger:
Clinical Application of Computer Assisted Continuous
Monitoring of Intracranial Pressure 378
W. Elies: Possibilities and Results by Using the Rhinosurgical
Approach in Cases of Anterior Cranial Fossa Injuries 382
A. Kühner and H. Penzholz: Experiences with Microvascular
Decompression in the Cerebellopontine Angle in Trigeminal
Neuralgia 386
M. Klinger: Spondylitis - A Complication Following Lumbar
Disc Operations 394

Subject Index 401

List of Editors and Senior Authors

Arnold, H.: Neurochirurgische Abteilung, Universitätskrankenhaus Eppendorf, Martinistraße 52, D-2000 Hamburg 20

Bockhorn, J.: Neurochirurgische Klinik und Poliklinik der Universität Würzburg, Josef-Schneider-Straße 11, D-8700 Würzburg

Bothe, H.W.: Neurochirurgische Klinik der Universität Mainz, Langenbeckstraße 1, D-6500 Mainz

Brandt, F.: Neurochirurgische Klinik und Poliklinik, Universitätsklinikum der Gesamthochschule Essen, Hufelandstraße 55, D-4300 Essen 1

Brandt, M.: Chirurgische Klinik und Poliklinik der Westfälischen Wilhelms-Universität, Jungeblodtplatz 1, D-4400 Münster/Westfalen

Brock, M.: Abteilung für Neurochirurgie, Neurochirurgische/Neurologische Klinik und Poliklinik, Universitätsklinikum Steglitz, Freie Universität Berlin, Hindenburgdamm 30, D-1000 Berlin 45

Dietrich, U.: Neurochirurgische Klinik, Medizinische Einrichtungen der Universität Düsseldorf, Moorenstraße 5, D-4000 Düsseldorf 1

Driesen, W.: Neurochirurgische Abteilung, Eberhard-Karls-Universität Tübingen, Calwer Straße 7, D-7400 Tübingen

Eggert, H.R.: Neurochirurgische Klinik, Albert-Ludwig-Universität Freiburg, Hugstetter Straße 55, D-7800 Freiburg

Elies, W.: Hals-Nasen-Ohrenklinik der Eberhard-Karls-Universität Tübingen, Silcherstraße 5, D-7400 Tübingen

Entzian, W.: Neurochirurgische Universitätsklinik, Sigmund-Freud-Straße 25, D-5300 Bonn-Venusberg

Gaab, M.R.: Neurochirurgische Klinik und Poliklinik der Universität Würzburg, Josef-Schneider-Straße 11, D-8700 Würzburg

Gilsbach, J.: Neurochirurgische Klinik, Albert-Ludwig-Universität Freiburg, Hugstetter Straße 55, D-7800 Freiburg

Grumme, Th.: Neurochirurgische Klinik im Klinikum Charlottenburg, Freie Universität Berlin, Spandauer Damm 130, D-1000 Berlin 19

Haßler, W.: Neurochirurgische Klinik, Albert-Ludwig-Universität Freiburg, Hugstetter Straße 55, D-7800 Freiburg

Heiß, E.: Neurochirurgische Klinik der Universität Erlangen-Nürnberg, Schwabachanlage 6 (Kopfklinikum), D-8520 Erlangen

Heller, W.: Chirurgische Klinik, Eberhard-Karls-Universität Tübingen, Calwer Straße 7, D-7400 Tübingen

Herter, Th.: Neurochirurgische Klinik und Poliklinik der Westfälischen Wilhelms-Universität, Jungeblodtplatz 1, D-4400 Münster/Westfalen

Heuser, D.: Institut für Anästhesie, Eberhard-Karls-Universität Tübingen, Calwer Straße 7, D-7400 Tübingen

Hoyer, S.: Institut für Pathochemie und Allgemeine Neurochemie im Zentrum Pathologie der Universität Heidelberg, Im Neuenheimer Feld 220-221, D-6900 Heidelberg

Hübner, B.: Neurochirurgische Abteilung der Berufsgenossenschaftlichen Unfallklinik, Friedberger Landstraße 430, D-6000 Frankfurt 60

Huk, W.: Neurochirurgische Klinik der Universität Erlangen-Nürnberg, Schwabachanlage 6 (Kopfklinikum), D-8520 Erlangen

Karimi-Nejad, A.: Neurochirurgische Universitätsklinik Köln, Joseph-Stelzmann-Straße 9, D-5000 Köln 41

Kempski, O.: Institut für Chirurgische Forschung der Universität München, Klinikum Großhadern, Marchioninistraße 15, D-8000 München 70

Klinge, H.: Neurochirurgische Universitätsklinik, Weimarer Straße 8, D-2300 Kiel-Wik

Klingelhöffer, G.: Neurochirurgische Klinik und Poliklinik der Universität Würzburg, Joseph-Schneider-Straße 2, D-8700 Würzburg

Klinger, M.: Neurochirurgische Klinik der Universität Erlangen-Nürnberg, Schwabachanlage 6 (Kopfklinikum), D-8520 Erlangen

Kluge, W.: Neurochirurgische Klinik im Klinikum Charlottenburg, Freie Universität Berlin, Spandauer Damm 130, D-1000 Berlin 19

Kretschmer, H.: Abteilung für Neurochirurgie der Eberhard-Karls-Universität Tübingen, Calwer Straße 7, D-7400 Tübingen

Kühner, A.: Neurochirurgische Abteilung des Chirurgischen Zentrums der Universität Heidelberg, Im Neuenheimer Feld 110, D-6900 Heidelberg

Kuhlendahl, H.: Hubbelrather Weg 14, D-4006 Erkrath

Lemke, J.: Neurochirurgische Universitätsklinik Kiel, Weimarer Straße 8, D-2300 Kiel

Leyendecker, K.: Neurochirurgische Abteilung der berufsgenossenschaftlichen Unfallklinik, Friedberger Landstraße 430, D-6000 Frankfurt 60

Lim, D.P.: Neurochirurgische Klinik, Medizinische Einrichtungen der Universität Düsseldorf, Moorenstraße 5, D-4000 Düsseldorf 1

Mauersberger, M.: Neurochirurgische Universitätsklinik, Sigmund-Freud-Straße 25, D-5300 Bonn-Venusberg

Mehdorn, H.M.: Neurochirurgische Klinik und Poliklinik, Universitätsklinikum der Gesamthochschule Essen, Hufelandstraße 55, D-4300 Essen 1

Menzel, J.: Neurochirurgische Abteilung des Chirurgischen Zentrums der Universität Heidelberg, Im Neuenheimer Feld 110, D-6900 Heidelberg 1

Moringlane, J.R.: Neurochirurgische Klinik im Krankenhaus Nordstadt der Landeshauptstadt Hannover, Haltenhoffstraße 41, D-3000 Hannover 1

Münch, F.: Institut für Anästhesiologie, Eberhard-Karls-Universität Tübingen, Calwer Straße 7, D-7400 Tübingen

Mundinger, F.: Abteilung Stereotaxie und Neuronuklearmedizin, Albert-Ludwig-Universität Freiburg, Hugstetter Straße 55, D-7800 Freiburg

Nahser, H.C.: Neurochirurgische Klinik und Poliklinik, Universitätsklinikum der Gesamthochschule Essen, Hufelandstraße 55, D-4300 Essen

Preger, R.: Neurochirurgische Universitätsklinik, Sigmund-Freud-Straße 25, D-5300 Bonn-Venusberg

Rama, B.: Neurochirurgische Universitätsklinik, Robert-Koch-Straße 40, D-3400 Göttingen

Rana, B.N.: Neurochirurgische Klinik, Katharinenhospital (Akademisches Lehrkrankenhaus der Universität Tübingen), Landeshauptstadt Stuttgart, Kriegsbergstraße 60, D-7000 Stuttgart 1

Ratge, D.: Abteilung für Klinische Chemie, Robert-Bosch-Krankenhaus, Auerbachstraße 110, D-7000 Stuttgart 50

Reinhardt, V.: Institut für Neuropathologie im Universitätsklinikum der Gesamthochschule Essen, Hufelandstraße 55, D-4300 Essen 1

Richard, K.E.: Neurochirurgische Universitätsklinik, Josef-Stelzmann-Straße 9, D-5000 Köln 41

Roosen, K.: Neurochirurgische Klinik im Universitätsklinikum der Gesamthochschule Essen, Hufelandstraße 55, D-4300 Essen 1

Schmitz, H.-J.: Neurochirurgische Abteilung, Neurochirurgische/Neurologische Klinik und Poliklinik, Universitätsklinikum Steglitz, Freie Universität Berlin, Hindenburgdamm 30, D-1000 Berlin 45

Schönmayr, R.: Zentrum für Neurologie und Neurochirurgie der Justus-Liebig-Universität Gießen, Klinikstraße 29, D-6300 Gießen

Schubert, R.: Neurochirurgische Klinik der Universität Mainz, Langenbeckstraße 1, D-6500 Mainz

Seibert, H.K.: Neurochirurgische Klinik, Medizinische Einrichtungen der Universität Düsseldorf, Moorenstraße 5, D-4000 Düsseldorf 1

Sprung, C.: Neurochirurgische Klinik im Klinikum Charlottenburg, Freie Universität Berlin, Spandauer Damm 130, D-1000 Berlin 19

Stolke, D.: Neurochirurgische Klinik der Medizinischen Hochschule Hannover, Karl-Wiechert-Allee 9, D-3000 Hannover 61

Thal, H.-U.: Neurochirurgische Klinik, Medizinische Einrichtungen der Universität Düsseldorf, Moorenstraße 5, D-4000 Düsseldorf 1

Tiyaworabun, S.: Neurochirurgische Klinik, Medizinische Einrichtungen der Universität Düsseldorf, Moorenstraße 5, D-4000 Düsseldorf 1

Voth, D.: Neurochirurgische Universitätsklinik Mainz, Langenbeckstraße 1, D-6500 Mainz 1

Wassmann, H.: Neurochirurgische Universitäts-Klinik, Sigmund-Freud-Straße 25, D-5300 Bonn-Venusberg

Wild, K. von: Neurochirurgische Klinik der Städtischen Kliniken Hannover, Haltenhoffstraße 41, D-3000 Hannover 1

Wintermantel, E.: Neurochirurgische Abteilung, Eberhard-Karls-Universität Tübingen, Calwer Straße 7, D-7400 Tübingen

Wismann, H.: Klinik und Poliklinik für Neurologie, Medizinische Einrichtungen der Universität Göttingen, Robert-Koch-Straße 40, D-3400 Göttingen

Patho-Biomechanik – die neue nosogenetische Dimension am Zentralnervensystem

Otfrid-Foerster-Gedenkvorlesung, Tübingen 24.4.1981

H. KUHLENDAHL

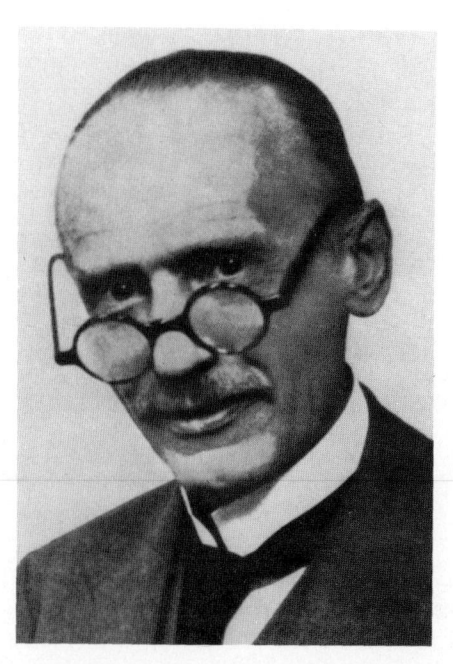

In wenigen Wochen jährt sich zum 40. Male der Todestag OTFRID FOERSTER's, der am 15. Juni 1941, noch nicht 68 Jahre alt, in Breslau starb. Eine wahrhaft einzigartige wissenschaftliche Laufbahn eines hochgebildeten überragenden Mannes, der ein ungewöhnlich umfangreiches wissenschaftliches Werk hinterließ, war zu Ende gegangen.

HUGHLINGS JACKSON's Devise: "Krankheit als Experiment der Natur" war auch die wissenschaftliche Grundeinstellung, von der aus OTFRID FOERSTER Forschung betrieb. Die funktionelle Morphologie des Nervensystems, die er subtil und souverän beherrschte wie kaum ein anderer, und die klinische Pathophysiologie standen für ihn immer im Mittelpunkt. So trug er während 4 Jahrzehnten wesentlich zur Erweiterung der damals noch verhältnismäßig jungen Wissenschaft der Neurologie bei. Es war für ihn dann eine zwingende Konsequenz, die von ihm gewonnenen neuen Erkenntnisse der Pathophysiologie eigenhändig – weitgehend als chirurgischer Autodidakt – in operative Behandlungsmöglichkeiten einer *neurologischen Chirurgie* zu übertragen. Für OTFRID

FOERSTER *war Neurochirurgie die Fortsetzung der Neurologie mit chirurgischen Möglichkeiten!*

Das Thema, das ich mir gewählt habe, befaßt sich ebenfalls - im Sinne OTFRID FOERSTERs - mit klinischer Pathophysiologie, ausgehend von der funktionellen Morphologie.

Die Komplexität der pathophysiologischen und klinischen Problematik der *Biomechanik des Nervensystems* wird meist unterschätzt und ist noch in vieler Hinsicht unerforscht. Über einige wesentliche Bereiche will ich versuchen einen systematischen Überblick zu geben.

Zunächst bedarf es aber einer Erläuterung bzw. Definition der Begriffe "Biomechanik" und "Patho-Biomechanik", mit denen - *nach* OTFRID FOERSTERs Zeit - ein neues Feld der Krankheitsentstehung im Bereich des Nervensystems erschlossen wurde. Grundsätzlich handelt es sich um das Zusammenwirken morphologisch-*morphogenetischer* und *dynamischer* Faktoren.

Als "Biomechanik" ist erst in jüngster Zeit eine neue Disziplin in der Medizin in rascher Entwicklung, die sich mit den physikalischen Eigenschaften der Körpergewebe und der Körperflüssigkeiten, mit der funktionellen Morphologie, physikalischen Grundlagen von Organfunktionen u.a. beschäftigt.

Für das Zentralnervensystem liegen ja nun augenfällige anatomische Gegebenheiten vor - seine totale Einschließung in knöcherne Hohlräume -, die es schon physiologisch zu einem *Musterfall der Biomechanik* machen, so daß es eigentlich erstaunlich ist, daß nicht schon viel früher das zwangsläufig darin gegründete vielfältige Krankheitspotential erkannt wurde; daß vielmehr erst so spät eine systematische Erforschung der damit gegebenen Problematik einsetzte.

Zwar waren schon im vorigen Jahrhundert wiederholt deformierende Veränderungen der Wirbelsäule als Ursache für mancherlei schmerzhafte Erkrankungen in Anspruch genommen worden (H. BRETSCHNEIDER, 1847: Versuch einer Begründung der Pathologie und Therapie der äußeren Neuralgien; Ch. SCHÜTZENBERGER, 1853: De l'arthrite rachidienne cervicale; J. BRAUN, 1875: Klinische und anatomische Beiträge zur Kenntnis der Spondylosis deformans. BARRÉ und LIEOU, 1925). Aber dabei handelte es sich um auf die äußeren Deformierungen der Wirbelsäule bezogene Hypothesen und zumeist Fehldeutungen. Erst Ende der 30er Jahre begann nach der Entdeckung der lumbalen Bandscheibenprotrusion als Ursache der Ischialgie eine systematische Erforschung dieser Problematik im Bereich des Wirbelkanals und der Nervenwurzeln, und danach wurde allmählich das übergreifende auf der Biomechanik gegründete nosogenetische System entwickelt. Hier war es vor allem ALF BREIG, dessen 1960 erschienene Monographie "Biomechanics of the Nervous System" einen ersten Meilenstein darstellt. Seine zahlreichen Arbeiten befassen sich aber (fast) ausschließlich mit dem Rückenmarkstrakt. Der Angelpunkt seiner Überlegungen und Untersuchungen sei mit folgendem Zitat gekennzeichnet: "Zusammen mit dem umgebenden Durarohr und den Ligg. denticulata bildet der Hirnstamm-Rückenmark-Cauda equina-Strang eine funktionelle Einheit dergestalt, daß unter normalen Verhältnissen bei zunehmender Verkürzung des Spinalkanals (nämlich bei Lordosierung (Ref.)) alle diese Weichteile zunehmend erschlaffen und daß sie bei zunehmender Verlängerung des Spinalkanals (d.h. bei Vorwärtsbeugen (Ref.)), zunehmend gespannt werden."

Unter Biomechanik des Nervensystems ist das Zusammenspiel von 3 Komponenten zu verstehen: (1) die plastische *Verformbarkeit* oder die Fähigkeit des nervösen Parenchyms zur elastischen Formveränderung; (2) dessen höchst differenzierter dynamischer *Kontakt* mit harten, meist knöchernen oder derb-elastischen Strukturen des Skeletts; sowie (3) *permanente Bewegungskräfte*. Als dynamische Einflußfaktoren resultieren vitale *Zug-, Spannungs-, Dehnungs- und Druckkräfte*.

Eine solche Konstellation findet sich in der Schädelhöhle und im Wirbelkanal, aber auch z.B. hinsichtlich der sog. "Engpaß-Syndrome" im Carpaltunnel, im Ulnariskanal am Ellbogen, in der Scalenuslücke usw. Es ist klar, daß die morphologisch und funktionell besonders komplizierten Verhältnisse des Spinalkanals und seines Inhaltes bei weitem die am meisten *komplexe Biomechanik* bieten und damit bevorzugt in eine Patho-Biomechanik führen, d.h. daß in der Funktionsgemeinschaft Wirbelsäule und Rückenmark/Nervenwurzeln/Cauda equina von vornherein ein Krankheitspotential vorgegeben ist. In der Wirbelsäule als einem kompliziert-beweglich gegliederten Organ mit der unendlichen Kette ständiger Makro- und Mikrobewegungen ist die Bewegungsdynamik des lebendigen Individuums gewissermaßen zentriert. Der Wirbelkanal und sein Inhalt bilden daher den Schwerpunkt dieses nosogenetischen Systems der Patho-Biomechanik des Zentralnervensystems.

Zunächst müssen wir aber für die Patho-Biomechanik als 4. Komponente den *Zeitfaktor* hinzunehmen. Natürlich gibt es durch akute Gewalteinwirkung auch akute Läsionen, gewissermaßen eine akute Pathobiomechanik: Musterbeispiel ist die Hirnerschütterung (OMMAYA, UNTERHARNSCHEIDT, GOLDSMITH, GURDJIAN u.a.); ferner die von RICHARD C. SCHNEIDER pathobiomechanisch analysierte 'zentrale Halsmarkschädigung' beim Hyperextensionstrauma; oder der komplizierte Vorgang des sog. Schleuder-Traumas, das deshalb immer noch kontrovers diskutiert wird. Hierzu wäre vieles zu sagen, aber wir wollen uns hier nur mit den *chronischen nicht-traumatischen* Prozessen biomechanischer Pathogenese befassen.

Kehren wir zurück zu den zuerst genannten 3 Komponenten der Biomechanik des Nervensystems. Der plastischen Verformbarkeit bzw. der elastischen Verformung des nervösen Gewebes kommt sowohl unter physiologischen Gegebenheiten wie erst recht unter pathologischen Bedingungen eine ganz erhebliche Bedeutung zu. Die Verformbarkeit ist selbstverständlich begrenzt. Aber denken wir einmal daran, welcher mechanischen Beanspruchung der N. ulnaris am Ellbogen ständig ausgesetzt ist. Vor allem aber das Rückenmark, insbesondere das Halsmark, wäre ohne eine physiologisch vorgegebene Verformbarkeit den durch die Beweglichkeit der Wirbelsäule bedingten mechanischen Beanspruchungen nicht gewachsen. Gegenüber der normal-physiologischen Formveränderung ist die pathologische Verformung aber von morphologischen Prozessen der umgebenden härteren (meist knöchernen) Gewebe sowie von Bewegungsvorgängen abhängig. Äußere und innere Bewegungen sind Angelpunkt der Biomechanik.

Zunächst einige Beispiele der pathologischen Verformung des nervösen Parenchyms, die jedoch nicht oder erst sehr spät zum Funktionsverlust führen. Haben Sie schon einmal überlegt, daß der N. facialis durch ein großes Akusticus-Neurinom eine ganz enorme Dehnung mit einer Verlängerung auf das 2 bis 3-fache erfährt und wie das möglich ist, ohne daß es zur Facialislähmung kommt?

Natürlich ist das *zeitabhängig*, vollzieht sich bekanntlich äußerst langsam im Verlauf von vielen Jahren und wird ermöglicht durch den ständigen Transport von Protein im Axon vom Zellkörper peripherwärts (etwa 20 mm pro Tag).

Oder denken wir an die starke Verformung bei der Verdrängung der Hirnsubstanz etwa beim parasagittalen Meningeom. Ebenso wenn das Rückenmark durch ein sehr langsam heranwachsendes spinales Meningeom zu einem platten Band zusammengedrückt, verformt ist, ohne daß es zu einer hochgradigen Parese kommt. Freilich: Handelt es sich nicht um Meningeome, sondern um rasch wachsende Metastasen, so kommt es in beiden Fällen sehr schnell zur Plegie. Es handelt sich also bei dem Verhältnis von Verformung und Funktion um ein Problem der *Adaptationsfähigkeit* des nervösen Parenchyms und damit um einen zeitabhängigen Grundfaktor der Patho-Biomechanik am Nervensystem. Hier sei auch gleich angefügt, daß hinsichtlich der Querschnittslähmung beim spinalen Meningeom noch zwei andere biomechanisch bedeutsame Umstände auch eine Rolle spielen: Sitzt das Meningeom nämlich ventral vor dem Mark, so kommt es früher zur pathologischen Dehnung des Markes und damit zur Funktionsschädigung der langen Bahnen, weil das Mark bei jedem Vorbeugen der WS über dem Tumor zusätzlich überdehnt wird. Andererseits sind die Verhältnisse hinsichtlich der Markschädigung bei thorakalem Sitz des Meningeoms günstiger, weil dort die äußeren Bewegungseinflüsse weniger gravierend sind.

Die Verformbarkeit des nervösen Parenchyms hat also als eine bestimmende Komponente im Rahmen der Biomechanik und erst recht der Patho-Biomechanik des ZNS zu gelten, und die zeitabhängige funktionelle Adaptation im Rahmen der Verformung ist ein entscheidend wichtiger Faktor in der Entwicklung der klinischen Symptomatologie.

Wenn auch der Spinalraum nicht nur in der Häufigkeit, sondern auch hinsichtlich der pathophysiologischen Komplexität durchaus im Mittelpunkt des Interesses steht, gibt es doch bedeutungsvolle pathobiomechanische Vorgänge auch im *intrakraniellen* Raum, auf die ich kurz eingehen will.

Hier sind biomechanisch-pathogene Prozesse eigentlich schon länger bekannt. Sie sind nur nicht aus der Perspektive eines allgemeinen nosogenetischen Systems gesehen worden. Hier sind es freilich keine äußeren Bewegungen, die den dynamischen Faktor darstellen.

Hauptsächlich handelt es sich um Begleit- bzw. Folgeerscheinungen der intrakraniellen Massenverschiebung und Drucksteigerung.

Die Tamponade der Cisternen, des Tentoriumschlitzes und des Foramen magnum mit ihren Folgen ist in der Neurochirurgie längst selbstverständliches Wissen seit den Arbeiten in WILHELM TÖNNIS' Institut für Hirnforschung in Berlin-Buch. Ich erinnere nur an die Arbeit von RIESSNER und ZÜLCH: "Über die Formveränderungen des Hirns ... bei raumbeengenden Prozessen" (1939) (Dtsch. Z. Chir.). Natürlich war OTFRID FOERSTER und HARVEY CUSHING (und den anderen älteren Neurochirurgen) die Tamponade der Cisterna magna durch die herabgepreßten Kleinhirntonsillen bekannt, und ich habe OTFRID FOERSTER oft vom "pressure conus" sprechen hören. Aber die Einklemmung des Uncus Gyri Hippocampi mit ihren Begleiterscheinungen und patho-biomechanischen Folgen wurde erst durch ZÜLCH und RIESSNER systematisch untersucht. Als klassischer biomechanischer Vorgang ist dabei auch die Entstehung der Oculomotoriuslähmung und der Abducenslähmung beim sog. Clivuskanten-Syndrom herauszustellen (WELTE und FISCHER-BRÜGGE).

Dazu gehört z.B. auch die Opticus-Druckschädigung beim Turmschädel. (Eine interessante Variante biomechanischer intrakranieller Pathogenese wird ferner morgen von Herrn PENZHOLZ für die Trigeminusneuralgie vorgestellt werden, wo möglicherweise der pulsierende Druck der A. cerebelli inf. von dorsal auf den Tractus spinalis trigemini in der Oblongata anzuschuldigen sein kann (in manchen Fällen).

Wenden wir uns nun dem eigentlichen Schwerpunktsbereich der Biomechanik des Nervensystems bzw. seiner Patho-Biomechanik zu: dem *Wirbelkanal mit dem Rückenmark-Nervenwurzel-Cauda equina-Strang*. Zunächst zur biomechanischen Normalsituation, die vor allem BREIG anatomisch, experimentell und klinisch untersucht hat. Aus dieser Perspektive wurde das umfassende biomechanisch-nosogenetische System entwickelt, das ich als die neue nosogenetische Dimension des Nervensystems bezeichne.

Der Anstoß kam aus der Entdeckung der Ätio-Pathogenese der Ischialgie als einer biomechanischen Nervenwurzel-Irritation bzw. "Kompression" durch MIXTER und BARR 1934/35 und der daraus in den folgenden anderthalb Jahrzehnten schrittweise entwickelten Erkenntnis: "Sciatica that means rupture of a disk" (LINDBLOM). Damals - um 1950 - herrschte noch die Konzeption von der entzündlichen "Neuritis" als Ursache aller solcher Schmerzleiden. Heute ist es selbstverständlich: Ischialgie und Brachialgie = mechanische Nervenwurzelreizung. Aber bis in die 50er Jahre war ebenso selbstverständlich: Ischialgie und Brachialgie = "Neuritis". War doch das Hauptwerk HEINRICH PETTE's: "Die entzündlichen Erkrankungen des Nervensystems", erst 1942 erschienen, worin auch die neuralgischen Affektionen - damals noch nicht als radikuläre Syndrome identifiziert - als entzündliche Erkrankung einbegriffen waren. Es bedurfte noch längerer Zeit, bis auch die Neurologen von entzündlicher "Neuritis" des peripheren Nerven auf biomechanische Irritation der Nervenwurzel umschalteten.

Fassen wir noch einmal die Grundtatsachen zusammen: Im Wirbelkanal ist das Rückenmark zwischen seiner Fixierung am kaudalen Hirnstamm bzw. am Hinterhauptsloch einerseits und durch das Filum terminale im Sakralkanal andererseits weniger "aufgehängt", wie man meist sagt, als vielmehr - mit begrenztem Bewegungsspielraum - ausgespannt, zusätzlich noch von Segment zu Segment durch die Zacken des Lig. dentatum und durch die Nervenwurzeln relativ fixiert. Der Durasack, in dem das Rückenmark also weitgehend fixiert ist, ist seinerseits durch zahlreiche band- und septenartige Strukturen und durch die Wurzelhüllen mit der Wand des Wirbelkanals nur mit geringem Bewegungsspielraum verbunden. Von der lordotischen Extension zur maximalen Ventralflexion verlängert sich aber der Wirbelkanal nach BREIG's Untersuchungen um immerhin 6 bis 7 cm, an seiner Dorsalseite gemessen. Der Rückenmark-Cauda equina-Strang, der diese Längenveränderung ja mitmachen muß, verformt sich zwischen Erschlaffung bei voller Lordosierung und Streckung bei Vorwärtsbeugung ebenfalls physiologischerweise mit einer axialen Längenänderung um 4,5 - 6,5 cm, wobei der Halsmarkabschnitt eine Längenänderung um 1,8 - 2,8 cm - immer gemessen auf der Dorsalseite - erfährt. Mit Recht muß man unter biomechanischen Gesichtspunkten von der funktionellen Einheit von Wirbelkanal, Durasack und Rückenmark-Cauda equina-Strang sprechen (BREIG). Die Fixierung der nervösen Anteile durch die Pia-Arachnoidea einschließlich des Lig. dentatum wird meist unterschätzt.

Unter normal-anatomischen und physiologischen Gegebenheiten reicht der Bewegungsspielraum freilich ohne weiteres aus. Aber es versteht sich ebenso von selbst, daß bestimmte pathologisch-morphologische Veränderungen zusammen mit chronisch einwirkenden *dynamischen Einflüssen*, d.h. *Bewegungskräften*, ohne scharfe Grenze in die Patho-Biomechanik führen und damit ein Krankheitspotential aufbauen.

Elastische Formveränderung zwischen Verkürzung = Erschlaffung und Verlängerung = Spannung ist ein physiologisches biomechanisches Grundprinzip im Nervensystem, wobei in der Entspannung/Verkürzung die axialen Elemente wie Nervenfasern (Axone) sich wellenförmig formieren und *bei Anspannung strecken*. BREIG hat das am Rückenmarkspräparat demonstriert.

Dasselbe Prinzip findet sich z.B. auch im Opticus, in welchem sich die Axone bei neutraler d.h. geradeaus gerichteter Bulbusstellung wellen, bei Seitbewegung des Bulbus strecken. -

Wenden wir uns nun zunächst im einzelnen den *Nervenwurzeln* zu. Die Ursache für die radikuläre Neuralgie, das sog. Wurzelkompressionssyndrom, liegt - wie wir alle wissen - im lumbalen Abschnitt praktisch ausschließlich in der elastisch-weichen Bandscheiben*protrusion*, dagegen im zervikalen Bereich meistens in der osteophytären spondylotischen Exostose am Zwischenwirbelloch. Dafür kennzeichnend ist u.a. der Altersunterschied der Patienten: Die zervikale radikuläre Neuralgie oder sog. Brachialgie findet sich bei im Durchschnitt um gut ein Jahrzehnt älteren Menschen als die Ischialgie.

(Übrigens ist für die große Mehrzahl der Fälle die Bezeichnung Bandscheiben-"prolaps" nicht zutreffend, sondern der Begriff der "Protrusion" richtiger).

Patho-biomechanisch gesehen dienen lumbale Protrusion wie zervikaler osteochondrotisch-ossärer Buckel als Hypomochlion, über welchem die Nervenwurzel reitend ausgespannt bzw. überdehnt wird. Mit BREIG stimme ich darin überein, daß das pathogenetische Grundprinzip, das principium irritans, weniger eine "Kompression" im eigentlichen Wortsinn als vielmehr die Dehnung/Überdehnung der Nervenwurzel ist.

Die *Elastizität* des rupturierten und dorso-lateral vordrängenden Faserknorpelgewebes der Bandscheibe ist übrigens ein spezieller biomechanischer Faktor, der in der Mehrzahl der Krankheitsfälle die Spontanheilung ermöglicht. Aber die Tendenz zur Spontanheilung wird heute vielfach zu gering eingeschätzt. Man ist zu schnell mit der Indikation zur Operation bei der Hand. Es werden zu viele Kranke operiert: ca. 20 000 Patienten pro Jahr, wie SCHIRMER ermittelt hat, allein in den neurochirurgischen Kliniken!
Wenn man sich nur vom Röntgen-Kontrastbild abhängig machte, sondern aus dem vertieften Verständnis der Biomechanik von klinisch-pathologischen Gesichtspunkten ausginge, würde weniger oft zum Messer gegriffen (und mancher unerfreuliche Schaden vermieden).

Eine durchaus interessante und problematische Frage ist nun aber, *warum* denn diese biomechanisch-pathologische Einwirkung auf die Nervenwurzel - oder allgemeiner gesagt: auf die afferente Nervenleitungsbahn - Schmerzempfindung hervorruft. Das ist nämlich durchaus nicht ohne weiteres selbstverständlich. Warum führt sie nicht zu Parästhesien oder gleich zur Lähmung?

Drücken Sie z.B. doch einmal kräftig und nachhaltig auf Ihren Nervus ulnaris im Sulcus nervi uln. am Ellenbogen: Sie werden keinen Schmerz distal im Ulnarisgebiet an der Hand hervorrufen, sondern nur Kribbelparästhesie und bei längerer Dauer Hypästhesie und Parese (wie bei der sog. Schlaflähmung). Warum also bewirkt der chronische biomechanische Kompressions- bzw. Dehnungsvorgang an der Nervenwurzel primär eine in das periphere Nervenwurzelgebiet projizierte Schmerzempfindung und nicht primär Hypästhesie? Denn die Funktion der Nervenbahn, die Erregungsleitung, wird dabei oft genug überhaupt nicht beeinträchtigt, und zudem ist die Schädigung meist vollständig reversibel.

Machen wir einen kleinen *Exkurs in die Neurophysiologie*.

Die Schmerzforschung beschäftigt sich seit jeher - mindestens seit GOLDSCHEIDER und v. FREY - eigentlich nur mit der Physiologie der Schmerz*perzeption*, d.h. mit den *Rezeptoren* (und in jüngerer Zeit mit der zentralen Sinnesverarbeitung). Seit jeher weiß man aber doch, daß Schmerzen nicht nur über die peripheren Rezeptoren perzipiert, daß also Schmerzempfindung nicht nur in der Peripherie erzeugt wird, sondern auch am Nerven, d.h. an der Leitungsbahn selbst; und seit bald 40 Jahren wissen wir, daß dem kein entzündlicher Prozeß im Nerven, wie lange Zeit geglaubt wurde, *keine* sog. "Neuritis" zugrundeliegt, sondern der biomechanisch angreifende Vorgang an der *Nervenwurzel*. Aber damit hat sich die Neurophysiologie bisher kaum befaßt.

Um mich einmal selbst zu zitieren: Ich habe deshalb schon vor 30 Jahren darauf hingewiesen, daß grundlegend unterschieden werden muß zwischen dem auf gewissermaßen *physiologischem* Wege, peripher über die Sinnes*rezeptoren* hervorgerufenen Schmerz, den man "Rezeptorenschmerz" nennen könnte und bei dem es sich um Schmerz*wahrnehmung* handelt; und andererseits dem "unphysiologisch" an der Leitungsbahn erzeugten Schmerz, der analog als "Traktusschmerz" zu bezeichnen wäre und für den der Begriff der Schmerz*empfindung* zutreffend ist. Zwar hat sich für letzteren der Begriff des "projizierten" Schmerzes eingebürgert. Aber der springende Punkt ist doch, daß es sich dabei - anders als beim Rezeptorenschmerz - um einen primär *unphysiologischen* Vorgang - man könnte sagen: abseits der eigentlichen Aufgabe des Schmerzsystems handelt, das ja *von außen* kommende Gefahr abwehren soll.

Kehren wir zurück zu der Frage, *wie* denn eine Schmerzempfindung seitens der afferenten Leitungsbahn, d.h. der Nervenfasern, erzeugt wird. Ich möchte dazu folgende Überlegungen vortragen, die sich auf Diskussionen mit Prof. HAASE, dem Neurophysiologen in Düsseldorf, stützen.

Von folgenden als mehr oder weniger gesichert geltenden Tatsachen kann ausgegangen werden:

a) Die differenzierte Spezifität der Rezeptoren gilt sehr wahrscheinlich auch für die Schmerzwahrnehmung. In jüngster Zeit wird jedenfalls von verschiedener Seite, insbesondere dem englischen Neurophysiologen IGGO die Spezifität eigener Schmerzrezeptoren im Bereich der sog. freien Nervenendigungen, hinter denen sich offenbar doch sehr differenzierte Mikrostrukturen verbergen, vertreten.

b) Unbezweifelt ist die Spezifität der afferenten Leitungsbahnen. D.h. alle Nervenfasern (Axone) haben ihre spezifische Leitungsfunktion für eine der verschiedenen sensiblen Wahrnehmungen. Es gibt also auch spezifische *Schmerzfasern* in der Hinterwurzel.

c) Mindestens die Hälfte aller Hinterwurzelfasern sind marklose langsam leitende C-Fasern, die spezifisch der Schmerzleitung dienen. Dazu kommen noch etwa 10 - 15% markhaltige A-delta-Fasern, die schnelleitende Schmerzfasern sind. Damit sind also ca. 2/3 aller afferenten Hinterwurzelfasern der Schmerzleitung vorbehalten. Dieses quantitative Übergewicht spricht für die große biologische Wertigkeit des Schmerzsinnes, von dem OTFRID FOERSTER immer als von dem *"nocifensorischen"* d.h. schadenabweisenden Sinnessystem gesprochen hat.

Hier könnte *eine* Antwort auf die Frage liegen, wieso die chronische mechanisch schädigende Einwirkung auf die Nervenwurzel zuerst und vor allem Schmerzempfindung hervorruft. Aber warum nicht auch taktile, Druck- und andere Empfindungen der epikritischen Sensibilität? Denn der Ischias-Kranke spürt eben - solange die Schädigung nicht so massiv ist, daß es zur Beeinträchtigung, gar Unterbrechung der Erregungsleitung kommt - *nur Schmerzen* und keine taktilen oder Temperatur-Sensationen. Es wäre denkbar, daß die unphysiologische Einwirkung auf die Hinterwurzel als *unspezifischer* Reiz an *allen* Fasern nur Schmerzempfindung auszulösen vermag.

d) Für die Funktion der Leitungsbahnen spielt die *Isolierung* der einzelnen Fasern mittels der Myelinscheide und der Schwann'schen Zellen eine entscheidende Rolle. - Schließlich

e) Der schuldige biomechanisch-pathogene Vorgang ist die *Überdehnung* der Nervenfaser.

Auf welche Weise erzeugt nun diese Überdehnung an der afferenten Bahn überhaupt elektrophysiologisch Erregung?

Zunächst: Die mechanische Einwirkung könnte zu einer ischaemischen Schädigung führen. Die Ischaemie führt aber doch nur überall dort zu Schmerzen, wo Rezeptoren vorhanden sind. Es ist offen, ob und ggfs. inwieweit eine ischaemische Schädigungskomponente mitspielt. Dies dürfte aber jedenfalls aus hier nicht zu erörternden Gründen gegenüber der direkten mechanischen Schädigung keine entscheidende Rolle spielen.

Vielmehr sind - soweit ich sehe - drei Vorgänge vorstellbar:

1. Die mechanische Einwirkung, also die (Über-)Dehnung, verändert die Ionen-Durchlässigkeit der Membran der Nervenfaser (die ja Träger der elektrophysiologischen Leitungsfunktion ist). Der dadurch provozierte Ionenstrom löst die elektrisch fortgeleitete Erregung am Ort der mechanischen Schädigung aus.

   Dabei wäre allerdings noch ein Problem zu bedenken, nämlich daß es wahrscheinlich eine *Spezifität der Membranen* gibt: *rezeptive* an den Synapsen und *konduktive* der Axone (Fasern). Der mechanische Reiz müßte also die Membranenspezifität durchbrechen.

2. In der Neurophysiologie gibt es den Begriff der sog. *"Quererregung"*.

   Wenn die Isolierung der Nervenfasern durch die biomechanisch-pathogene Einwirkung zerstört oder mindestens geschädigt ist, kann Erregung zwischen den Fasern überspringen, also von erregten zu in Ruhe befindlichen. Es entsteht eine sog. "künstliche Synapse" (GRANIT/KUGELBERG, ZOTTERMAN).

   Es ist gut vorstellbar, daß die Aufhebung bzw. Schädigung der Isolierung an den marklosen Hinterwurzelfasern (die, wie gesagt, mehr als die Hälfte aller Hinterwurzelfasern ausmachen) *leichter und früher* eintritt als an den markhaltigen Fasern, und damit sowohl Erregung durch den Ionenstrom induziert als auch *Quererregung* provoziert und damit eine sehr niederschwellige "künstliche Synapse" erzeugt wird.

3. Schließlich ist zu bedenken, daß die markhaltigen Fasern der epikritischen Qualitäten eine niedrigere Erregungsschwelle haben und daß es beim Drucksinn keine Adaption gibt, so daß in den Axonen (Fasern) der Druckrezeptoren *ständig* ein Erregungsstrom fließt. Im Falle der Zerstörung der Isolierung kann dieser ständige Erregungsstrom von den Axonen der Druckrezeptoren im Sinne der Quererregung auf die Schmerzfasern überspringen, die an sich eine höhere Erregungsschwelle haben.

4. Für Anhänger der "gate-control-Theorie" (zu denen ich nicht gehöre) könnte ein weiterer Faktor in Betracht gezogen werden: Die biomechanische Störung der afferenten Erregungsleitung auch in den markhaltigen Nervenfasern der taktilen und Drucksensibilität (deren isolierende Markscheide ebenfalls geschädigt ist) stört oder behindert auch den gate-control-Mechanismus, so daß die Impulse in den schmerzleitenden Bahnen unkontrolliert und ungebremst (im Sinne der gate control) den Cortex erreichen. Die Schmerzempfindung würde dadurch mindestens verstärkt, weil die supranukleäre Hemmung i.S. der gate-control-Theorie beeinträchtigt ist.

Die Antwort bleibt also hypothetisch, *warum* an der Nervenbahn, die in ihrem natürlichen Zustand ja gar nicht so empfindlich bzw. von außen nicht so leicht erregbar ist - sonst müßten wir viel mehr und alltäglich unter Nervenschmerzen leiden! -, im Zustand der *chronischen* biomechanischen Schädigung so intensive projizierte Schmerzempfindung erzeugt wird.

Zum Abschluß dieses Kapitels möchte ich formulieren:

Das pathogenetische Prinzip der Neuralgie als einer projizierten Schmerzempfindung ist gesetzmäßig eine chronische biomechanische Irritation der afferenten sensiblen Leitungsbahn, erzeugt vor allem durch die Schädigung der Isolierung der Axone und damit überspringende Quererregung.

Wenn es mir für das Kapitel der radikulären Neuralgien eigentlich nur darum ging, den theoretischen und pathophysiologischen Hintergrund zu erhellen, so geht es bei dem jetzt noch offenen Kapitel der *zervikalen Myelopathie* zusätzlich um aktuelle klinische Probleme. Da dieses Thema jedoch vor 1 1/2 Jahren auf unserem Essener Kongreß bereits diskutiert wurde und ich selbst dazu ein Referat gehalten habe, will ich mich hier kurz fassen.

Die *chronische spondylotische zervikale Myelopathie* ist natürlich das klinisch bedeutsamste Krankheitsbild auf dem Boden einer sehr komplexen patho-biomechanischen Krankheitsentstehung. Hierbei wirken eine ganze Anzahl sowohl morphologischer wie dynamischer Faktoren, eine *biomechanische Ursachenkette*, zusammen, um zu der mehr oder weniger massiven, mehr oder weniger progredienten Halsmarkschädigung zu führen (Tabelle 1). Das Halsmark hat normalerweise verhältnismäßig viel Bewegungsspielraum im Halswirbelkanal. Es muß daher immer wieder darauf hingewiesen werden, daß die Einengung eines normal weiten Kanals durch Protrusionen auf der Ventralseite keineswegs ohne weiteres zu einem Myelopathie-Syndrom führt. Eine der *obligaten Voraussetzungen* ist vielmehr die vorgegebene Enge, eine nicht seltene konstitutionelle Variante, die maßgebliche Vorbedingung zur Entstehung einer chronischen biomechanischen Schädigung des Halsmarkes. Bei einem sagittalen Durchmesser unter 13 - 14 mm, sicherlich aber unter 12 mm, muß es bei Hinzutreten spondylotisch deformierender Veränderungen früher oder später zur Rückenmarksschädigung kommen.

Aber auch dabei ist die Krankheitsentwicklung absolut abhängig von der Einwirkung der permanenten Bewegungskräfte, die die chronische Irritation bewirken: Die kyphosierende Beugebewegung, die zur Dehnung des Halsmarkes führt, während die Lordosierung eine Kompression im Sinne des Kneifzangenmechanismus durch die Einwölbung des Lig. flavum bewirkt. Zu den äußeren Bewegungen kommen aber die *inneren Bewegungen* im engen Halswirbelkanal hinzu: Die blutpulsatorische und die atmungsabhängige axiale Eigenbewegung des Halsmarkes, die pulsierende Volumenschwankung transversal. *Überdehnung, Reibung,*

Tabelle 1. Synopsis des biomechanisch/pathobiomechanischen Ursachenfaktoren-Komplexes bei der zervikalen Myelopathie

A. Morphogenetische Faktoren	B. Dynamische Faktoren
I. Primär/konstitutionell	I. Exogen
a) Enger Wirbelkanal (!) b) Gestreckter bzw. kyphotischer Wirbelsäulenaufbau	a) Bewegung des Kopfes und der Halswirbelsäule verschieben Rückenmark gegen den Wirbelkanal axial b) Beugebewegung bewirkt Zugspannung im Rückenmark, Reklination bei engem Kanal Kompression des Halsmarkes
II. Prozeßabhängig/sekundär	II. Innere (endogene)
c) Chondro-ossäre Protrusion(en) d) Lokale adhäsive Pia-Arachnoidea Fibrose, besonders ventral e) Altersbedingte Verminderung der Plastizität des Markparenchyms	c) Rhythmische Eigenbewegung des Markes mit der Blutpulsation (transversal) mit der Atmung (longitudinal) d) Rhythmische Volumenschwankung des Markes e) (Venöse) Zirkulationsbeeinträchtigung

Folgen: Überdehnung, Reibung, Kompression; Ischaemie, Strangdegeneration

Kompression sind die mechanisch schädigenden Kräfte. Die eingangs dargestellte Situation der "Funktionseinheit Rückenmark-Nervenwurzeln-Cauda equina-Strang und Wirbelsäule" machen das verständlich. Eine ischaemische Komponente spielt sicherlich zusätzlich eine Rolle.

Es handelt sich um eine *Kombination von direkter biomechanischer Parenchymschädigung* und *vasculärer Ischaemie*, wobei aber der direkten mechanischen Parenchymschädigung die entscheidende Rolle zukommt.

Auf eine bisher offenbar zu wenig beachtete Konsequenz der biomechanischen Analyse für die Durchführung des operativen Vorgehens sei besonders hingewiesen. Um eine zusätzliche intraoperative Schädigung zu vermeiden (die nicht ganz selten vorgekommen ist), muß auf dem Operationstisch eine Ventralflexion von Kopf/Hals auf jeden Fall strikt vermieden werden beim dorsalen Eingriff, auch wenn damit die Laminektomie etwas schwieriger wird. Ebenso ist aber auch beim ventralen Zugang eine stärkere Lordosierung obsolet. Eine postoperativ verstärkte oder gar totale Querschnittslähmung ist ein vermeidbares Unheil!

Wenn wir den so vielfältigen Komplex der Patho-Biomechanik am Nervensystem überblicken, so mag es nützlich sein, noch einmal daran zu erinnern, daß alle diese Krankheitsbilder bis vor nicht sehr langer Zeit - kaum mehr als 20 Jahre - unter vielfältig falscher Ätiopathogenese eingeordnet wurden. Die Neurochirurgie war auf diesem Gebiet Vorreiter, während die Neurologie nur zögernd folgte. Das bedeutet aber nicht, daß jetzt alles nur auf operative Behandlung hinausliefe. Das tiefere Verständnis der biomechanischen nosogenetischen Zusammenhänge sollte der Indikation zur operativen Therapie die angemessenen Schranken setzen. -

Erlauben Sie mir zum Schluß noch ein paar Bemerkungen, wie man sie sich wohl in meinem Alter leisten darf, ohne damit als überheblich gelten zu müssen - höchstens als anachronistisch!

Der Beruf des Arztes lebt - zwar nicht unbedingt in der täglichen Routine, aber doch im Grunde in einem wesentlichen Maße - aus einer *zweifachen Faszination* (wie vergleichbar nur in wenigen Berufen): Einmal, wenn dem Arzt eine nicht gerade einfache Diagnose gelingt (in den meisten Fällen sollte die Diagnose eine eigene geistige Leistung sein); zum anderen wenn seine therapeutischen Bemühungen mehr oder weniger erfolgreich sind.

Beides gilt für den Neurochirurgen in besonderem Maße.

Inzwischen aber ändert sich im diagnostischen Bereich einiges grundlegend. Der Einsatz der technisch teils so großartigen Apparaturen, die gerade dem Neurochirurgen weithin die Anstrengung medizinisch-kriminalistischen Spürsinns ersparen, beraubt ihn leider zugleich eben der Faszination einer selbst erarbeiteten schwierigen diagnostischen Leistung - sofern er nicht wenigstens vor dem Einsatz der Technik seine klinisch-diagnostischen Möglichkeiten ausspielt. Gerade darum geht es.
Denn dies ist keine Philippica gegen den technischen Fortschritt in der Medizin. *Es geht vielmehr um das Bemühen um die richtige, angemessene Einordnung des technischen Fortschritts.*

Und wer wollte es leugnen: *Der Sog der technischen Möglichkeiten* ist gewaltig. Liefert doch z.B. das CT-Bild eine mehr oder weniger perfekte Diagnose ohne sonstiges Zutun, gewissermaßen auf dem Präsentierteller. Auch das ist in gewisser Weise faszinierend - aber ohne eine besondere geistige Leistung abzufordern. Es geht nicht um ein Zurück in die "gute alte Zeit", keine Maschinenstürmerei! Es geht um die ständige Bewußtmachung, daß das Übergewicht der technischen Möglichkeiten allzu leicht den Blick für das grundlegende Verständnis der klinischen Pathophysiologie verstellt und damit die Einsicht in - ich möchte sagen - das "Lebendige" am kranken Menschen. Sich allzu sehr abhängig zu machen von technisch - in unserem Fach natürlich überwiegend neuroradiologisch - gewonnenen Befunden, führt in eine Einbahnstraße, die oft genug eine Sackgasse ist.

Ich sage das nicht so pathetisch ohne konkreten Grund. Es ist vielmehr die immer häufigere erschreckende Erfahrung (mir jetzt vorwiegend im Gutachtenbereich zufließend) einer manchmal geradezu bestürzenden Hilflosigkeit von Ärzten, die gewissermaßen nur am Kontrastbild kleben und keiner originären diagnostischen Leistung mehr fähig zu sein scheinen, weil sie die grundlegende patho-physiologisch-klinische Analyse nicht mehr beherrschen.

Deshalb immer wieder mein ceterum censeo: Mehr Pathophysiologie (d.h. für uns auch Neurologie) und weniger Radiologie!

Es ist zudem der Verlust der - oder der Verzicht auf die intellektuelle Befriedigung, ja eine Art intellektuellen Vergnügens der persönlichen diagnostischen Leistung, wie ich das schon einmal bei anderer Gelegenheit gesagt habe.

Noch einmal: Nichts gegen die Anwendung und volle Ausschöpfung der - oft genug absolut unentbehrlichen - technischen Möglichkeiten, aber nur im Zusammenhang mit oder in Ergänzung der "klinischen" Diagnostik.

Die Neurochirurgie war jedenfalls zu OTFRID FOERSTERs Zeit noch höchst spannend (was nicht heißen soll, daß sie es heute nicht mehr ist). Aber sie ist heute doch hier und da langweilig geworden, z.B. an der Wirbelsäule: Schmerzen - Myelographie - Operation. Aber 20 000 Bandscheibenoperationen pro Jahr - ich sagte es schon - allein in den neurochirurgischen Kliniken: Wer wollte ernsthaft bestreiten, daß das ein paar tausend zu viel sind, besonders wenn man die Ergebnis-Statistik unter die Lupe nimmt.

Es hängt von jedem von uns ab, daß die Neurochirurgie weiterhin in allen Bereichen interessant und spannend bleibt:

Nämlich als Fortsetzung der Neurologie (und zwar einer voll ausgeschöpften Neurologie und Pathophysiologie) mit chirurgischen Mitteln - im Sinne OTFRID FOERSTERs.

Literatur

1. Barré, J.A., Lieou Yong Choen: Troubles radicularies et pyramideaux par arthrite cervicale ou tumeurs de cette région. Rev. Neurol. 663 (1925)

2. Braun, J.: Klinische und anatomische Beiträge zur Kenntnis der Spondylitis deformans als einer der häufigsten Ursachen mannigfacher Neurosen. Hannover 1875

3. Breig, A.: Biomechanics of the central nervous system. Stockholm: Almquist & Wiksell 1960

4. Breig, A.: Die Biomechanik des Rückenmarks und seiner Häute im Wirbelkanal. Verh. Anat. Ges. Ergänz. d. Anat. Anzeigers Heft 3, Band 115 (1965)

5. Breig, A., El-Nadi, A.F.: Biomechanis of the cervical spinal cord. Acta radiol. (Diagn.) $\underline{4}$, 602-624 (1966)

6. Casey, K.L.: The neurophysiologic basis of pain. Postgrad. Med. $\underline{53}$, 58-64 (1973)

7. Denny-Brown, D., Brenner, Ch.: Paralysis of nerve induced by direct pressure and by tourniquet. Arch. Neur. $\underline{51}$, 1-14 (1944)

8. Denny-Brown, D., Brenner, Ch.: Lesion in peripheral nerve resulting from compression by spring clips. Arch. Neur. $\underline{52}$, 1-19 (1944)

9. Duus, P.: Die Einengung der Foramina intervertebralia infolge degenerativer Wirbelsäulenprozesse als Ursache von neuralgischen Schmerzzuständen. Nervenarzt $\underline{19}$, 489 (1948)

10. Fischer-Brügge, E.: Das Clivuskanten-Syndrom. Zbl. Neurochir. $\underline{11}$ (1951)

11. Foerster, O.: Die Leitungsbahnen des Schmerzgefühls. Berlin, Wien: Urban & Schwarzenberg 1927

12. Goldsmith, W.: Biomechanics of head injury. In: Biomechanics. Its foundations and objectives. In: Fung, Y.C., Perrone, N., Anliker, M. (eds.). Englewood Cliffs, N.Y.: Prentice-Hall, Inc. 1972

13. Granit, R.: Nerve fiber interaction in the roots. Acta psychiat. (Kopenh.) Suppl. $\underline{46}$, 14 (1947)

14. Granit, R., Leksell, L., Sloglund, C.R.: Fibre interaction in injured or compressed region of nerve. Brain $\underline{69}$, 310 (1946)

15. Gurdjean, E.S., Webster, J.E., Lissner, H.R.: Observations on the mechanism of brain concussion, contusion and laceration. Surg. Gyn. Obstet. $\underline{101}$, 680-690 (1955)

16. Hensel, H.: Schmerz und der Begriff der Spezifität. In: Schmerz. Janzen, R. et al. (Hrsg.). Stuttgart: Thieme 1972

17. Iggo, A.: Beweise für die Existenz von "Schmerz"-Rezeptoren. In: Schmerz. Janzen, R. et al. (Hrsg.). Stuttgart: Thieme 1972

18. Klensch, H.: Serienentladungen an druckparabiotischen Nervenstellen. Pflüg. Arch. $\underline{252}$, 369-380 (1950)

19. Klensch, H.: Parabiotische Nervenstelle als Modell eines Mechano-Receptors. Pflüg. Arch. $\underline{253}$, 87-90 (1950)

20. Kugelberg, E.: Injury activity and Trigger zones. In: Human nerves. Brain $\underline{69}$, 310 (1946)

21. Kuhlendahl, H.: Zur Problematik des Schmerzgeschehens. Das neuralgische Syndrom. Ärztl. Forschg. $\underline{5}$, I/4-10 (1951)

22. Kuhlendahl, H.: Cervical Myelopathy. In: Advances in Neurosurgery, Vol. 8. Berlin, Heidelberg, New York: Springer 1980
23. Kuhlendahl, H.: Versuch einer Begründung der Pathologie der Neuralgien. Habilitations-Schrift Düsseldorf 1953
24. Mixter, W.J., Barr, J.S.: Rupture of the intervertebral disc with involvement of the spinal canal. New Engl. J. Med. 221, 210-215 (1934)
25. Ommaya, A.K.: Mechanical properties of tissues of the nervous system. J. Biomech. 1, 127-138 (1968)
26. Ommaya, A.K., Rokoff, S.D., Baldwin, M.: Experimental Concussion. J. Neurosurg. 21, 249-265 (1964)
27. Riessner, D., Zülch, K.J.: Über die Formveränderungen des Hirns. Dtsch. Z. Chir. 253, 1-61 (1939)
28. Schirmer, M.: Untersuchungsbogen bei Lumboischialgie. Dtsch. Ärztebl. 77, 755-758 (1980)
29. Schneider, D.: Die Dehnbarkeit der markhaltigen Nervenfaser des Frosches in Abhängigkeit von Funktion und Struktur. Ztschr. Naturforsch. 7b, 38-48 (1952)
30. Schützenberger, M.Ch.: De l'arthrite rachidienne cervicale. Gaz. Méd. de Strasbourg 6, 461-471 (1853)
31. Sunderland, S., Bradley, K.C.: Stress-strain phenomena in human peripheral nerve trunks. Brain 84, 102-119 (1961)
32. Unterharnscheidt, F.: Experimentelle Untersuchungen über gedeckte Schäden des Gehirns. Fortschr. Med. 80, 369-378 (1962)
33. Welte, E.: Zur formalen Genese der traumatischen Mydriasis. Zbl. Neurochir. 8, 217-234 (1943)
34. Wolf, B.S., Khilnani, M., Malis, L.: The sagittal diameter of the bony cervical spinal canal and its significance in cervical spondylosis. J. Mt. Sinai Hosp. New York 23, 283-292 (1956)
35. Zotterman, Y.: Schmerz und Juckreiz - Elektrophysiologische Studien an Hautnerven. In: Schmerz. Janzen, R. et al. (Hrsg.). Stuttgart: Thieme 1972

Computerized Tomography

Has Computed Tomography Led to Earlier Diagnosis of Brain Tumors?

W. KLUGE and C. SPRUNG

Introduction

Development of new diagnostic techniques proceeds on the assumption that early diagnosis of a brain tumor and exact knowledge of its location, size and probable histological classification will improve the patient's prognosis.

Since the introduction of computed tomography (CT) (by AMBROSE and HOUNSFIELD) in 1973 many authors have emphasized the technique's superiority over conventional radiological methods in the diagnosis of virtually all types of brain tumor (1).

However, no study has been published to date dealing with the question whether the advantage of CT - its simplicity and negligible risk and discomfort for the patient - have in fact been associated with a measurable reduction in the period between onset of symptoms and definitive diagnosis of brain tumors.

Material

Retrospective analysis of approximately 200 case histories allowed calculation of the mean interval between onset of symptoms and definitive diagnosis in patients with glioblastoma, astrocytoma, oligodendroglioma and meningeoma treated in the neurosurgery department of Klinikum Charlottenburg before the introduction of CT in 1975 (Table 1). These cases were compared with a collection in which diagnosis was made by means of computed tomography. Patients were selected at random. The interval was calculated in months for glioblastoma and in years for the other tumors. Results were expressed in terms of percentages of all diagnosis of a given tumor at defined intervals after the onset of symptoms.

Table 1. Number of patients (with one of each of 4 types of brain tumors

	Without CT (n)	With CT (n)
Glioblastoma	52	50
Astrocytoma	50	47
Oligodendroglioma	50	46
Meningioma	52	52
Total	204	195

Results

Improved diagnosis with CT is evident in glioblastoma (Table 2). Diagnosis was made within a month of the onset of symptoms in only 27% of cases before the introduction of CT, as compared to 52% of cases with CT studies. Intervals are longer in cases of astrocytoma, but the advantage of CT over conventional methods is evident in this group of tumors as well (Table 3). 81% of diagnosis were made in the first year, compared to 40% before the introduction of CT. By comparison, there was no significant reduction in the symptomatic interval before diagnosis of oligodendroglioma or meningeoma with CT studies. Diagnosis was made more than 1 year after the onset of symptoms in 50% or more of cases, both before and after the introduction of CT (Tables 4, 5).

Table 2. Glioblastoma statistics. Diagnosis (as a percentage of all tumors) in relation to duration of the symptomatic interval

	Without CT (%)	With CT (%)
< 1 month	27	52
< 2 months	15,3	22
< 3 months	15,3	8
> 3 months	42,4	18
	100,0	100,0

Table 3. Astrocytoma statistics. Diagnosis (as a percentage of all tumors) in relation to duration of the symptomatic interval

	Without CT (%)	With CT (%)
< 1 year	40	81
< 3 years	20	6,3
> 3 years	40	12,7
	100,0	100,0

Table 4. Oligodendroglioma statistics. Diagnosis (as a percentage of all tumors) in relation to duration of the symptomatic interval

	Without CT (%)	With CT (%)
< 1 year	50	52
< 3 years	22	26
> 3 years	28	22
	100	100

Table 5. Meningioma statistics. Diagnosis (as a percentage of all tumors) in relation to duration of the symptomatic interval

	Without CT (%)	With CT (%)
< 1 year	46	48
< 3 years	29	29
> 3 years	25	23
	100	100

Discussion

Interpretation of these results is difficult. A larger collection might demonstrate a shift in the percentages. Exact definition of the onset of symptoms, especially discrete psychological or neurological disorders, is extremely difficult in some cases. The shortest interval to diagnosis was estimated in these patients. There was no significant correlation between tumor-size and location or specific symptoms and the interval until diagnosis was made. This was true of all 4 tumor groups. Earlier diagnosis in glioblastoma was probably related to the morphology of these tumors and their high growth rate. Extensive perifocal edema usually results in early and rapidly progressing symptoms which lead the patient to seek medical attention. The chief complaint was a psychological disorder in 50% of cases, often accompanied by additional neurological deficit at a later date. Earlier diagnosis was possible for different reasons in cases of astrocytoma. Although our collection was relatively small, our results were virtually identical with those reported by KUHLENDAHL (1973) for astrocytomas of brain, with seizures as the chief complaint in 60 - 70% of cases. Such an event almost always leads the patient to seek medical attention, usually from a neurologist, who prescribes the appropriate diagnostic procedures. In addition, it has been shown that CT studies are capable of demonstrating regions of decreased density in astrocytomas which have a normal appearance in angiographic studies.

Although morphologically different, oligodendrogliomas and meningiomas have similarly low growth rates. This determines the gradual development of symptoms which may be so uncharacteristic that neither the patient nor his family physician is led to suspect an organic lesion. Headache was the initial symptom in 40% of our patients with meningioma, and the history ranged from weeks to months and even up to 10 years in these cases. Seizures were observed in 20% of patients, while the remaining symptoms and signs were related to location of the tumor and include disorders of vision and olfactory sensation and paralysis.

Seizures were observed in 50% of patients with oligodendroglioma, a high percentage, though less than that found in astrocytoma. These are often psychomotor seizures, and genuine epilepsy may be suspected in these cases if other deficits are not evident, with the result that additional diagnostic studies are deferred. Headache was the chief complaint in 25 - 30% of cases in this group.

Conclusion

Half of all slow-growing brain tumors are still diagnosed more than 1 year after the onset of symptoms, even with the help of CT studies. We believe that this fact is related to the insufficient use of the technique. Continuing education programs should inform primary care physicians of the exceptional diagnostic potential for the method. This well necessarily lead to an increase in the number of CT studies performed, but we believe that the indication for the procedure must be expanded to include uncharacteristic or persistent headache. We shall deal with the significance of headache as the chief complaint in cases of brain tumor in an additional study.

References

1. Wende, S., Aulich, A., Kretzschmar, K., Grumme, Th., Meese, W., Lange, S., Steinhoff, H., Lanksch, W., Kazner, E.: Eine Sammelstudie über 1658 Tumoren. Radiologe 17, 149-156 (1977)
2. Kuhlendahl, H., Miltz, H., Wüllenweber, R.: Die Astrocytome des Großhirns. Acta Neurochirurgica 29, 151-162 (1973)

Conflicting Neuropathological and Computertomographic Findings in Cases of Suspected Brain Tumors or Retrobulbar Tumors

H.-U. Thal, A. Wanis, U. Pasch, and M. Weizsäcker

Introduction

CUSHING's monography includes 2000 histologically verified intracranial tumors, 1031 cases of suspected and 859 histologically unverified tumors during a period of 30 years. We report 12 cases among 520 space-occupying lesions seen during the last two years in whom the diagnosis of a tumor could not be proven histologically. 4 patients are already excluded where the clinical course or the second operation finally proved the diagnosis of a tumor. It seems that this number remains too high with respect to the improved diagnostic methods including CT scanning.

Material and Method

All patients were under outpatient surveillance up to 20 months (mean 10 weeks) before hospitalisation. Progression of symptoms which lasted for years in several cases (mean 31 weeks) and neuroradiological signs led to hospitalisation and operation. In the history, headache occurred with one patient, focal seizures with 3 patients, generalized seizures with 5, and hemiparesis with 3 patients. With 3 patients protrusio bulbi progressed despite corticosteroid therapy. Papilloedema occurred only with one patient. Except the patients with retrobulbar lesions, all had pathological EEG-findings demonstrating dysrhythmia in 3 cases, focal signs in 5 cases, general disorders in 2 cases, and epileptic signs in 2 cases. CT scans were performed 54 times, and in all cases the suspicion of tumor was mainly based on CT scan findings. In addition to the 3 lesions with retrobulbar location, 3 frontal, 1 temporal, 3 parietal, 1 occipital, and 1 infratentorial lesion could be localized. As seen in Table 1, six cases demonstrated low-density areas, 5 cases high-density areas, both with positive contrast enhancement. 1 case showed a low-density area with negative contrast enhancement. In this case and two others the lesions were space occupying. Radionuclide scans remained negative in almost all cases even after multiple controls. Therefore, ischemic lesions of the brain had to be excluded diagnostically. 9 patients had angiograms which were repeated with 2 patients. The results showed normal findings in 4 cases, poorly vascularized lesions in 4 cases, of which one was space-occupying. Tumor vessels within a space-occupying lesion were found in 1 angiogram. With another patient, occlusion of the aqueduct could be demonstrated by ventriculography as the cause of hydrocephalus and papilloedema.

Table 1. Computertomographic findings in 12 patients with suspected brain tumors or retrobulbar tumors

No. of patients	Density according to brain tissue	No. of patients with signs of space-occupying lesions
6	Hypodensity with enhancement	3
5	Hyperdensity with enhancement	2
1	Hypodensity without enhancement	1

Results

Including shunt operation and ventriculography 16 surgical interventions were done on the 12 patients. 13 specimens were taken for neuropathological diagnosis. In 7 cases tumors were suspected macroscopically, in 6 cases the macroscopical diagnosis remained unsure. The neuropathological evidence has been listed in Table 2. With 8 specimens, only signs of acute to chronic blood brain barrier disturbances were found neuropathologically including two, in which diffuse gliomas (grade I) were diagnosed. One biopsy showed multiple old brain abscesses. With 3 biopsies taken from the orbital lesions 2 showed chronic non-specific inflammation, and 1 normal fatty tissue. Brain infarction could be excluded for all specimens.

Table 2. Neuropathologic evidence in cases of suspected brain or retrobulbar tumors

No. of patients	
5	Acute to subacute brain edema
1	Chronic brain edema
2	Chronic brain edema with diffuse gliomatous reaction (gliom grade I)
1	Multiple brain abscesses
2	Unspecific inflammatory disease
1	Lipomatous tissue
12	

Postoperative CT scans verified that the surgical fields included the pathological areas, as seen in Figs. 1 and 2. One patient deteriorated during the course of the disease. Unfortunately, with reoperation no further diagnostic or clinical improvement could be achieved. This patient died at home, and no autopsy was performed. Another patient who died in hospital from an intercurrent infection was autopsied including histopathological investigation at our clinic.

Discussion

While false negative CT scans have been reported frequently (2, 4-6, 8, 9) false positive findings are rarely reported (6, 9). Only DAVIS and TAVERAS (4) reported on two patients in whom suspected brain tumors were not found during the operation. While 1 of these patients had radiation necrosis, no pathological findings were made with the other.

Of course, there is a preference to report positive results, but cases as reported above seem to exist. The diagnoses which have to be addressed in these cases did change slightly since the times of CUSHING (1, 3, 7): While syphilis, tuberculosis, or parasitoses of the brain became rare, diseases of the blood vessels now dominate the diagnostic considerations (2, 4, 5). Brain abscesses, bleeding disorders, trauma, aneurysms, or encephalitis play a minor role. Among our cases some groups can be separated.

The retrobulbar lesions: In 2 out of 9 retrobulbar lesions we found inflammatory pseudo-tumors exceeding the percentage reported by WENDE (10).

Only the patient presenting with papilloedema can be compared to the pseudo-tumors with or without hydrocephalus as reported by NONNE (7) and BAILEY (1). Also the patient reported by DAVIS and TAVERAS (4) has been operated upon false positive CT scan and ventriculography.

One patient demonstrated multiple old calcified brain abscesses which had been misinterpreted by us as oligodendroglioma preoperatively.

The remaining 7 cases with neurological signs and symptoms of hemisphere tumors demonstrated pathological findings in the CT scans and in one half of the angiograms. However, except in one case, radionuclide scans were negative. Especially, ischemic infarctions could not be verified by clinical, neuroradiological, and neuropathological findings. Meanwhile, 2 patients have died, and 1 patient's brain revealed diffuse gliomatosis of one hemisphere at autopsy. Whether the remaining 5 cases can be classified as "pseudo-tumor cerebri" according to NONNE with curative outcome (7) only the future will reveal.

Conclusion

12 cases are reported where the neuropathological findings of biopsy material could not prove the existence of tumors which were suspected preoperatively. The false positive CT scans in connection with progressive neurological status, and neuroradiological findings led to surgical intervention. In some of the 5 cases which remained diagnostically unclear only the clinical course may finally lead to the diagnosis. However, because autopsies frequently cannot be obtained, these cases may remain undiagnosed. For the responsible surgeon, these patients demonstrate that under certain circumstances neither the clinical investigation nor CT scans or neuroradiological findings can avoid negative results at operation.

References

1. Bailey, P.: Contribution to the histopathology of "pseudotumor cerebri". Arch. Neurol. and Psych. 4, 401-416 (1920)
2. Bradac, G.B., Simon, A.S., Grumme, T., Schramm, J.: Limitations of computed tomography for diagnostic neuroradiology. Neuroradiology 13, 5, 243-247 (1977)

3. Cushing, H.: Intrakranielle Tumoren. Berlin: Springer 1935
4. Davis, K.R., Taveras, J.M., Roberson, G.M., Ackerman, R.H.: Some limitations of computed tomography in the diagnosis of neurological diseases. Am. J. Roentgenol. 127, 111-123 (1976)
5. Kazner, E., Wende, S., Meese, W.: Reliability and limitations of cranial computerized tomography. In: Cranial Computerized Tomography. Lanksch, W., Kazner, E. (eds.), pp. 463-470. Berlin, Heidelberg, New York: Springer 1976
6. Mori, H., Lu, Ch., Chiu, L.C., Cancilla, P.A., Christie, J.H.: Reliability of computed tomography: Correlation with Neuropathologic Findings. Am. J. Roentgenol. 128, 795-798 (1977)
7. Nonne, M.: Über Fälle vom Symptomenkomplex "Tumor cerebri" mit Ausgang in Heilung (Pseudotumor cerebri). Dt. Ztschr. f. Nervenheilk. 27, 169-216 (1904)
8. Tentler, R.L., Palacios, E.: False-negative computerized tomography in brain tumor. Jama 238, 339-340 (1977)
9. Wende, S., Aulich, A., Lange, S., Lanksch, W., Schmitt, E.J.: Computerized tomography in diseases of the orbital region. In: Cranial Computerized Tomography. Lanksch, W., Kazner, E. (eds.), pp. 207-211. Berlin, Heidelberg, New York: Springer 1976
10. Wende, S., Aulich, A., Kretschmar, K., Grumme, Th., Meese, W., Lange, S., Steinhoff, H., Lanksch, W., Kazner, E.: Die Computer-Tomographie der Hirngeschwülste. Eine Sammelstudie über 1658 Tumoren. Radiologe 17, 149-156 (1977)

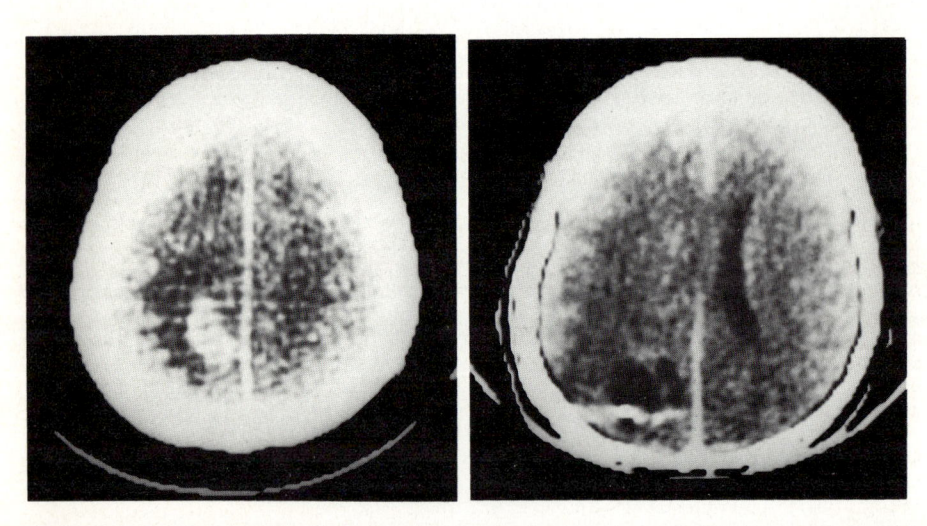

Fig. 1 *(left)*. Preoperative CT of patient M.K. with contrast enhancement

Fig. 2 *(right)*. Postoperative CT of patient M.K. after application of Angiografin

Computer Tomographic Findings of Brain Tumors Projected on X-Rays and Scalp

W. HASSLER, J. GILSBACH, W. BIRG, H.-R. EGGERT, and W. SEEGER

Introduction

Using computed tomography, it is possible in almost every case to directly establish the diagnosis of tumors, including their size and their relation to neighboring structures. CT scans have become more and more precise, enabling neuroradiologists to detect even very small tumors. This sometimes makes it difficult for the neurosurgeon to find the tumor at surgery. Only after section scans, which up to now have usually been horizontal, are transferred exactly onto X-rays and then onto the scalp can trepanation be so centred as to afford aid in localizing the tumor. A typical example is the parasagittal tumor, in which case major errors can occur if the plane of the layer is unknown.

Transferring Computer Tomographic Findings Onto the X-Ray

External Marking

A barium impregnated tube or a metal wire is placed over the shaved head of the patient and is fastened at each ear (4-9). Ideally it should lie in the parietal region over the assumed site of the tumor. A lateral skull scan is then taken. After this, with the marking tube still in place, computed tomography of the skull is carried out. The positional relation between the tumor and the outer tubes can be seen on the CT scan. Usually the tubes are not exactly on one place so that in the lateral scan, the front or back portion of the tube can be put in relation to the localization of the tumor (Figs. 1, 2).

Reference points of the skull on the X-ray - such as nasion, bregma, lambda, inion, and external auditory meatus - make it possible to transfer the size of the trepanation onto the X-ray.

Reconstruction of CT Layers on the X-Ray

A second possibility to transfer tumors onto the X-ray is to reconstruct the CT plane with the layer thickness and the layer angle (2, 10). Reconstruction is done using CT planes close to the base (Fig. 2). For this purpose, bony structures, which can be put in relation to the X-ray, are primarily used. These structures include the frontal sinuses, the orbital roofs, the sphenoid plane, the clinoid processes, the dorsum sellae, the surface of the petrous bone, the inion, and, in the upper layers of the ventricular sections, the foramina of Monro, the pinealis, and the posterior edge of tentorium (Table 1).

Table 1. Distances of inner cerebral structures from brain surface or skull inner surface

Frontal pole	Genu corporis callosum	30 - 35 mm
Frontal pole	Foramina of Monro	60 - 65 mm
Temporal pole	Occipital horn tip	40 mm
Occipital pole	End of corpus callosum	60 mm
Convexity (parietal region)	Corpus callosum	40 mm
Bregma	Foramina of Monro	60 mm

If one of the basal CT layers is transferred onto the X-ray, the CT scan is constructed layer by layer on the X-ray, according to the projective distortion. The distance from the bone is derived in the CT from the layers on which the tumor is demonstrated and is then transferred onto the X-ray.

Computational Transfer of the CT-Findings onto the X-Ray

A further possibility of transferring the CT-findings onto the X-ray is by computation. This has been proposed by BIRG, KREPPER, and MUNDINGER (1). This method involves scanning the frontal and occipital skull periphery points with a plotter into the individual axial CT sections and then feeding them into the computer (Fig. 2). After the desired X-ray distortion and the distance between the axial tomographic layers have been fed in, the computer, with the aid of the plotter, can then draw in a lateral reconstruction of the skull periphery and of the tumor borders. The drawing of the reconstruction is produced on a transparent stencil and is then superimposed on the corresponding X-ray. An advantage of this method is that after the skull points have once been fed in, a new stencil can be made up in any X-ray distortion scale. Thus a drawing can be constructed and adjusted for other X-ray methods such as angiography, ventriculography, and X-ray native scans. Modern CT-devices may provide a lateral or coronal reconstruction of the relevant brain areas; however, in contrast to this method, they yield only the relation skull convexity - brain contour - tumor contour, and not the relation skull convexity-tumor contour - brain vessels.

Transfer of the Tumor Localization from the X-Ray onto the Scalp

In transferring the tumor localization from the X-ray onto the scalp, reference points have to be used that are identical on the X-ray and on the external skull surface and scalp surface (Fig. 3).

The bregma is situated 13 cm from the nasion and can be recognized by its slight curvature. 12 cm behind the bregma in the midline is the point where the lambdoid and sagittal sutures meet. This point is seen as a small dent and can also be measured at 7 cm from the protuberantia occipitalis externa (Table 2).

Situated laterally on the skull is the fronto-zygomatic point which is the external protruding part of the orbital arch. In the X-ray it is not displayed but is an important reference point when the scalp has been opened. On the side of the skull, it is possible to identify

Table 2. Distances in the area of the skull convexity

Nasion	Bregma	13 cm
Bregma	Lambda	12 cm
Lambda	For. parietale	3 cm
Lambda	Inion	7 cm

Lambda = point where lambdoid and sagittal sutures meet

the sutures, the linea temporalis superior, and the beginning of the zygomatic arch. The zygomatic arch lies 1,5 cm in front of the external auditory meatus, which is not visible at operation (11-13).

Reference points on the head (scalp unopened) are nasion, bregma, inion, external auditory meatus, orbital arch, fronto-zygomatic point and midline (Table 3).

Examples

Frontal Tumors. The distance from the midline is measured in the a.p.-X-ray. In the case of fronto-polar tumors, we additionally measure the height above the orbital arch in order to determine the center of the tumor. With fronto-dorsal and fronto-lateral tumors, a line is drawn through the marked center of the tumor to the auditory meatus (alemannic obliquity). The other side of the line intersects the convexity of the skull. The distance to the bregma is measured from this point of intersection. With fronto-lateral tumors we measure the distance from the auditory meatus. It only makes sense, however, to take measurements of the distances from the tumor center up to 10 cm, since the curvature of the skull becomes too large at distances of more than 10 cm from the auditory meatus. The same procedure is used in the case of pre-central tumors.

Table 3. Reference points for brain tumor projection

	Skin	Skull	X-ray
Nasion	+	+	+
Bregma	+	+	+
Inion	+	+	+
Orbital Arch	+	+	+
Meatus acousticus ext.	+	+	+
Midline	+	+	+
Sutures	-	+	(+)
Fronto-zygomatic point	+	+	-
Beginning of zygomatic arch	-	+	-
Point where lambdoid and sagittal sutures meet	(+)	+	+
Linea temporalis superficialis	-	+	-

Temporal Tumors. The tumor can be constructed either as with fronto-lateral tumors or starting from the external auditory meatus. If the scalp has been opened, one can orientate oneself on the zygomatic arch, which is 1,5 cm in front of the auditory meatus.

Parietal Tumors. In the parietal region, particularly up to the lambdoid, the starting line bregma/auditory meatus is very suitable (alemannic obliquity) (Fig. 3). With tumors close to the convexity measurement is taken from the bregma or from the inion. If the tumors are situated in the area of the largest curvature of the skull cap, additional measurement is taken from the midline.

Occipital Tumors. Occipital tumors are constructed from the midline or from the base line of the external auditory meatus/inion. With tumors close to the midline additional measurement is taken from the midline.

Deep-Seated Tumors. Deep-seated tumors, whose position can also be determined in relation to ventricles, the foramina of Monro, and the pinealis, are projected onto the skull surface by the shortest distance. If during this procedure functionally important areas or large cerebral veins are hit, we shift the approach. The projective displacements that occur thereby are drawn in on the a.p.- and lateral X-ray.

Surgical Procedure. When the center of the tumor and its outer border is drawn on the scalp, the pedicle graft is placed around the tumor towards the base. The fact that the center of the tumor is situated in the middle of the graft provides an additional point of orientation.

Conclusion

The methods described above are useful albeit not as precise as stereotactic procedures. Minor errors can occur due to the position of the head during the operation and because of the various axis settings of the microscope.

A definitive advantage of these methods, however, is that the exact trepanation above the center of the tumor facilitates establishing points of orientation in cases of intracerebral tumors.

In a few years these methods might possibly be obsolete: the patient will then leave CT with a mark on his skin above the center of the tumor.

References

1. Birg, W., Krebber, L., Mundinger, F.: Ein einfaches Verfahren für die Übertragung von Tomographie-Scan-Schichten auf das Röntgenbild, insbesondere für die funktionelle Neurochirurgie. Fortschr. Neurol. Psychiat. 47, 637-640 (1979)
2. Cail, W.S., Morris, J.L.: Localization of intracranial lesions from CT scans. Surg. Neurol. 11, 35-37 (1979)
3. Galicich, J.H., Deck, M.: Surgical localization of small lesions demonstrated by CT scan. Neurosurg. 2, 170 (1978)
4. Hayman, L.A., Evans, R.A., Hinck, V.C.: Scalp markers for precise craniotomy siting, using computed tomography. Comput. Assist. Tomogr. 3, 701-702 (1979)

5. Hinck, V.C., Clifton, G.V.: A precise technique for craniotomy localication using computerized tomography. J. Neurosurg. 54, 416-418 (1981)
6. Lee, S.H., Villafana, T., Lapayowker, M.S.: CT intracranial localization with a new marker system. Neuroradiology 16, 570-571 (1978)
7. Levinthal, R., Winter, J., Bentson, J.R.: Technique for accurate localization with the CT scanner. Bull Los Angeles. Neurol. Soc. 41, 6-8 (1976)
8. Moseley, J.I., Giannotta, S.L., Renaudin, J.W.: A simple, inexpensive technique for accurate mass localization by computerized tomography. J. Neurosurg. 52, 733-735 (1980)
9. Norman, D., Newton, T.H.: Localization with the EMI scanner. Am. J. Roentgenol. 125, 961-964 (1975)
10. O'Leary, D.H., Lavyne, M.H.: Localization of vertex lesions seen on CT can. J. Neurosurg. 49, 71-74 (1978)
11. Seeger, W.: Atlas of topographical anatomy of the brain and surrounding structures. Wien, New York: Springer 1978
12. Seeger, W.: Microsurgery of the brain, Vol. 1: Anatomical and technical principles. Wien, New York: Springer 1980
13. Seeger, W.: Microsurgery of the brain, Vol. 2: Anatomical and technical principles. Wien, New York: Springer 1980

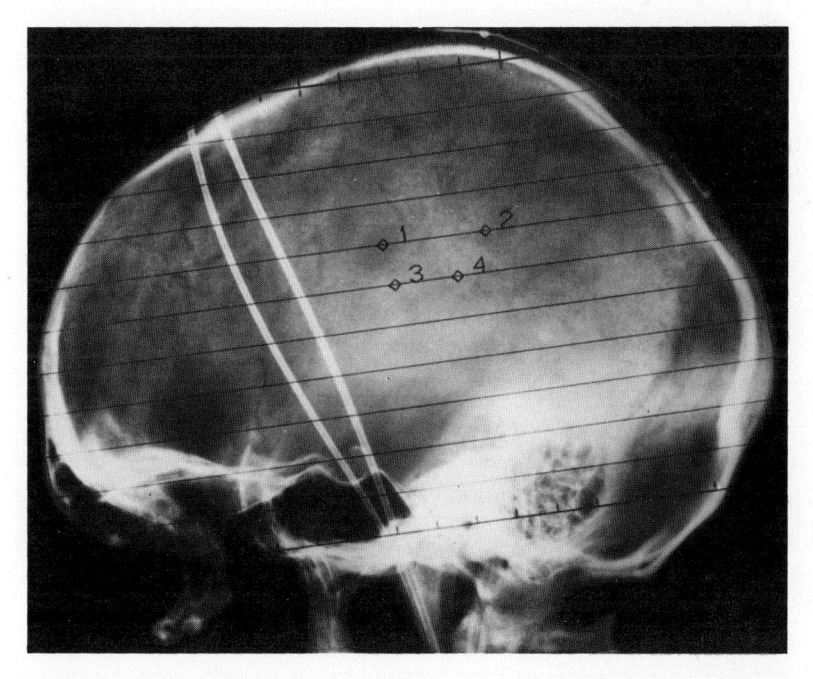

Fig. 1. CT with marking tube

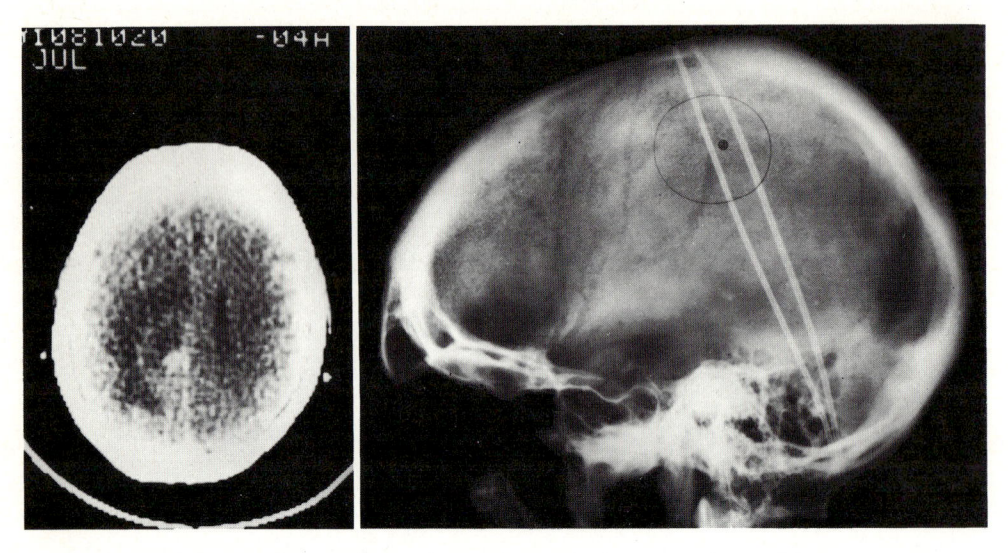

Fig. 2. Synopsis of the 3-marking-method (external marking, reconstruction of the CT-scan, computational transfer)

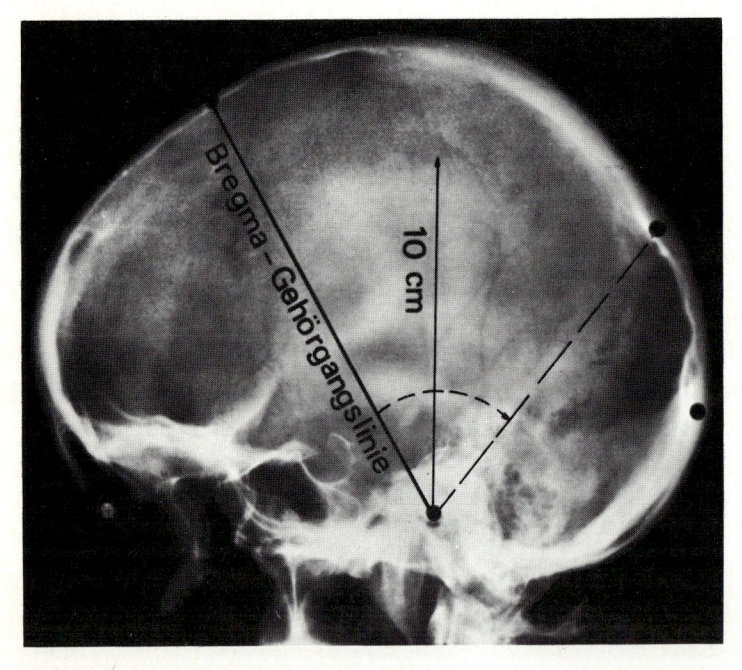

Fig. 3. Important marking points for construction of the tumor on the X-ray and scalp; alemannic obliquity: line bregma - external auditory meatus

Stereotactic Brain Surgery with the Aid of Computed Tomography (CT-Stereotaxy)

F. MUNDINGER and W. BIRG

Computer stereotaxy (2, 3) can be combined with modern computer tomographic systems to achieve directly, without the aid of invasive neuroradiological techniques, a precise presentation and targetting of the morphological structure (1, 4-7). We have now further developed our own procedure, based on the fact that with modern CT scanners it is possible to obtain from the CT scans the coordinate information necessary for the stereotactic operation.

A simple procedure for determining the target points for functional indications (Parkinson syndrome, extrapyramidal hyperkinesia, spasticity, epilepsy, intractable pain) and for non-functional indications (puncture and resection of tumors, cysts, foreign bodies, abscesses, the implantation of catheter and electrode systems and radioisotopes) is made possible with our stereotactic device (RIECHERT and MUNDINGER [7, 10, 11], MUNDINGER and BIRG [2, 3]). For it is one of the very few on the market today that works on the polar coordinate principle. This stereotactic device principle can be easily adapted to any CT device with a large gantry (> 40 cm).

The target point is the vertical tip of the cartesian spatial coordinates, which are established in the center of the base ring (= 0 point) fastened on the head. It is therefore only necessary to make the 0-point of the base ring identical with the 0-point of the coordinate system of the CT-scanner gantry and to establish the x-y-axis position. In this respect there are no changes to be made on our stereotactic device.

1. Procedure

The procedure is carried out as follows: the patient's head, which is placed securely with special fixers in a base ring developed for our stereotactic system is scanned in the CT gantry (Fig. 1). We have constructed a holder which makes it possible to achieve an exact relation between the coordinates represented on the scanner and the 0-point of the base ring; or to convert the CT coordinates into the base ring coordinates.[1]

(1) A frontal and sagittal scout view CT scan is taken (Fig. 2).

(2) CT scans are taken, parallel to the stereotactic base ring, with a gantry angle of 0° and a distance between layers of 5 - 10 mm. The lowest CT layer is in the 0 plane of the stereotactic base ring (z = 0) (see Fig. 2).

---

[1] These additional parts, like the stereotactic device, are manufactured by F.L. Fischer Hospital Equipment, D-7800 Freiburg/Br., West Germany

(3) Thin sections of 0.5 - 1.5 mm are made in the area of the relevant structures (diencephalon, tumor, etc.) in order to facilitate reconstruction in the coronal and sagittal plane.

(4) The sagittal and coronal reconstructions are calculated using the pixel size, according to the site of the target (1 - 20 = 1.1 - 22 mm). For time-saving purposes, these reconstructions are limited to the target area.

2. Evaluation

(1) Functional Stereotaxy: The thin section areas of the target range (diencephalon, internal capsules, amygdala, etc.) are measured with the CT computer or with an external computer. To determine the foramen of Monro - commissure posterior, which we usually take as the intracerebral base line (3, 9), the following structures are measured:

a) Foramen of Monro: The x and y coordinates are taken from the respective axial CT scans. The z coordinate is, in each case, given by the position of the section relative to the middle of the base ring (= 0-point).

b) Commissure Posterior: The coordinates are taken from the CT scans as with a).

c) The target point is determined in relation to the base line.

(2) If the software for reconstruction is available, the base line and the target point are taken from the sagittal and coronal (vertical) reconstruction of thin sections (1.5 mm) (Fig. 3). This is done according to the procedure carried out before in contrast ventriculograms. The structures are related to the coordinate system.

(3) Trepanation Point: The coordinates of the trepanation point are measured on the scout view scan. The y and z coordinates are taken from the sagittal scans, the x coordinate from the coronal scout view scan (Fig. 4). It must be taken into account in all evaluations of the scout view scan that only the plane containing the scanner axis is free of X-ray distortion. The measuring errors that arise from this, however, can be ignored in determining the trepanation point. The coordinates of the target point are measured from the sagittal and coronal reconstruction (Fig. 3).

(4) The electrode appraoch at a required angle to the target point (e.g., 65° to the zona incerta of the subthalamus) and the coordinate can be established in the reconstructions (sagittal, coronal) as well as in the scout view scans. The pertinent trepanation point is obtained in the same manner.

3. Non-Functional Neurosurgery

For non-functional neurosurgery, tumor biopsy, cyst drainage, catheter and radioisotope implantation, etc., coronal and sagittal reconstructions of the pathological process are made. The coronal projection of the tumor is taken from the coronal reproduction. The axial CT section is examined in which the greatest extension of, e.g., the tumor is manifested.

(1) The x and y coordinate of the tumor's "target point" are measured using the CT computer. The z coordinate is the level of the examined CT section (Fig. 4).

(2) The tumor is marked as "region of interest" and the mean X-ray density and the tumor surface in this section is established.

(3) The trepanation point is determined as under 2.(3)-(4).

All the coordinate information necessary for the stereotactic puncture with the aid of CT is thus at hand. There is no further need for contrast ventriculography. For economic and aseptic reasons, the operation takes place in the operating room. In the holder of the base ring an additional full size radiograph is built in a.p. and laterally. The setting parameters (angles, electrode) for the stereotactic device can be calculated using the coordinate information. The stereotactic computer program (2, 3) can be integrated into the CT computer software.

The 28 cases (March 31, 1981) treated by us so far, show that the stereotactically established target points are hit by probe or electrode with a deviation of less than 1 mm. This increase in precision is a result of the direct measuring of the anatomical and pathological structures - without a transferring process (ventriculography, angiography) or a special head fixation device (1, 5, 6) - and also of the direct use of the stereotactic coordinates.

The fact that no invasive neuroradiological methods are applied in functional neurosurgery makes it possible to use our methods on a wide range of indications, as far as age and relative contraindications are concerened (Tables 1 - 3). Our method also enabled us to treat small tumors with a diameter of only a few millimeters.

Table 1. Functional intracerebral indications for CT-stereotaxy

Pyramidal-, extrapyramidal motor disorders

Intractable pain (electrode stimulation system, DBS)

Epilepsies

Psychosurgery

Table 2. Non Functional intracranial indications for CT-stereotaxy

Biopsy

Puncture of cysts, abscesses

Implantation of radioisotopes, catheters

Extraction of foreign bodies

Resection of small tumors (metastasis)

Clipping, embolization of a.v.-malformations, aneurysms (combined open-stereotactic approaches)

Table 3. Advantages of CT-stereotaxy

Direct pathological anatomical morphological visualization of structures

Direct destination of targets

Less need of indirect invasive neuroradiological methods e.g. ventriculography (i. art. angiography)

Less complications

Wider range of indications (age, relative contraindications)

Better results

Abstract

Computed tomography (CT) - stereotaxy is presented as a new method of stereotactic neurosurgery. With the polar coordinate - stereotactic device developed by RIECHERT and MUNDINGER in the computer compatible modification by MUNDINGER and BIRG, the target points and their coordinates for functional indications (hyperkinesias, intractable pain, epilepsy, etc.) and non-functional indications (tumor biopsy, radioisotope and catheter implantation, etc.) are taken directly from the CT scan. The CT's are produced with a stereotactic base ring which is fastened on the head. Using a special adjustable holder, the 2 coordinate systems can be made to coincide. Invasive neuroradiological transfer procedures - indirect and secondary - (frame-constructions) are not necessary. The indication span is thus broadened and the precision of the stereotactic surgical procedure (> 1 mm) is further enhanced.

References

1. Bergström, M., Greitz, T.: Stereotactic computed tomography. A.J.R. 127, 167-170 (1976)
2. Birg, W., Mundinger, F.: Computer calculations of target parameters for a stereotactic apparatus. Acta neurochir. 29, 123-129 (1973)
3. Birg, W., Mundinger, F., Klar, M.: Computer assistance for stereotactic brain operations. Adv. Neurosurg. 4, 287-291 (1977)
4. Brown, R.A.: A computerized tomography-computergraphies approach to stereotaxic localization. J. Neurosurg. 50, 715-720 (1979)
5. Greitz, T., Bergström, M., Boethius, J., Kingsley, D., Ribbe, T.: Head fixation system for integration of radiodiagnostic and therapeutic procedures. Neuroradiology 19, 1-6 (1980)
6. Huk, W., Baer, U.: A new targeting device for stereotaxic procedures within the CT scanner. Neuroradiology 19, 13-17 (1980)
7. Koslow, M., Abele, M.G., Griffith, R.C., Mair, G.A., Chase, N.E.: A computerized tomographic controlled stereotactic surgical system (in press)
8. Mundinger, F.: Stereotaktische Operationen am Gehirn. Grundlagen-Indikationen-Resultate. Stuttgart: Hippokrates 1975
9. Mundinger, F., Riechert, T.: Die stereotaktischen Hirnoperationen zur Behandlung extrapyramidaler Bewegungsstörungen (Parkinsonismus und Hyperkinesen) und ihre Resultate. Fortschritte der Neurologie-Psychiatrie 1, 1-120 (1963)

10. Riechert, T., Mundinger, F.: Beschreibung und Anwendung eines Zielgerätes für stereotaktische Hirnoperationen (II. Modell). Acta Neurochir. 3, 308-337 (1956)

11. Riechert, T., Mundinger, F.: Ein kombinierter Zielbügel mit Bohraggregat zur Vereinfachung stereotaktischer Hirnoperationen. Arch. Psychiat. Nervenkr. 199, 377-385 (1959)

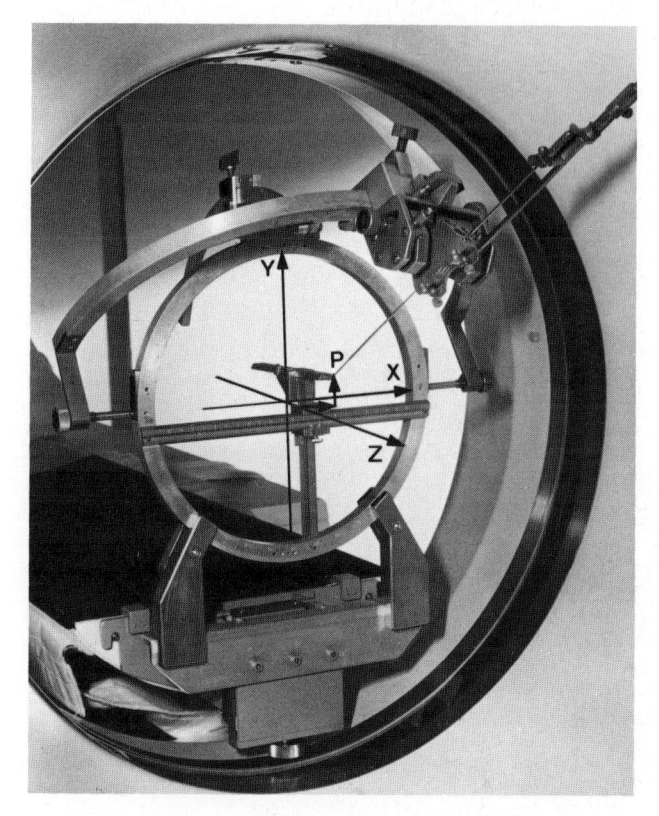

Fig. 1. Presentation of the CT scanner gantry with the stereotactic device developed by RIECHERT and MUNDINGER in the computer compatible modification by MUNDINGER and BIRG. The cartesian target point coordinates of the stereotactic device are identical with the coordinates of the CT scanner when the 0-point of the stereotactic device is in the origin of the CT scanner

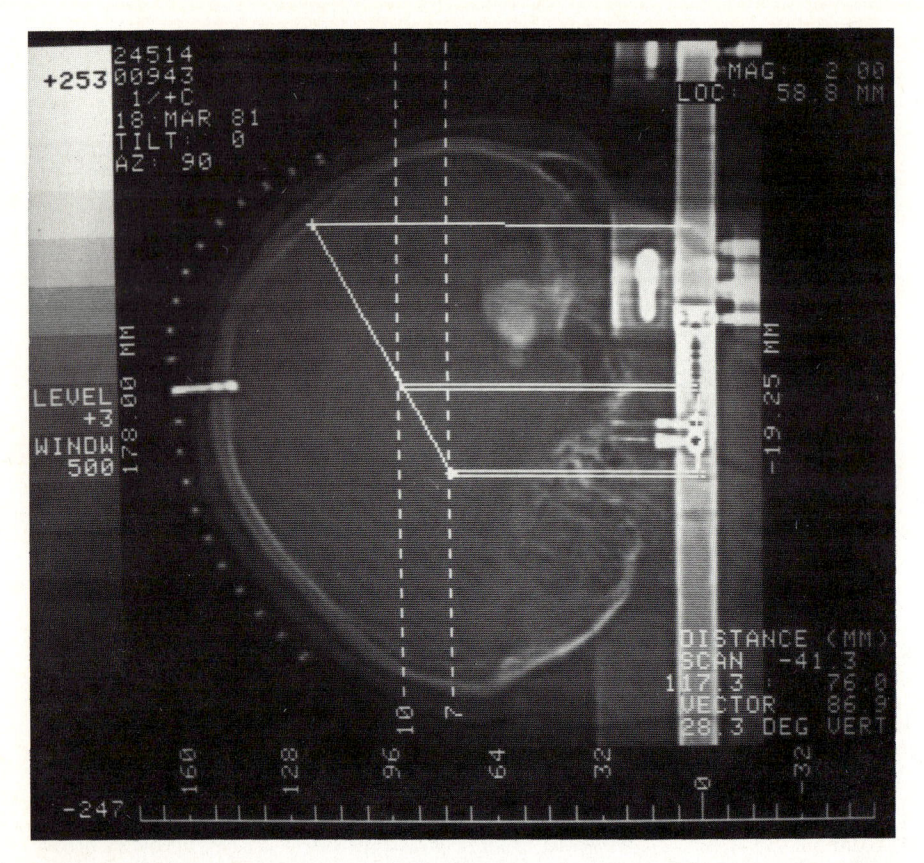

Fig. 2. Lateral scout view. CT scan taken parallel to the stereotactic base ring with a gantry angle of 0° and a distance between layers of 1,5 - 10 mm. The lowest CT layer is in the 0 plane of the stereotactic base ring (z = 0). The y- and z-coordinates of the trepanation point are measured on the scout view scan is taken from the x-coordinate from the coronal scout view scan (see Fig. 4)

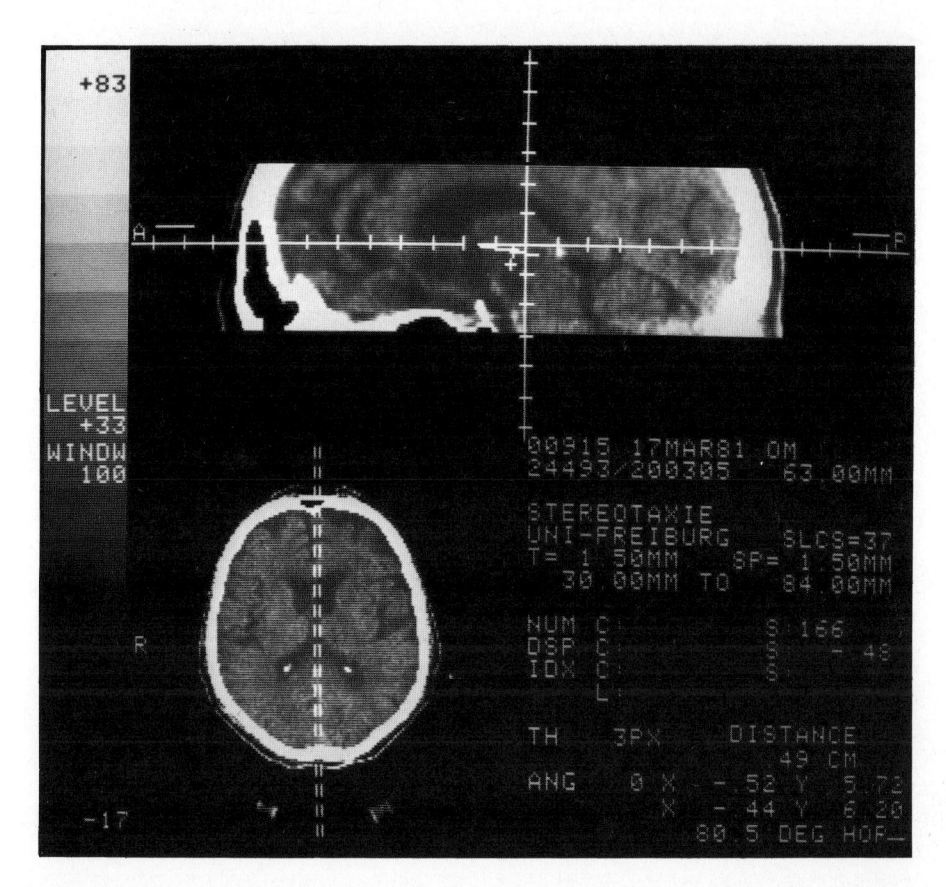

Fig. 3. Sagittal reconstruction of thin sections of 1,5 mm. The foramen of Monro and commissure posterior base line is marked. The target point (zona incerta in this case of parkinsonism) is determined in relation to the base line. The coordinates of the target point are calculated using the CT-computer

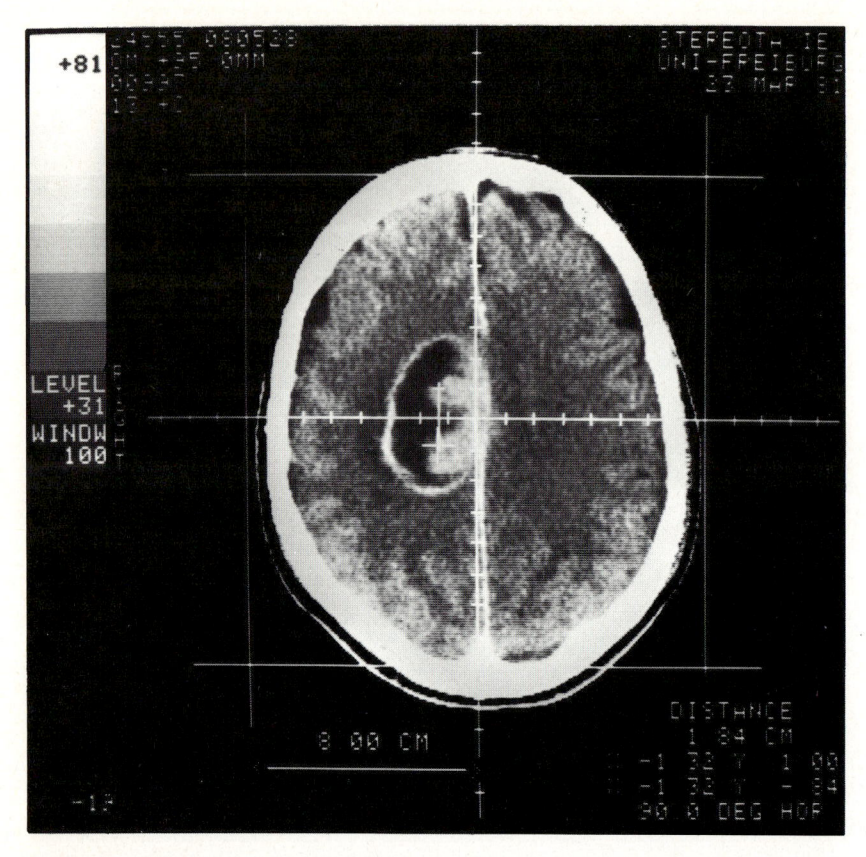

Fig. 4. Glioblastoma multiforme for interstitial iodine-125 Brachy-Curie-therapy. The two target points for the implantation are determined and the x- and y-coordinates are calculated using the CT-computer (see right lower corner). The z-coordinate corresponds with the CT level (in this case 95 mm above the middle of the base ring) (coronal scout view scan)

Necessity for Biopsy After the Introduction of Computerized Tomography

H. C. NASHER, H.-E. NAU, L. GERHARD, W. GROTE, and V. REINHARDT

Introduction

Computertomography has brought about an impressive improvement of localisation (and specifying) of cerebral diseases as well as the present improvement in radiological and chemical therapy. Therefore the opinion has increased that non-operative diagnosis is already sufficient (5, 12) in many patients for the decision for a specific therapy (like in cases of midline tumors the risk of biopsy seems to be much greater for some authors than the value of biopsy for diagnostic and therapeutical procedures). In our opinion, however, the comparison of neuroradiological and histological findings enables clinicians to discuss a more accurate way of therapy and avoid possible diagnostic errors. We would like to demonstrate this in a number of cases and point to possible sources of diagnostic errors.

The most frequent discrepancies between clinical and histological diagnosis - in special regard to computertomography - is demonstrated in Table 1. On the one hand there is a misinterpretation of circulatory disturbances and inflammations as gliomatous tumors (3), on the other hand a wrong estimation of the kind of the underlying tumorous process. That is why a tumor may be thought of as being malignant, but during operation it proves itself as a relative benign one (11). Also metastasis and gliomatous tumors sometimes cannot be differentiated without the help of biopsy (7). This differentiation, however, is nowdays necessary following the introduction of very diverse radio- and chemotherapeutic procedures or for the successful control of such management. So the radiation of a benign tumor can be the consequence of the non-operative clinical diagnosis. The misinterpretation of circulatory disturbances as inflammatory (8) or tumorous processes can be called an extremely bad mistake. In these cases the therapy of the underlying disease is impossible or may be seriously delayed. For example the administration of cortisone and derivatives is contraindicated in inflammatory processes as well as the suppression of the endogenous defence mechanisms by chemotherapy and irradiation.

Case Reports

Case 1: Differential diagnosis: tumor - vascular disease.
45-year-old diabetic patient developed grand mal attacks. CT scan showed hypodense and hyperdense areas in the native scan, spotted enhancement in the head of caudate nucleus, putamen, pallidum and the right parietal lobe after application of contrast medium. Angiography confirmed a space-occupying process without pathological vessels in the right parietal area.

Table 1. Possible misinterpretations by CT

Clinical diagnosis	Biopsy diagnosis
Primary brain tumor	Ischaemia, infarction, hematoma, primary vascular disease
Primary brain tumor	Inflammation, abscess, encephalitis, demyelinating processes (multiple sclerosis)
Metastatic tumor	Primary brain tumor
Malignant primary brain tumor	Benign intracranial tumor

Histology demonstrated cortical areas with large hemorrhages and fibrous tissue which has started an organizing reaction from the leptomeninges. Elastica - van GIESON revealed no tumor at all. HE stain demonstrated mainly older hemorrhages (Fig. 1).

Case 2: Differential diagnosis: malignant primary tumor - benign intracranial tumor.

47-year-old patient with decompensated renal insufficiency. After the first generalized seizure CT scan: hypodense space occupying lesion in the left frontal lobe, extending into the right hemisphere via the genu of corpus callosum. Renal insufficiency permitted only low dose application of contrast medium.
Histology showed two aspects of this tumor. In addition to a characteristic portion of a meningiotheliomatous meningioma histology revealed a complete fatty degeneration of meningioma cells in 90% of the tumor. This might be the cause for a partly non-typical picture of the CT scan.

Case 3: Differential diagnosis: benign intracranial tumor - malignant primary brain tumor.

74-year-old male with hypacusis and facial paresis on the left side, disturbed labyrinthine function and incoordination. In the scan homogenous enhanced area with low grade perifocal oedema in the left cerebellopontine angle and without fourth ventricle.
Histology revealed small to medium sized cells with very scanty cytoplasm arranged in lines between argophylic fibres. Typical picture for a lymphoma or reticulum cell sarcoma (Fig. 2).

Case 4: Differential diagnosis: metastasis - benign intracranial tumor.

42-year-old female with non-Hodgkin lymphoma IV in complete remission after chemotherapy. After developing a left hemiparesis focal radiation therapy of the intracranial tumor without success.
CT scan showed a polycyclic homogenous enhanced area extending to the lateral ventricle.
Histology confirmed a typical meningioma (Fig. 3).

Case 5: Differential diagnosis: metastasis - malignant primary brain tumor.

69-year-old female with progressive aphasia and hemiparesis. Radiological signs of renal tumor.
CT scan showed a left parietal hypodense area with ring blush.
Histology revealed only small areas with undifferentiated glious cells among large areas of nearly complete necrosis of a glioma or a glioblastoma.

Case 6: Differential diagnosis: benign intracranial tumor - malignant primary brain tumor.

53-year-old female with hemianopsia and cerebellar symptoms.
CT demonstrated a nearly homogenously enhanced structure in the right occipital lobe. Operative diagnosis: meningioma of the tentorium.
Histology of the biopsy material had a very polymorphic appearance with giant cells, many spindle cells of different sizes and strands of connective tissue suggesting some sarcoma with a possible metastatic or meningeal origin. The autopsy proved a glioblastoma extending mainly in the arachnoid space and invading the dura mater. A cortical field from the occipital lobe showed typical tumorous glia cells (Fig. 4).

Conclusion

The examples demonstrate the initially mentioned problems. Clinical mistakes in diagnosis may have different causes, but the most frequent cause is misinterpretation of the CT scan. The pseudospecificity of the computerized picture can be imitated by etiologically very different processes in the single case. This statement can even be proven by the interpretation of ring structures in the CT scan and the underlying morphological processes (1, 4, 6, 9, 10). In cases of obvious CT diagnosis other clinical procedures are not performed for reasons of risks and costs; there we would remind you of angiography, cytology of CSF as well as diagnostic laboratory measurements. Our experience demonstrates that the place of clinical procedures is more and more taken over by detailed CT diagnosis only (in contrast to this comparison of detailed CT and biopsy findings can even elucite the morphological diagnosis which would remain uncertain, at least without the CT).

In this regard the enormous difficulty to differentiate between reactive, secondary or perifocal glial alterations - also in cases of stereotactic biopsy (2) and the central metastatic tumor or a nonglial tumor has been diminished by the comparison of CT scans - also in the course of the disease - for the histologist. It has to be stressed however that the biopsy has to contain enough material for histological examination. This cannot be achieved by stereotactic biopsy.

References

1. Baker, H.L., Houser, O.W., Campbell, J.K.: National cancer institute study: Evaluation of computed tomography in the diagnosis of intracranial neoplasms. I. Overall results, Radiology 136, 91-96 (1980)
2. Bosch, D.A.: Indications for stereotactic biopsy in brain tumors. Acta Neurochirurgica 54, 167-179 (1980)
3. Foy, P.M., Leandro, L., Shae, M.D.: Vascular malformation simulating a glioma on computerized tomography. J. Neurosurg. 54, 125-127 (1981)
4. Kendall, B.E., Jakubowski, J., Pullicino, P., Symon, L.: Difficulties in diagnosis of supratentorial gliomas by CT scan. J. Neurolog., Neurosurg. and Psychiatry 42, 485-492 (1979)

5. Latchaw, R.E., Payne, J.T., Loewenson, R.B.: Predicting brain tumor histology: Change of effective atomic number with contrast enhancement. AJR 135, 757-762 (1980)

6. Nahser, H.C., Nau, H.-E., Reinhardt, V., Löhr, E.: Computertomographische Befunde und Verlaufskontrolle bei konservativ und operativ behandelten intracerebralen Blutungen nicht traumatischer und nicht aneurysmatischer Genese. Radiologie 20, 122-129 (1980)

7. Nahser, H.C., Gerhard, L., Reinhardt, V., Nau, H.-E., Bamberg, M.: Diffuse and multicentric brain tumors - correlation of histological, clinical and CT-appearance. Acta Neuropathol. (Berl.), Suppl. VII, 101-104 (1981)

8. Nahser, H.C., Gerhard, L., Flossdorf, R., Clar, H.C.: Development of brain abscess - computerized tomogram compared with morphological studies. In: Advances in neurosurgery, Vol. 9, pp. 32-35. Heidelberg, New York: Springer 1981

9. Potts, D.G., Abott, G.F., Snydern, J.V. van: Evaluation of Computed tomotraphy in the diagnosis of intracranial neoplasms. III. Metastatic tumors. Radiology 136, 657-664 (1980)

10. Pullicino, P., Kendall, B.E.: Contrast enhancement in ischemic lesions. Neuroradiology 19, 235-239 (1980)

11. Pullicino, P., Kendall, B.E., Jakubowski, J.: Difficulties in diagnosis of intracranial meningiomas by computed tomography. J. Neurol., Neurosurg. and Psychiatry: 43, 1022-1029 (1980)

12. Zülch, K.J.: Principles of the New World Health Organization (WHO) Classification of brain tumors. Neuroradiology 19, 59-66 (1980)

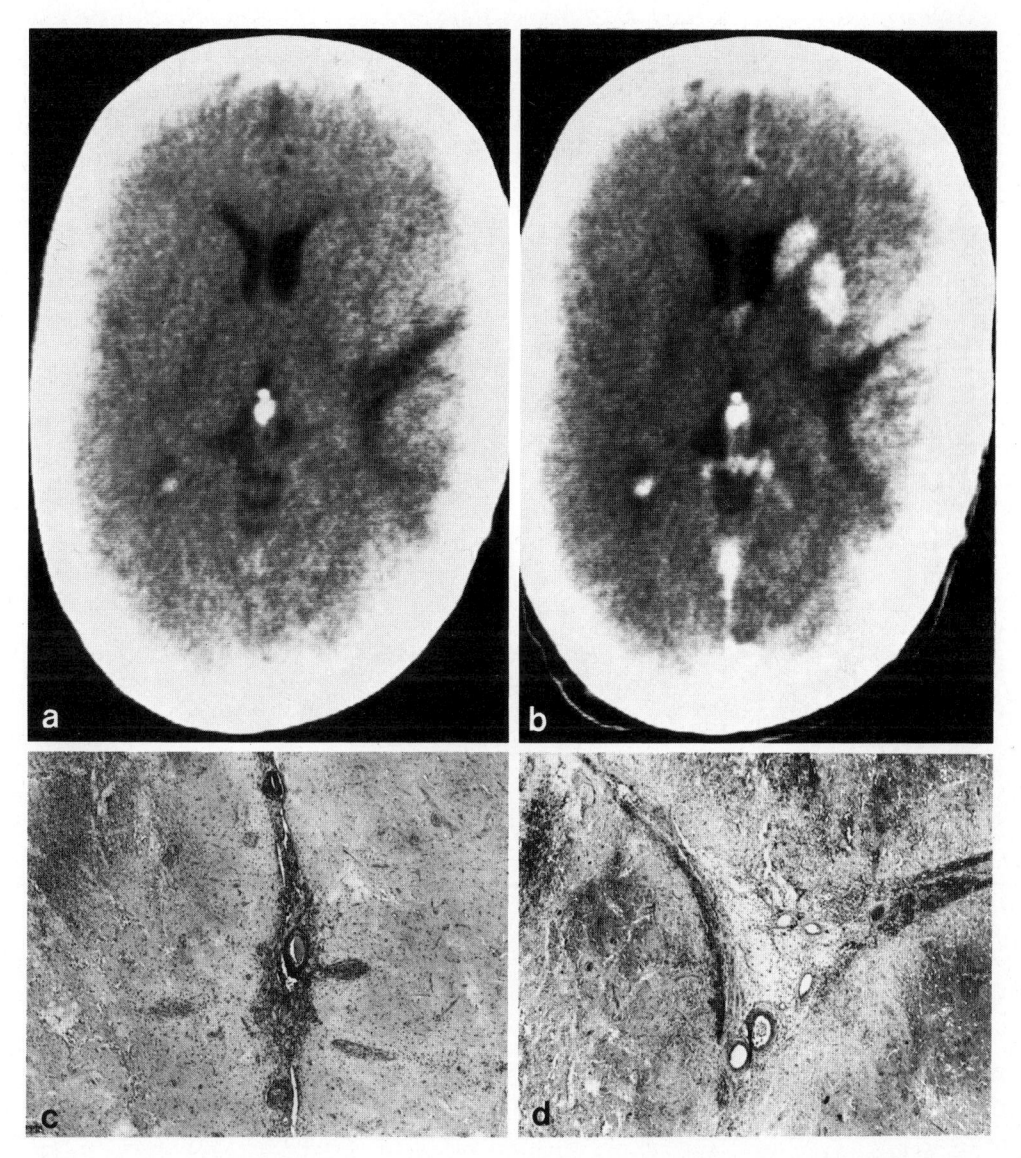

Fig. 1 a-d. CT diagnosis: gliomatous tumor. a Scan without contrast. b Postcontrast scan. Histological diagnosis: hemorrhagic necrosis. c Elastica v. GIESON stain (38:1). d HE stain (38:1)

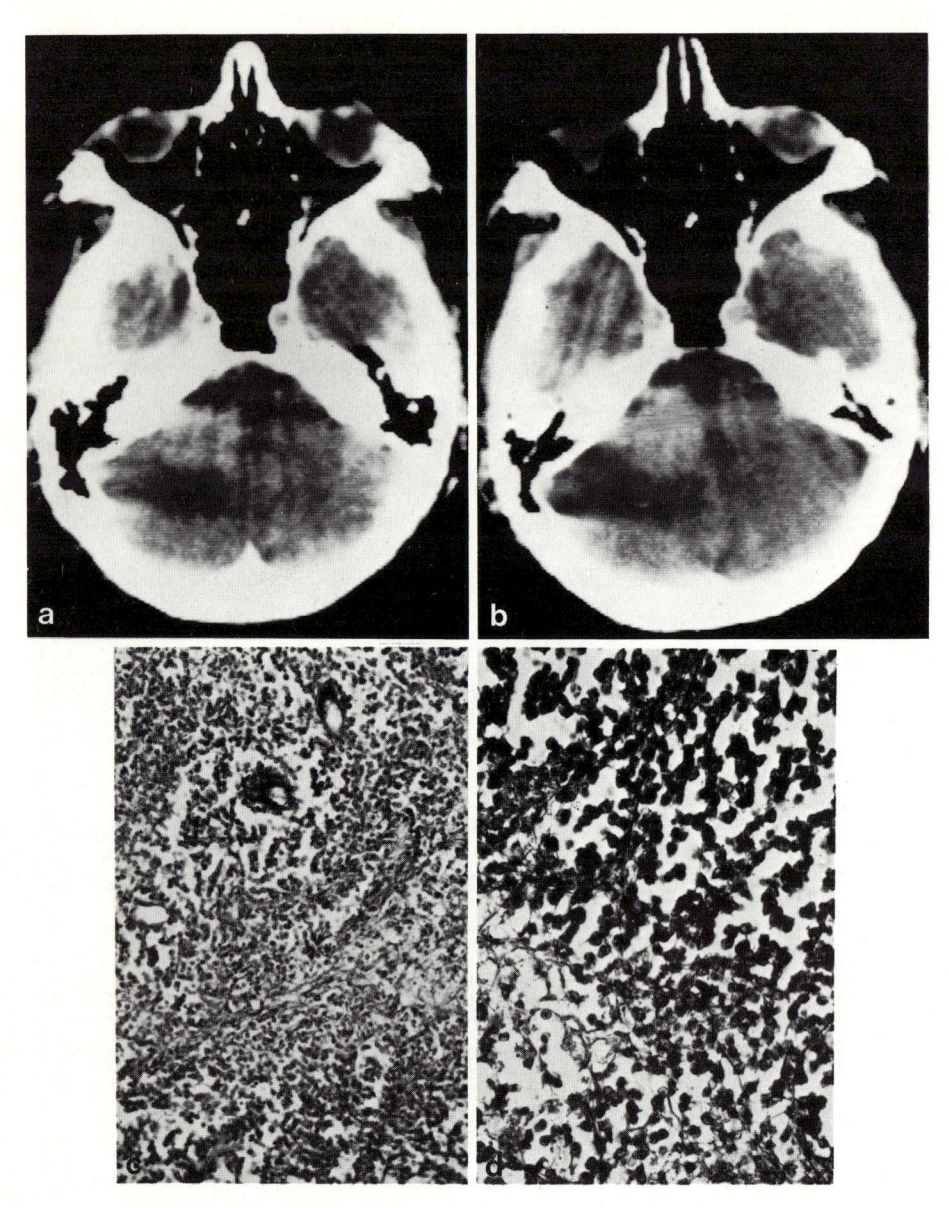

Fig. 2 a-d. CT diagnosis: tumor of cerebellopontine angle. a, b Postcontrast scan. Histological diagnosis: lymphoma or reticulum cell sarcoma. c PAS-reaction (175:1). d Gomori stain (400:1)

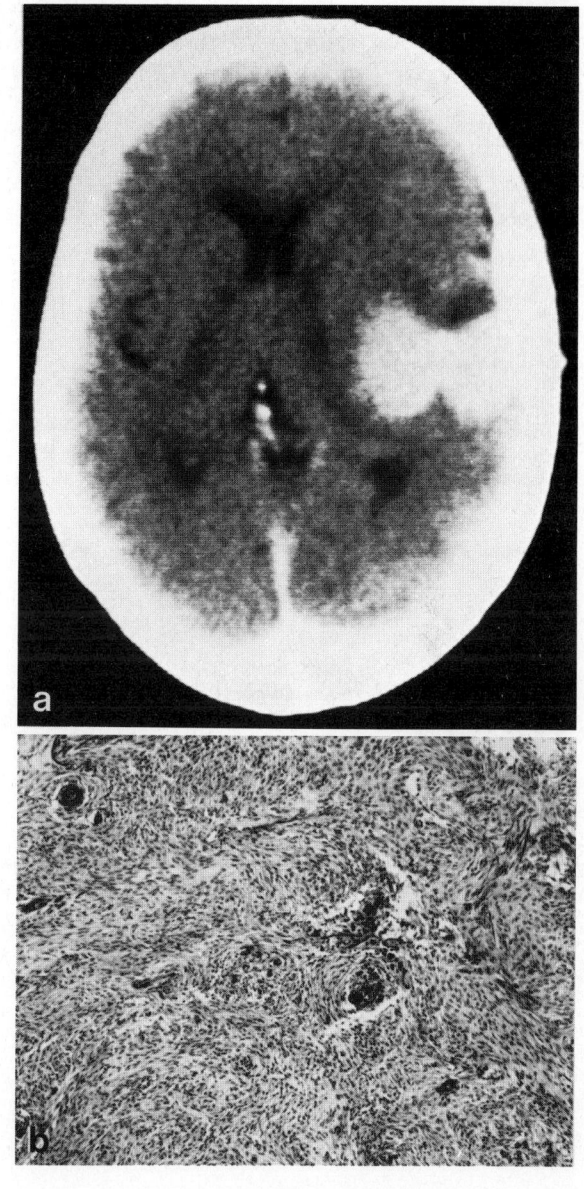

Fig. 3 a, b. CT diagnosis: metastasis of non-Hodgkin lymphoma. a Postcontrast scan. Histological diagnosis: meningioma. b Elastica v. GIESON stain (90:1)

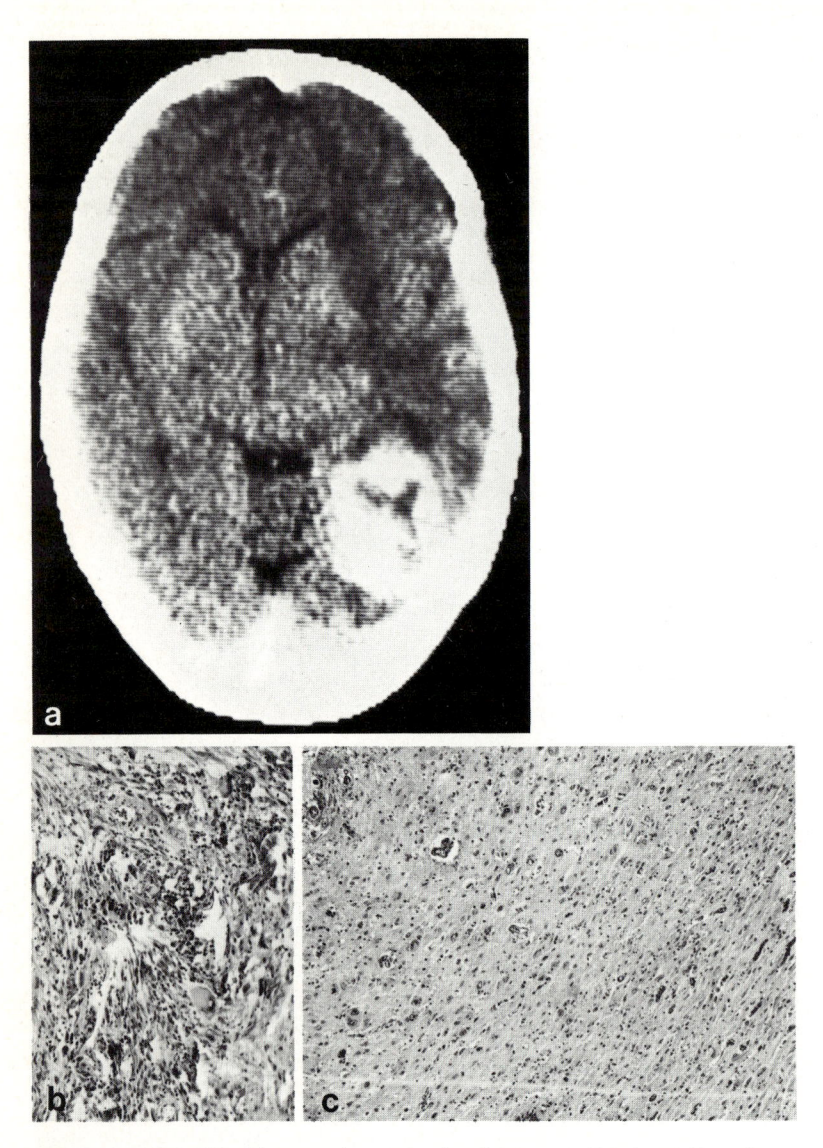

Fig. 4 a-c. CT diagnosis: meningioma. a Postcontrast scan. Histological diagnosis: b Bioptic material: sarcoma-like picture, Elastica v. GIESON stain (70/1). c Autoptic material: occipital lobe with tumorous glia cells, HE stain (70:1)

The Value of Computerized Tomography in the Preoperative Diagnosis of Brain Tumors

W. Huk and M. Klinger

The reliability of CT-findings in establishing the preoperative diagnosis of the various kinds of intracranial tumors has been discussed since computerized tomography (CT) was introduced into neuroradiology. In the meantime experience with a larger number of tumors allows a more realistic evaluation of the significance of CT images of brain tumors than in the beginning.

In Table 1 the most important measurable and visual parameters of brain tumors in the CT-image are listed. As the measurable parameters are of little value in routine diagnosis, we have concentrated only on the visual features. In a number of cases some of these lead to the identification of intracranial neoplasms. Among these characteristics the localisation of brain tumors is of major diagnostic importance, for example in tumors of the pituitary fossa, pineal gland and the cerebellopontine angle. Specific density values, which are another quality of similar significance are much less frequent. These include lipomas (Fig. 1) and epidermoid cysts.

In the great majority of brain tumors, however, no criteria of sufficient diagnostic reliability are known. This group includes gliomas, meningiomas, metastases and others.

In a series of 703 tumors, the eight most common neoplasms were studied (Table 2): Meningiomas were accurately recognized in 90% of the cases. Differentiation of histological subgroups and proof of the rare malignancy of meningiomas was not possible (Fig. 2).

Table 1. CT-parameter of brain tumors

1. Measurable parameters
a) Mean density
b) Density distribution (histogram, density profile)

2. Visual parameters
a) Localisation
b) Signs of space occupation
c) Density distribution
d) Density distribution
e) Regularity and definition of borderline
f) Degree of enhancement
g) Perifocal edema

Table 2. Diagnostic accuracy of CT in the diagnosis of brain tumors

Type of tumor	No. of cases	Diagnosed by CT	Diagnostic accuracy (%)
Astrocytoma I + II	40	28	70
Glioblastoma	117	85	73
Meningioma	156	142	91

There is a danger of misinterpretation in cases of lymphomas, gliomas, solid angioblastomas, neurinomas and metastases.

Among 40 histologically verified astrocytomas grade I and II of our series 70% showed a "typical" CT-image. In six tumors with similar features, however, higher grades of malignancy were detected (Fig. 3). Differential diagnostic considerations should include all hypodense lesions of neoplastic and non-neoplastic origin such as encephalitis and brain infarction.

Calcifications were seen in 15% of the astrocytomas and 75% of the oligodendrogliomas (Table 2).

In more malignant gliomas and in glioblastomas, increasing and pathological vascularity was observed with blood-brain-barrier dysfunctions and regressive changes. CT-findings showed iso- or hyperdense areas of solid tumor tissue with positive contrast enhancement and hypodense zones of necrotic tissue and perifocal edema. After enhancement vital tumor parts may appear as ring-shaped (48,1%), irregular (30,2%) or nodular (19,7%) structures. Glioblastomas on the other hand may also be seen as merely hypodense areas or cysts.

The differential diagnosis of these tumors therefore includes all benign and malignant tumors of the central nervous system, as well as non-neoplastic lesions such as abscesses and cerebral infarctions. In our series diagnostic problems existed in 34 out of 106 cases (27%).

This means that the CT-image of glioblastomas is much less significant than that of meningiomas. Nevertheless, a ring-shaped tumor in the age group from 40 - 60 years indicates a "glioblastoma" as the most probable diagnosis. Not because of its unmistakable CT-image, however, but because of its relatively high incidence in this age group.

The CT-findings of cerebral metastases were variable and offered no significant information as to the underlying matrix. Single metastases, which we saw mainly in cases of bronchial, hypernephroid and GI-tract carcinomas, may be mistaken for primary intracranial tumors (Fig. 4). This diagnostic problem is not completely eliminated in multiple lesions, since multilocular growth is also seen in glioblastomas, meningiomas, lymphomas, abscesses and even encephalomyelitis.

The *diagnostic reliability of CT images* of less frequent kinds of brain tumors according to the literature and our own findings was 50%.

In the beginning of the CT-era ELKE and co-workers had the impression that every brain tumor may be mistaken for every other brain tumor. This statement seems to be valid even today. However, experience has taught us to differentiate between the various kinds of brain tumors. Together with the patient's history and the clinical information, CT enables us to establish the diagnosis of many brain tumors with sufficient reliability, so that therapeutic decisions can be made. CT-findings still do not provide the conclusiveness of histological examinations. In cases, where a histological diagnosis is necessary, a - stereotaxic - biopsy should therefore be made.

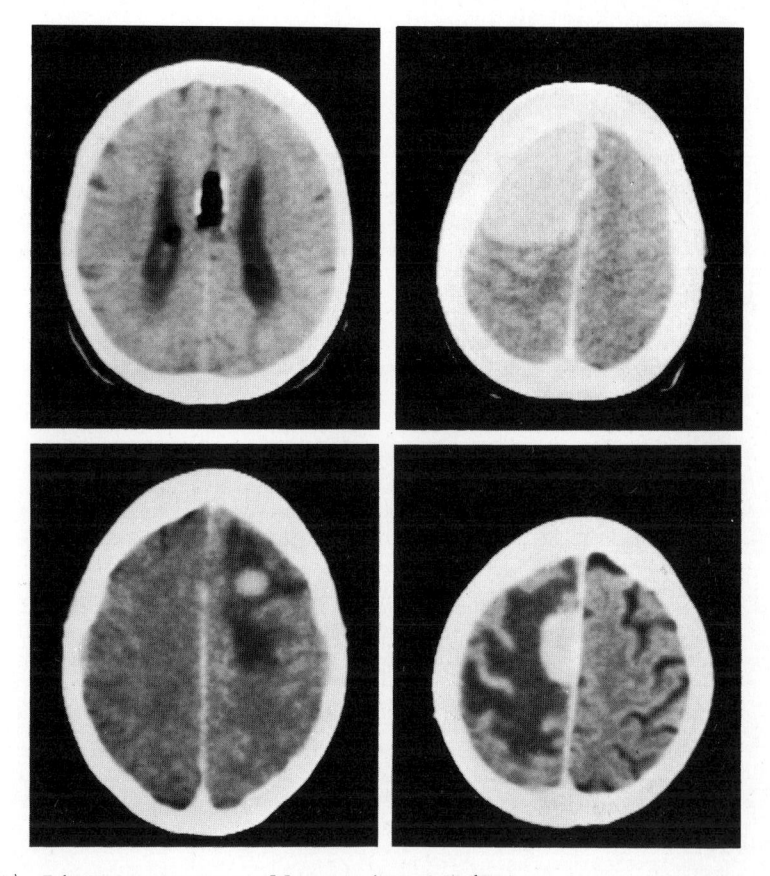

Fig. 1 (above left). Lipoma corpus callosum (CT 169/79)

Fig. 2 (above right). Malignant meningioma (CT 3548/78)

Fig. 3 (below left). Astrocytoma, not a metastasis with perifocal edema (CT 3671/79)

Fig. 4 (below right). Solitary metastasis of breast cancer, not a meningioma of the falx (CT 3824/79)

Metrizamide CT for Diagnosis of Intracranial Cystic Lesions

H. Arnold and D. Kühne

For the recognition of cystic intracranial abnormalities, CT has made it possible to avoid invasive procedures such as pneumoencephalography, ventriculography and angiography. Moreover it provides more precise information than the invasive methods regarding anatomical relationships of those lesions. Whenever necessary, CSF enhancement by intrathecal metrizamide can be performed in order to narrow the differential diagnostic possibilities and to complete information needed for pretreatment and preoperative planning.

During the period from 1976 to 1981 more than 40 cystic intracranial lesions were recognized by CT scan, in 18 of which metrizamide enhancement has been thought to be of diagnostic use.

Normally, large temporal arachnoidal cysts can be diagnosed by CT scan due to the typical intracranial alterations caused by them: enlargement of the temporal fossa, sharp boundary against the surrounding brain, shift of the midline structures. Occasionally the cyst is less pronounced, and shifting of the midline structures to the opposite side is not seen though some bulging of the temporal bone can be observed. In those cases, free communication of the cystic formation with the normal subarachnoid space is to be supposed, the proof of which can be provided by metrizamide CT cisternography (Fig. 1). Most of supratentorial midline cysts can be recognized as communicating or noncommunicating formations from their site, shape, and effect on the surrounding structures and the ventricular system. Generally, additional investigations are superfluous. Metrizamide CT is helpful, if the question whether the cystic lesion communicates with the ventricular system cannot be answered by normal CT scan. In case 2, a communication between the frontomedial cystic lesion and the ventricular system was proved by very discrete ventricular CSF and equal cyst fluid enhancement that was not visible on the photographs but recognizable by measuring the CT units. Paracollicular cysts produce typical alterations almost always excluding doubts in diagnosis.

Only rarely difficulties will arise in deciding if there exists an enlarged chiasmatic cistern or an intracisternal cystic lesion not visible in normal CT scan. CSF contrast enhancement allows one to visualize intracisternal cysts. In case 3 (Fig. 2) an explanation for amenorrhoea was searched for, and a suprasellar cyst was detected. In contrast, in case 4 (Fig. 3) CT cisternography did not contribute to the diagnosis of a large supra- and retrosellar cyst.

Dandy-Walker malformation exhibits typical pathological features on CT scan. The abnormally high position of the torcular Herophili and lateral sinuses, absence of the cerebellar vermis, wide separation of the cerebellar hemispheres, dilatation of the ventricular system, and a large infratentorial midline cyst permit one to make the diagnosis. An additional procedure is not required. Extra-axial posterior fossa cysts may mimic Dandy-Walker malformations, but by means of CT scan one can readily differentiate them from each other. The fourth ventricle can be identified. It is mostly pushed forward or shifted laterally.

By chance, the question may be raised, whether a connection between an arachnoidal cyst and a cistern or ventricle brought about by operation continues to be patent. CSF contrast enhancement makes it possible to prove patency by means of CT scan (Fig. 4).

Metrizamide enhancement may be helpful in recognizing the limits of the cysts in relation to the cisterns and to identify the fourth ventricle. Generally, however, CSF enhancement will be dispensable since the shape of the lesion and the shifting of the surrounding structures is evidence of the cystic nature of the space-occupying lesion. At a first glance, a large cisterna magna can sometimes be mistaken for either of the two entities mentioned above. It is a variant, however, that is thought to be normal in infants or young children and can be readily differentiated from a Dandy-Walker malformation and extra-axial infratentorial cysts. CT demonstrates a large or giant cisterna magna presenting with a normal fourth ventricle and a ventricular system which is not dilated.

Metrizamide CT cisternography can provide additional information concerning cystic intracranial lesions. A skilful analysis of the CT scan, however, renders metrizamide application dispensible in most instances. Critical re-evaluation of 18 cases which were given metrizamide for CSF enhancement revealed, that additional information useful for planning therapeutic procedures was gathered in only 5 cases.

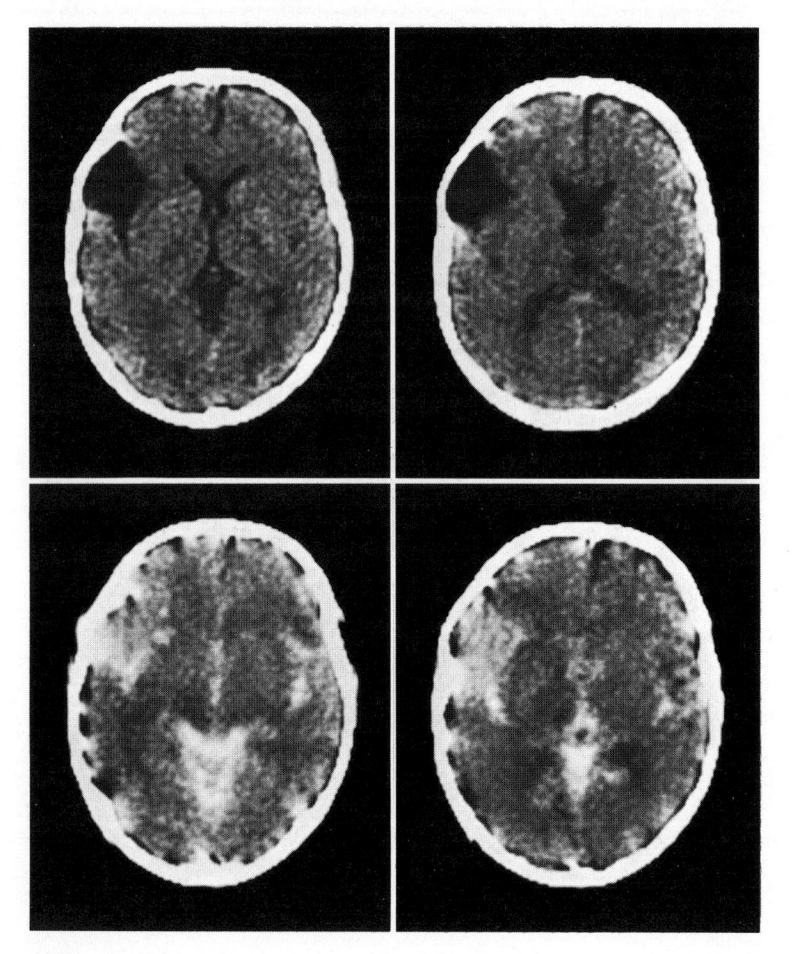

Fig. 1. Left temporal cyst without shifting of the midline structures. Slight bulging of the temporal bone. Metrizamide enters the cyst proving free communication to the basal cisterns

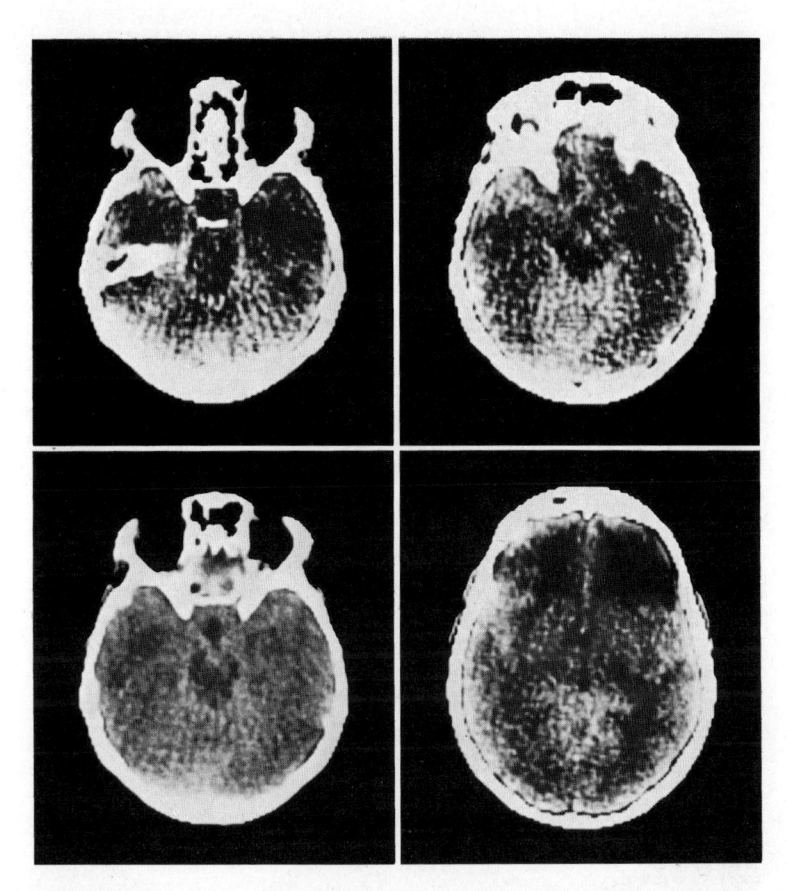

Fig. 2. Small suprasellar cyst not visible in normal CT scan. After metrizamide application a suprasellar sparing turns out proving the presence of a cyst

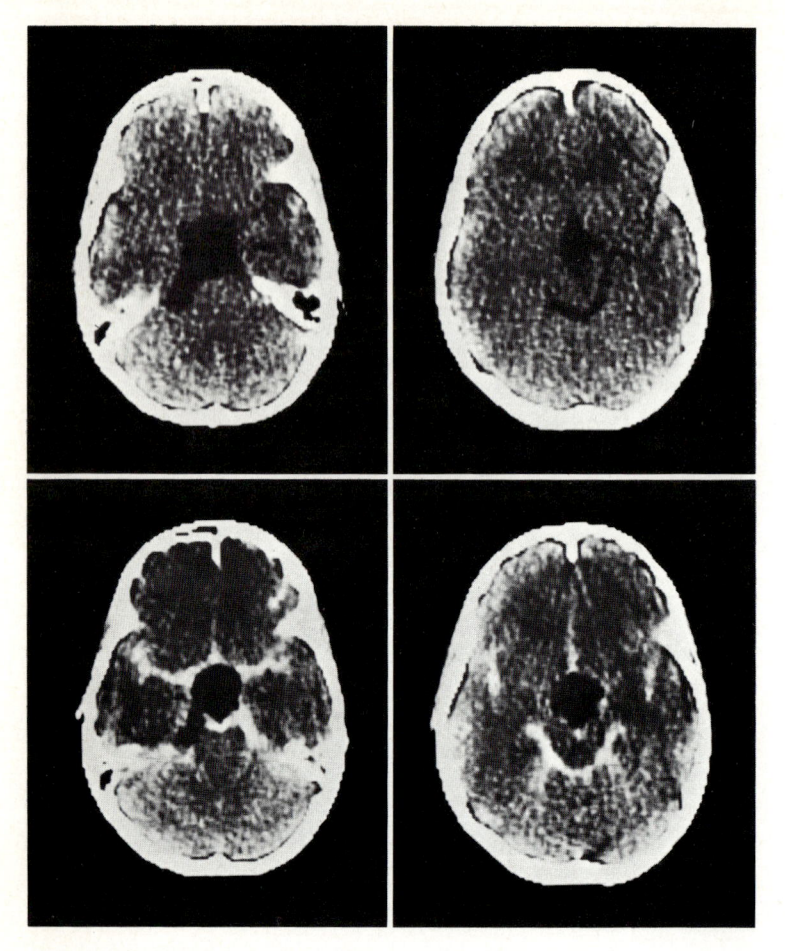

Fig. 3. A large supra- and retrosellar cyst presents in normal CT scan. CSF contrast enhancement provides little additional information

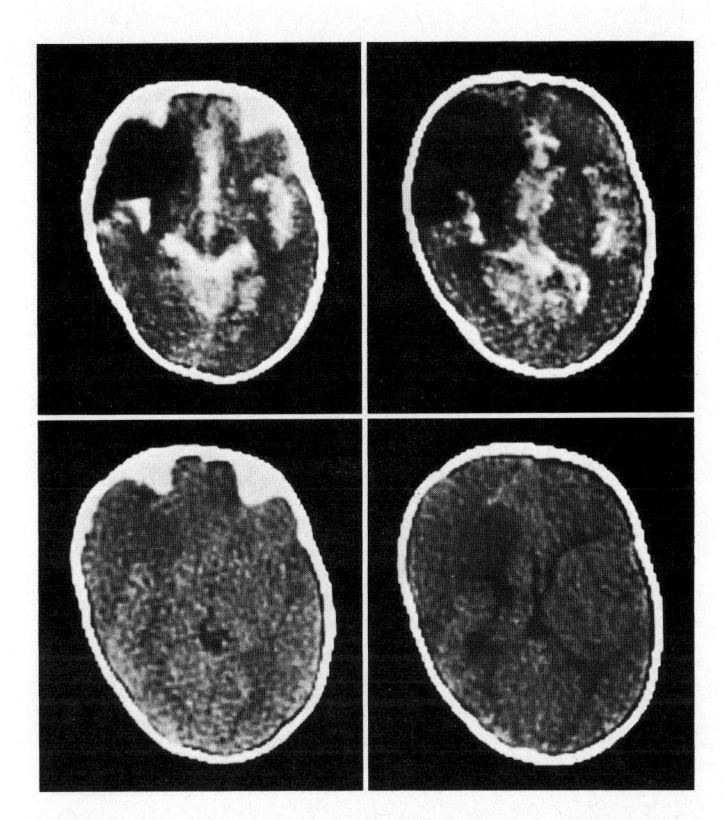

Fig. 4. A ventriculostomy was performed from the extensive fronto-temporal cyst. 6 months later, CT cisternography (inferior range) proves patency of the ventriculostomy

The Effect of Computed Tomography on Diagnosis, Operative Techniques and Prognosis of Tumors of the Middle Cranial Fossa (Petrous Apex)

J. Menzel and U. Schmidt-Gayk

Tumors of the base of the middle cranial fossa are problematical both from a diagnostic and a therapeutic point of view. In the analysis of the clinical symptomatology, we see that this results from the relationship of the tumor to the cranial nerves in the cavernous sinus and the trigeminal nerve on the one hand and the auditory and balance apparatus on the other hand (Figs. 1, 2). Accordingly, we find complete and incomplete cavernous sinus-syndromes, trigeminal neuralgias and disturbances of hearing and balance. In diagnosing the nature of the condition, one must reckon primarily with primary cholesteatomas, meningiomas and metastases (Table 1).

Since the introduction of computed tomography, we have had a total of 12 cases with tumors of the middle base of the skull. They are diagnosed by plain X-rays, angiography, cisternography and computed tomography. It is to be observed that the computed tomography of the brain differs in some points from that of the base of the skull. The wide application of this technique in investigations of the brain is known to be based on the fact that symmetrical structures are involved which only display slight differences in density (1, 4). Density differences of 0.5 - 1% are already detected when the lesion displays a sufficient mass (3, 6). Finally, the diagnostic accuracy is raised by the effect of the pathological process on the cerebrospinal fluid spaces, the concomitant edema and by its own density (2).

On the other hand, the structures of the base of the skull are heterogenous. The density values within the same layer vary substantially, since spaces filled with air, fat, musculature and bone are registered. If one uses narrow windows which display low density differences, these structures cannot be visualized on one diagram. With application of wide windows, the pictures become blurred and slight differences in density are not detected. Moreover, outside the brain the tumor is visualized merely via its vessel pool and possibly via the distribution of the contrast medium into the extracellular space.

Table 1. Differential diagnosis of petrous apex lesions (according to the References)

1. Primary cholesteatoma	8. Carotid aneurysm
2. Cartilaginous tumor	9. Giant cell tumor
3. Schwannoma	10. Large air cell
4. Meningioma	11. Cholesterol granuloma
5. Petrositis	12. Histiocytosis
6. Glomus jugulare tumor	13. Lymphoma
7. Metastatic tumor	14. Mucocele

With regard to the recording technique, it can be stated that the base of the middle cranial fossa can be best visualized with the orbito-meatal line -15° (7).

Our series reports on 12 tumors of the middle cranial fossa floor: 6 primary cholesteatomas, 1 neurinoma, 4 meningiomas and 1 aneurysm of the internal carotid artery (Table 2). In the analysis of the diagnostic value of the individual diagnostic techniques in epidermoid, a destruction of the pyramidal tip was found in four cases (Table 3). Angiographic criteria for space occupation existed in two cases, and the tumor was visualized by computed tomography in five cases. In a 30-year-old female patient with typical trigeminal neuralgia, the computer tomogram was normal. The pyramid comparison in conventional tomography also did not reveal any pathological finding, just like the angiography. Only the Pantopaque cisternogram showed a recess at the pyramidal tip. Intraoperatively, an epidermoid of 2 cm diameter reaching up to the trigeminal impression was found. This had to be radically extirpated. In another case, a 19-year-old female patient suffered from a typical dextrolateral trigeminal neuralgia. Various computed tomography investigations had first of all revealed no pathological findings.

Plain X-rays and angiography were normal. Only the repetition of computed tomography showed the epidermoid located at the pyramidal tip up to the trigeminal impression: this could be radically extirpated.

Four cases involved meningiomas of the middle cranial fossa floor (Table 4). All tumors were detected by computed tomography. Angiographically, the tumor was demonstrated in one case by the appreciable displacement of the internal carotid artery. The size of the tumors varied between 2 and 4 cm in diameter. The largest meningioma with a diameter of 4 cm derived from the dura of the anterior pyramidal surface. Radical extirpation was performed via the temporal intradural and transtentorial route. Another case involved a typical trigeminal neuralgia which had already been treated several times with thermocoagulations. Plain X-rays and angiography did not reveal any special features. Only computed tomography showed a meningioma located at the trigeminal impression. This could be extirpated from the posterior fossa. The neurinoma of the middle cranial fossa and the aneurysm of the internal carotid artery were detected with every diagnostic technique employed (Table 5).

Table 2. Differential diagnosis of petrous apex lesions (according to the own cases, n = 12)

1.	Primary cholesteatomata	6
2.	Neurinoma	1
3.	Meningioma	4
4.	Carotid aneurysm	1

Table 3. Diagnostic evidence in primary cholesteatomata (n = 6)

1.	Conventional tomography	4 +
2.	Angiography	2 +
3.	Computerized tomography	5 +

Table 4. Diagnostic evidence in meningiomas (n = 4)

1. Conventional tomography	2 +
2. Angiography	1 +
3. Computerized tomography	4 +

Table 5. Diagnostic evidence in neurinoma and carotid aneurysm

1. Neurinoma	Conventional tomography + Angiography + Computerized tomography +
2. Carotid aneurysm	Conventional tomography + Angiography + Computerized tomography +

The pyramidal tip can be approached by three routes (Fig. 3). The temporal extradural or intradural access will be used when the tumor has affected the base of the middle cranial fossa, the anterior pyramidal surface and the pyramidal tip. With localisation at the pyramidal tip and spreading to the posterior surface of the pyramid, one proceeds suboccipitally. The transcochlear route must be practised by ENT (ear-nose-throat) surgeons (5).

Summary

1. Of 12 tumors of the middle cranial fossa floor (petrous apex) an epidermoid of the pyramidal tip which was 2 cm in diameter was not detected by computed tomography
2. The small meningiomas of the pyramidal tip which are otherwise difficult to diagnose were all shown up by computed tomography
3. Computed tomography has proved to a very important criterion concerning the question of the operability of a tumor and the approach to be chosen
4. Computed tomography enables the radicality of the surgical procedure to be assessed objectively
5. The costs and radiation exposure from computed tomography are less than in conventional tomography.

References

1. Ambrose, J.: Computerized transverse axial scanning (tomography) Clinical applications. Brit. J. Radiol. 46, 1023-1047 (1973)
2. Caillé, J.M., Dop, A., Constant, P., Renaud-Salis, J.L.: C.A.T. studies of tumors of the skull base and face. In: Computerized axial tomography in clinical practice. Du Bouley, G.H., Moseley, I.F. (eds.). Berlin, Heidelberg, New York: Springer 1977
3. Dop, A., Constant, P., Renaud-Salis, J.L., Caille, J.M.: Intérêt de la tomodensitométrie en pathologie tumorale de la base du crâne et du massif facial. J. Neuroradiol. 3, 193-214 (1976)
4. Hounsfield, G.N.: Computerized transverse axial scanning (tomography). Description of the system. Brit. J. Radiol. 46, 1016-1022 (1973)

5. House, W.F., Hitselberger, W.E.: The transcochlear approach to the skull base. Arch. Otolaryngol. 102, 334-342 (1976)
6. Kramer, R.A., Janetos, G.P., Peristein, G.: An approach to contrast enhancement in computed tomography of the brain. Radiology 116, 641-647 (1975)
7. Vignaud, J., Aubin, M.L.: CT of the skull base. In: Computerized tomography. Caille, J.M., Salamon, G. (eds.), pp. 41-47. Berlin, Heidelberg, New York: Springer 1980

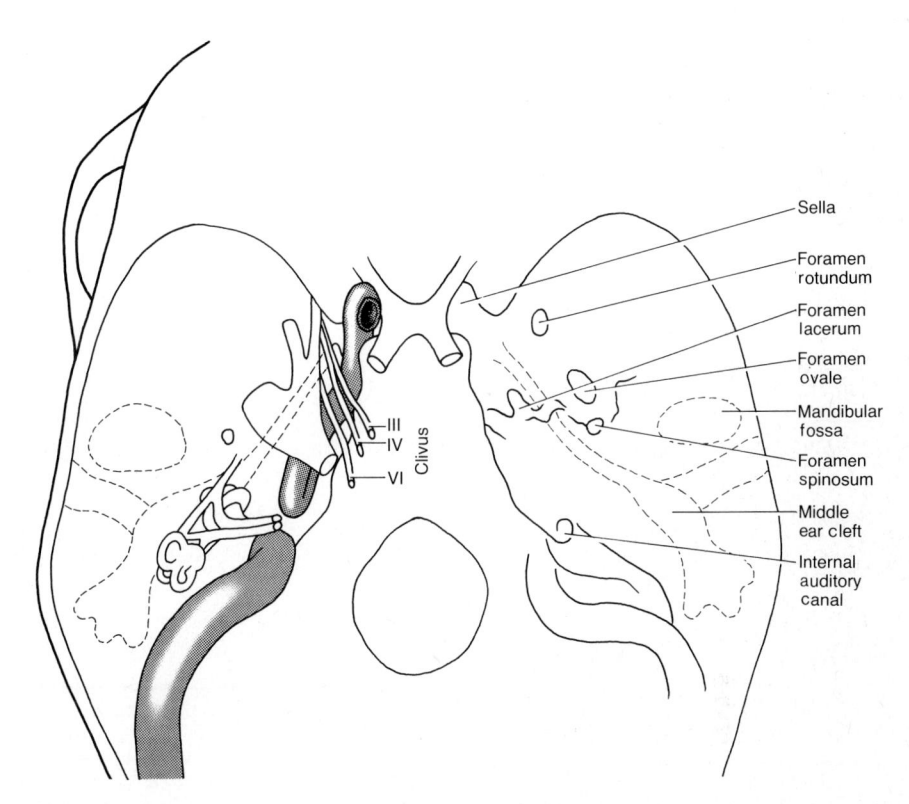

Fig. 1. Schematic representation of the structures of the base of the middle cranial fossa (from above)

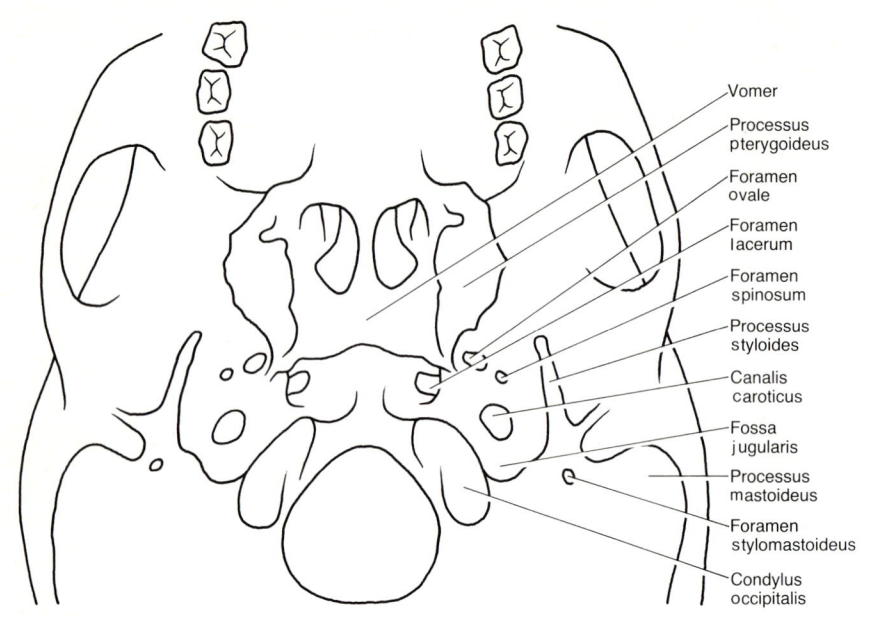

Fig. 2. Schematic representation of the structures of the base of the middle cranial fossa (from below)

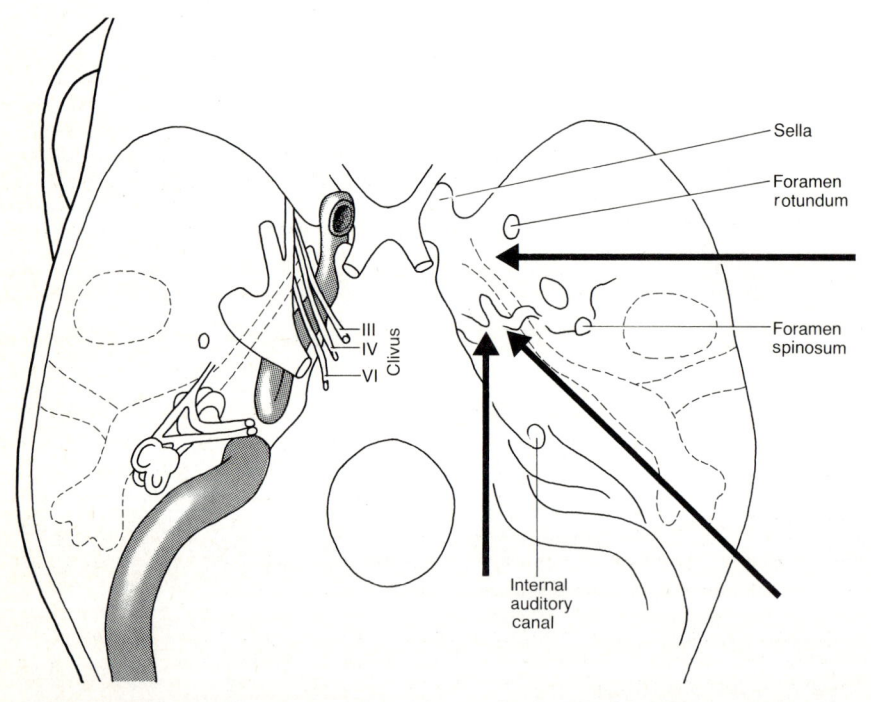

Fig. 3. Schematic representation of the different approaches to the pyramidal apex. *Upper great arrow:* temporal approach; *middle great arrow:* transcochlear approach; *lower great arrow:* suboccipital approach

Spontaneous Brain Stem Lesions. CT-Findings and Clinical Data in Respect to Morbidity

R. SCHÖNMAYR, A. LAUN, A. L. AGNOLI, and O. BUSSE

Introduction

The differential diagnosis of vascular brainstem lesions - especially haemorrhages and infarctions - has been made possible through computerized tomography. The visualization of the lesion may be difficult because of artefacts in the lower brain stem sections or because its size falls below the scope of the CT-scan.

In cases which show a haemorrhage or a brain stem infarction in CT, a direct correlation between the CT detectable density changes and the actual tissue damage need not be necessarily present.

In acute supratentorial infarctions it is often not possible to differentiate between the area of actual tissue damage and the surrounding edema. Only the permanent defect, demonstrable in repeated examinations, will reflect the extent of the actual lesion. On the other hand our serial examinations in brainstem infarctions showed that in these cases no appreciable change in the size of the lesion occurs.

The extent of an acute haemorrhage is clearly recognizable in the CT. In serial CT examinations a transition from an initially increased density zone to an isodense area can be seen. This however does not indicate the resorption of the haematoma. This was shown by post mortem examinations in patients who died at the time, when the damaged area was isodense. The change in density most likely depends on the chemical alterations of the haematoma (1, 4).

Lesions at the borderline of the resolution power of the scan can in some cases be identified with the support of soft-ware programs such as enlargement, density measurements, histograms, high-light-program or digital printing.

Out of 16 patients with spontaneous brain stem haemorrhages demonstrated in CT, 13 died (Table 1). In these cases extensive haemorrhage was present (Fig. 1). The haematoma for the most part extended in a longitudinal direction from pons to midbrain, and in at least one section occupied the greater part of the brain stem diameter. In 8 patients an additional perforation of the haematoma into the 4th ventricle and in 1 case into the 3rd ventricle was present.

With the exception of 2 patients all those, who died, were admitted in a deep comatous state. 3 patients had bulbar syndromes, the others were in decerebrate condition when admitted.

A good correlation between the location of the haematoma in the CT-scan and the neurological deficit was found only in patients with

Table 1. Etiology of vascular brain stem lesions and mortality

| | Haemorrhage | | | Infarction | |
Etiology	Total No. of cases	Deaths	Etiology	Total No. of cases	Deaths
Hypertension	9	8	Basilar or bilateral vertebral occlusion	6	5
A-V-malformation	3	3			
Coagulopathy	2	—	Others	8	2
Unknown	2	2			
	16	13		14	7

small haemorrhages as in the case of the 3 surviving patients. One patient suffered from a circumscribed small haemorrhage in the region of the lamina quadrigemina which led to a paralysis of vertical ocular movements (Fig. 2). The second suffered from a haemorrhage located in the ventral section of the midbrain. He also showed a paralysis of vertical eye movements, with additional weakness of convergent gaze, gait disturbances and head and arm tremor. These symptoms remained persistent on repeated examinations. The third, a haemophilic child, after a minor head injury suffered from a small haemorrhage within the lateral part of the lamina quadrigemina and had no neurological deficits.

In comparison to haemorrhages, the brain stem infarctions are more difficult to demonstrate, especially when very small lesions are delt with, or when the lower parts of the brainstem are involved such as in the relatively frequent WALLENBERG syndrome.

The presence of infarction is therefore not excluded by negative CT-findings. In larger infarctions - as in basilar artery occlusion - the hypodensity can affect the entire brain stem section. In this case, just as in large haemorrhages, a differentiated topic correlation is impossible. In some cases the CT may be normal (Table 2). If, however, CT-findings are positive, in minor infarctions a close topic correlation to the neurological deficit can be seen (2, 3).

For example: in a patient a left paramedian pontine infarction with slight extension to the right side was found on CT examination (Fig. 3). Upon admission the patient was drowsy, showed dysarthria, a supranuclear paralysis of tongue and swallow-reflex, a paresis of horizontal ocular movements to the left, a rightsided sensomotor hemiparesis, leftsided hemiataxia and bilateral BABINSKI responses.

All positive CT-findings are backed up by repeated control examinations. Standardized investigations however were not possible, because the patients were admitted for treatment at widely varying times after the infarction.

Table 2. Visualization of brain stem infarctions in CT

	Haemorrhage	Infarction
Positive	16	14
Uncertain	--	13
Negative	?	29

Conclusion

In regard to brain stem haemorrhages the extent of the haematoma as seen in CT is the decisive factor for the prognosis. In no case of spontaneous haemorrhages were we able to detect an occlusion of the perimesencephalic cisterns which is in sharp contrast to brainstem haemorrhages secondary to supratentorial lesions (5).

No abnormalities in CT were found in some brainstem infarctions, even in patients with severe neurological deficit due to angiographically confirmed basilar artery occlusion. Patients with negative CT-findings showed a lower mortality rate than patients with positive CT-findings (Table 3), even if we take into account that the group with negative CT-includes in addition to patients with basilar artery occlusion patients with the WALLENBERG syndrome.

In spite of the small number of cases, it seems that in patients with brain stem infarction and comparable neurological deficits as positive CT suggests a more adverse prognosis as far as mortality and morbidity are concerned.

Table 3. Visualization of brain stem infarctions in CT and mortality

	No. of cases	Deaths
Recognizable in CT	14	8
Unascertainable or negative CT	42	4

References

1. Arseni, C., Stancin, M.: Primary haematomas of the brainstem. Acta Neurochir. 28, 323-330 (1973)
2. Busse, O., Agnoli, A.L., Feistner, H.: Beziehungen zwischen neurologischen Ausfällen und CT-BEfund bei Hirnstamminfarkten. Verh. Dtsch. Ges. Neurol. 1. Mertens, H.G., Przuntek, H. (eds.). Berlin, Heidelberg, New York: Springer 1980
3. Feistner, H., Busse, O., Agnoli, A.L.: Computertomographische Befunde bei Hirnstamminfarten. Nervenarzt 52, 163-166 (1981)
4. Jacobs, L., Kinkel, W.R., Heffner, R.R.: Autopsy correlations of computerized tomography: Experience with 6.000 CT scans. Neurology 26, 1111-1118 (19)
5. Johnson, R.T., Yates, P.O.: Brainstem haemorrhages in expanding supratentorial conditions. Acta Radiol. 46, 250-256 (1956)
6. Watanabe, R.: Clinicopathological study on primary massive pontine haemorrhage. Clin. Neurol. 3, 94-112 (1963)

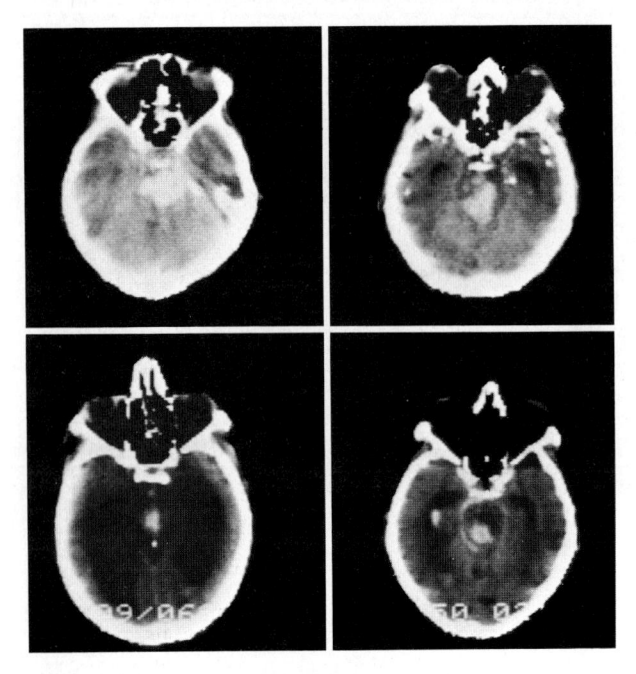

Fig. 1. Four cases of massive brain stem haemorrhage

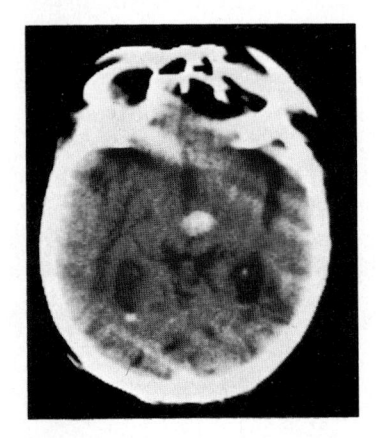

Fig. 2. Circumscribed brainstem haemorrhage (anticoagulant therapy). Paralysis of vertical ocular movements, no other neurological deficits

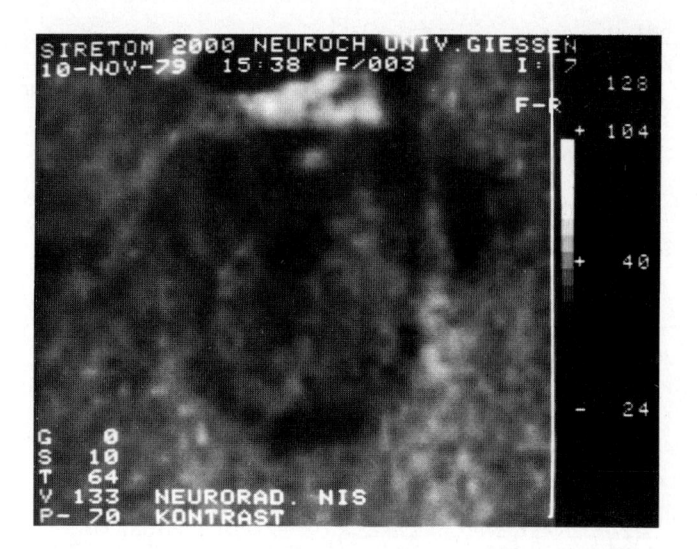

Fig. 3. Left paramedian pontine infarction

CT Localization and Operative Approaches in Posterior Fossa Lesions

J. Gilsbach, H. R. Eggert, Ch. Ostertag, and W. Seeger

Introduction

With the help of the computed tomography more than 90% of the tumors and av-malformations of the posterior fossa can be positively shown. With the first generation computers only the geometrical position of the tumor could be determined in relation to the bony structures. With the most modern scanners which have a thin section and reconstruction possibilities, the relationship to each cerebellar lobe and brain stem structures can be recognized.

By the knowledge of the precise position of the tumor and its relationship to neighbouring structures, large openings, punctures, and splitting procedures because of diagnostic uncertainties, are a thing of the past. In the following paper we discuss the approaches which we have used in the last three years routinely in lesions of the posterior fossa which were detected by the computed tomography.

Principles

We operate in the sitting position using the Doppler sonographic aeroembolism check, use only longitudinal skin incisions, split the muscles longitudinally, trepan osteoplastically whenever possible, remove not routinely the posterior rim of the foramen magnum and the arch of C1, use external drainage only exceptionally, and prefer the preoperative shunt. At the beginning of the operation we open the dura as short as possible, centered over the tumor, we do not resect the cerebellum and try to reduce first the tumors, also the gliomas, internally, then advance to the boundary. With the above mentioned measures, disorders in the healing process, C.S.F. leaks from the wound, subcutaneous CSF collection, unsightly osteoclastic defects with slipped masses of muscle, and unnecessary cerebellar lesions become rare. As always, infections and hemorrhage into the tumor bed cause problems.

Lateral Suboccipital Trepanation (Fig. 1)

Lesions in the cerebellopontine angle, which amount to a surprisingly great number, we operate on a lateral suboccipital osteoplastic approach which has last been improved by YASARGIL. Besides the classic extracerebellar tumors we have also operated upon tumors of the lateral aspect of pons and lobulus biventer.

Unilateral Suboccipital Trepanation (Fig. 2)

We prefer the unilateral exposure after a paramedian longitudinal incision if a tumor is located mainly in the area of the lobulus biventer or the lobuli semilunares, even if it extends to the fourth ventricle, the cerebellopontine angle or to the lobulus quadrangularis.

With the lesions in the anterior aspect of the lobulus quadrangularis or unilaterally in the region of the quadrigeminal plate, we widen the trepanation supratentorially in order to enlarge the approach by lifting the tentorium.

Median Suboccipital Trepanation (Fig. 3)

From an osteoplastic median approach we operate on processes in the region of the vermis, the hemispheres, in the fourth ventricle and the dorsal brain stem. The foramen magnum and the arch of C1 are only resected in cases of a basal extension of the tumor.

Lesions near the midline of the quadrigeminal region or if the culmen is to be handled, we trepan over the transverse sinus in order to gain a better view by lifting the tentorium.

Basal Trepanation (Figs. 2, 4)

If we want to reach the medial part of the cerebellomedullary system we widen the foramen magnum osteoclastically and resect the arch of C1, while for unilateral procedures in the paramedullar region an unilateral enlargement of the foramen magnum and a one-sided resection of the arch of C1 are sufficient. For manipulations far ventrally in the paramedullar space, an additional resection of medial parts of the condylus atlantis and occipitalis up to the tuberculum jugulare is useful.

Conclusions

The conclusions we draw from five years experience with computed tomography and posterior fossa lesions are:

1. The applied trepanations of the posterior fossa are not new, but the preoperative knowledge of the tumor localization facilitates the choice of the approach and saves an unnecessarily wide resection of the bone.

2. The procedures in the region of cisterns and in the fourth ventricle have become more simple, sure, and specific because of the exact preoperative knowledge about size, location, and neighbouring structures, in addition to the fact that we are informed preoperatively about intra- or extracerebellar tumor.

3. The way through the substance in intracerebellar lesions has become more protective, differentiated, and functional.

4. Unnecessary attacks on primarily inoperable, diffuse brain stem tumors are avoidable.

References

1. Adson, A.W.: A straight lateral incision for unilateral suboccipital cranitomy. Surg. Gynec. Obst. 72, 99-100 (1941)
2. Böhm, B., Mohadjer, M., Hemmer, R.: Preoperative continous measurements of ventricular pressure in hydrocephalus occlusus with tumors of the posterior fossa: the value of ventricular shunt. In: Advances in neurosurgery, Vol. 5. Berlin, Heidelberg, New York: Springer 1978
3. Dandy, W.E.: Results of removal of acoustic tumors by the unilateral approach. A.M.A. Arch. Surg. 42, 1026-1033 (1941)
4. Foerster, O.: Das operative Vorgehen bei Tumoren der Vierhügelgegend. Wien. Klin. Wschr. 41, 986-990 (1928)
5. Frazier, C.H.: The midline bloodless approach to the posterior fossa. Tr. Ann. S.A. 44, 229-247 (1926)
6. Krause, F.: Operative Freilegung der Vierhügel nebst Beobachtungen über Hirndruck und Dekompression. Zentralbl. J. Clin. 53, 2812-2819 (1926)
7. De Martle, T.: La thérapeutique des tumeurs cerebrales. Technique chirurgicale. Rapp. Congr. Soc. Internat. Chir. 1, 803-846 (1926)
8. Naffziger, H.C.: Brain surgery with special reference to exposure of the brain stem and posterior fossa, the principle of intracranial decompression and the relief of impactions in the posterior fossa. Surg. Gynec. Obst. 46, 240-248 (1928)
9. Rand, R.W., Kurze, T.: Facial nerve preservation by posterior fossa transmeatal microdissection in total removal of acoustic tumors. J. Neurol. Neurosurg. psychiat. 28, 311-316 (1965)
10. Torkildsen, A.: A new palliative operation in case of inoperable occlusion of the Sylvian aquaeduct. Acta Chir. Scand. 82, 117-124 (1939)
11. Unsöld, R., Ostertag, Ch., de Groot, J., Newton, T.H.: Computed tomography and computer refoemation of the brain and skull base. Berlin, Heidelberg, New York: Springer (in press)
12. Yasargil, M.G., Smith, R.D., Gasser, J.C.: Microsurgical approach to acoustic neurinomas. In: Advances and technical standards in neurosurgery. Krayenbühl, H. Ted.). Vol. 4. Wien, New York: Springer 1977
13. Zapetal, B.: Ein neuer operativer Zugang zum Gebiet der Incisura tentorii. Zbl. Neurochir. 16, 64-69 (1956)

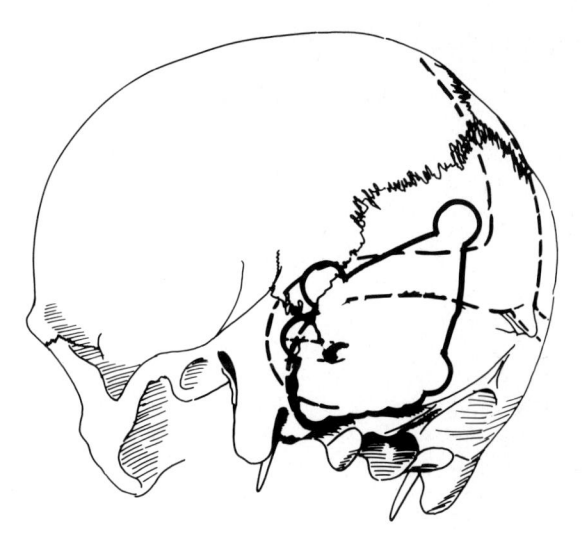

Fig. 1. Lateral approach
Cerebellopontine cistern 52
Cerebellopontine and prepontine cistern 6
Prepontine cistern 1
Lateral cerebellar cistern 8
Lobulus biventer (lateral) 4

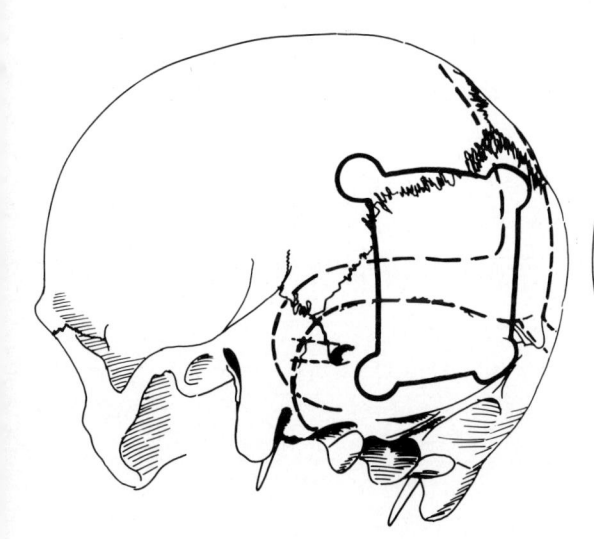

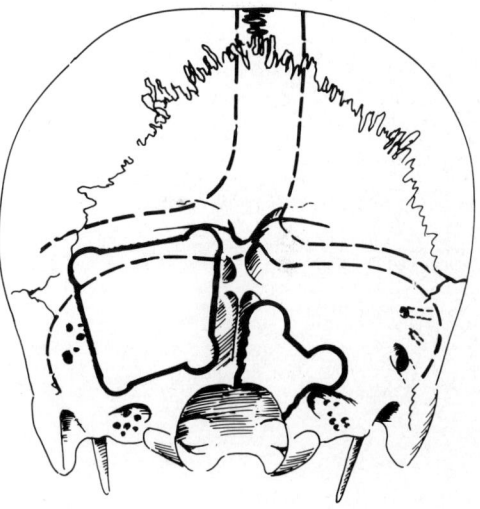

Fig. 2. Unilateral approach (n = 20)
Suboccipital lobulus quadrangularis
biventer
semilunaris 17
Suboccipital and occipital tentorium 1
quadrigeminal plate
(infratentorial
supracerebellar) 2

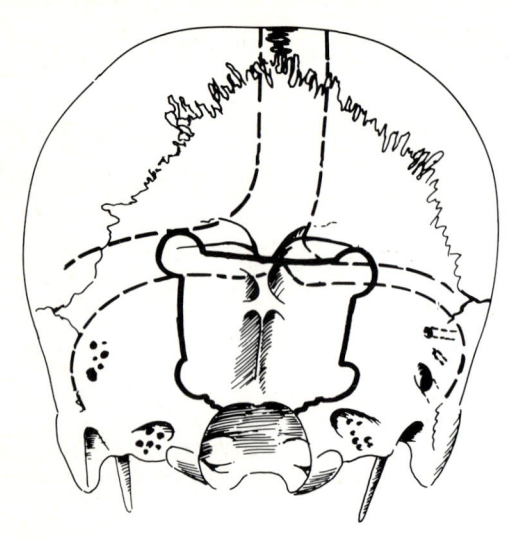

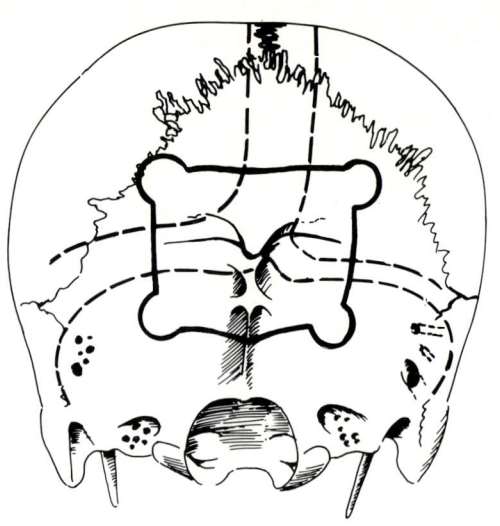

Fig. 3. Medial approach (n = 47)
Suboccipital hemisphere/vermis
              fourth ventricle, medulla   44
Suboccipital and occipital quadrigeminal plate/culmen
                         (infratentorial/supracerebral)   2
                         tentorium   1

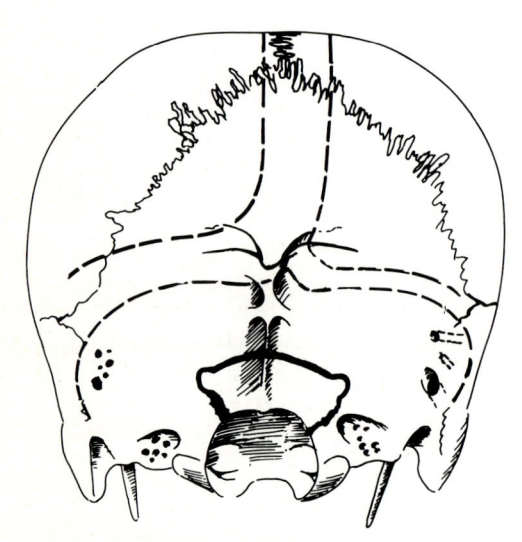

Fig. 4. Basal approach
Cerebellomedullary cistern
Medial   1
Lateral 1

Local complications		+
Hematoma: Tumor bed	10	(6)
Epidural	3	(0)
Subdural (frontal)	1	(0)
Intracerebral (frontal)	1	(1)
Meningitis	11	(4)
CSF leak (→eustachian tube)	6	(0)

Operative Approaches to the Rostral Brain Stem According to the CT-Findings

H. R. EGGERT, J. GILSBACH, and W. SEEGER

Introduction

Computed tomography has, in recent years, considerably broadened our knowledge of the localisation and extension of intracranial processes. This has come from more and more refined resolutions in every plane. Surgical procedures are more easily planned because of this. Thereby, better adapted approaches can be used including lesions of the medial skull base.

Approaches

YASARGIL's (6, 12, 13) *pterional approach* (Fig. 1) to aneurysms of the circle of Willis provides an survey of the planum sphenoidale, both optic nerves, and the optic chiasma, the hypophysial stalk, and the diaphragma with both posterior clinoid processes, and the anterior parts of both tentorial edges. With the exception of the lateral side of the contralateral carotid artery with the posterior communicating and anterior choroidal artery almost all of the circle can be seen. The prerequisite for this view is the trepanation up to the frontal and temporal base and up to at least the lateral margin of the superior orbital fissure and the broad opening of the arachnoid of the Sylvian fissure, from the internal carotid up to the bifurcation of the middle cerebral artery. This method prevents tension at the temporal lobe. The opening of the lateral fissure should be accompanied by a careful exposure of the superficial Sylvian veins, which can often, but not always, be coagulated without complications. The typical pterional approach with its wide opening of the Sylvian fissure, allows in principle three ways to the prepontine space: Behind the internal carotid artery and under the posterior communicating artery, between the carotid artery and the optic nerve, and between both optic nerves. The way one has to choose depends on the topographical relationships in each case and can lastly be decided only after the opening of the dura because neither computerized tomography nor angiography provide satisfactory information.

The typical pterional approach allows only an oblique view between both nerves. If, mainly with suprasellar lesions, based on the computed tomography, an approach through both optic nerves must be assumed, we widen the frontal part of the trepanation up to the middle of the orbita.

Thereby the chiasm can be seen from a smaller angle. The opening of the sinus which is often inevitable, makes a plastic cover necessary. Nevertheless, as we observed in one case, rhinorrhoea with fatal meningitis can be the result.

If the computed tomography shows a dominant expansion of the process in the area of the tentorial edge, we widen the trepanation in the temporal direction. After separating the uncus from the carotid artery and the third nerve, the tentorium fold can be viewed up to the peduncle if the uncus is slightly retracted laterally. Preserving the Sylvian veins is, however, often not possible.

Lesions in the area of the free tentorium margin (Fig. 2), of the upper clivus up to the origin of anterior inferior cerebellar artery, the peduncle and the lower parts of the interpeduncular cistern can be shown by a *subtemporal approach* according to DRAKE's description for basilar aneurysms (1). This approach between the basal aspect of the temporal lobe and the petrous bone is considerably obstructed by the veins belonging to the vein of Labbé and the superior petrosal sinus.

Because the coagulation of these vessels can lead to swelling and infarction of the temporal lobe, as we observed in four cases, we only use this approach if the lesions cannot be reached by a pterional approach, if they are localized either laterally in the peduncle area or in the posterior fossa, so that the tentorium must be split parallel to the petrous bone. With the enlargement towards the temporopolar region, the subtemporal approach permits an survey of the internal carotid and the lateral parts of the optic chiasm, the optic tract, and the suprasellar space.

Especially with the help of coronal and sagittal projections, we can differentiate with the help of computed tomography in most cases between lesions which originate from the base and implicate the hypothalamus and the third ventricle from below and between lesions which originate primarily in the third ventricle. In these latter processes we use *an interhemispheric approach* (Fig. 3) (4, 8), whereas we seldom use a transfrontal way (5, 7, 11). Thereby the brain, dependent on the bridging veins is retracted up to 15 mm from the falx. The exposure of the longitudinal fissure up to the corpus callosum requires exact knowledge of the variations of the venous (anterior) system. The opening of the corpus callosum amounts to 1 - 2 sq.cm.

Depending on the width of the foramen of Monro, the floor of the third ventricle can be surveyed from the recussus infundibuli up to the corpora mamillaria. With the opening of the floor we can see the region from the diaphragma to the interpeduncular cistern. Parts of the roof of the third ventricle directly in front of and behind the foramen of Monro, cannot be overlooked exactly.

Conclusion

Altogether there are only three different operative approaches with modifications - adapted to each individual case - which we, in the last five years (Table 1), have found to be satisfactory for the treatment of space-occupying and vascular lesions in the area of the rostral brain stem. All three approaches utilize the natural brain clefts. (In all a small reclination of the brain is sufficient). In all the veins are a fundamental problem.

Table 1. Approaches to the rostral brain stem used from 1976 to 1980

	Pterional	Pterional and frontal	Pterional and frontal	Subtemporal	Transcallosal	
Aneurysms	114	1	2			117
(Hypophyseal) Pituitary adenomas	3	37				40
Craniopharyngiomas	9	6	5	3	7	30
Sphenoidal ridge meningiomas	18	2	4			24
Tuberculum sellae meningiomas	10	6				16
Tentorial meningiomas	4	2	6	2		14
Angiomas				5	1	6
Diaphragma sellae meningiomas		5				5
Gliomas				2	3	5
Clivus meningiomas	1			2		3
Chordomas	1			2		3
Other	11	6	2	1	3	23
	171	65	19	17	14	286

References

1. Bonnal, J., Louis, R., Combalbert, A.: L'abord temporal transtentorial de l'angle ponto-cérébelleuse et du clivus. Neuro-Chirurgie 10, 3-12 (1964)
2. Drake, C.G.: Surgical treatment of ruptured aneurysms of the basilar artery. Experience with 14 cases. J. Neurosurg. 23, 457-473 (1965)
3. Drake, C.G.: Further experience with surgical treatment of aneurysms of the basilar artery. J. Neurosurg. 29, 372-392 (1968)
4. Harper, R.L., Ehni, G.: The anterior transcallosal approach to brain tumors. In: Advances in neurosurgery, Vol. 7. Marguth, F., Brock, M., Kazner, E., Klinger, M., Schmiedek, P. (eds.), pp. 91-96. Berlin, Heidelberg, New York: Springer 1979
5. Hirsch, J.F., Zouaoui, A., Renier, D., Pierre-Kahn, A.: A new surgical approach to the third ventricle with interruption of the striathalamic vein. Acta Neurochir. 47, 135-147 (1979)
6. Krayenbühl, H.A., Yasargil, M.G., Flamm, E.S., Tew, J.M.: Neurosurgical treatment of intracranial saccular aneurysms. J. Neurosurg. 37, 678-686 (1972)
7. Little, J.R., MacCarty, C.S.: Colloid cysts of the third ventricle. J. Neurosurg. 40, 230-235 (1974)
8. Long, D.M., Chou, S.N.: Transcallosal removal of craniopharyngiomas within the third ventricle. J. Neurosurg. 39, 563-567 (1973)
9. Perlmutter, D., Rhoton, A.L.: Microsurgical anatomy of the distal anterior cerebral artery. J. Neurosurg. 49, 204-228 (1978)
10. Sugita, K., Kobayashi, S., Shintani, A., Mutsuga, N.: Microneurosurg. 51, 615-620 (1979)
11. Viale, G.L., Turtas, S.: The subchoroid approach to the third ventricle. Surg. Neurol. 14, 71-76 (1980)
12. Yasargil, M.G., Fox, J.L., Ray, M.W.: The operative approach to aneurysms of the anterior communicating artery. In: Advances and technical standards in neurosurgery, Vol. 2. Krayenbühl, H. (ed.), pp. 115-128. Wien: Springer 1975
13. Yasargil, M.G., Antic, J., Laciga, R., Jain, K.K., Hodosh, R.M., Smith, R.D.: Microsurgical pterional approach to aneurysms of the basilar bifurcation. Surg. Neurol. 6, 83-91 (1976)

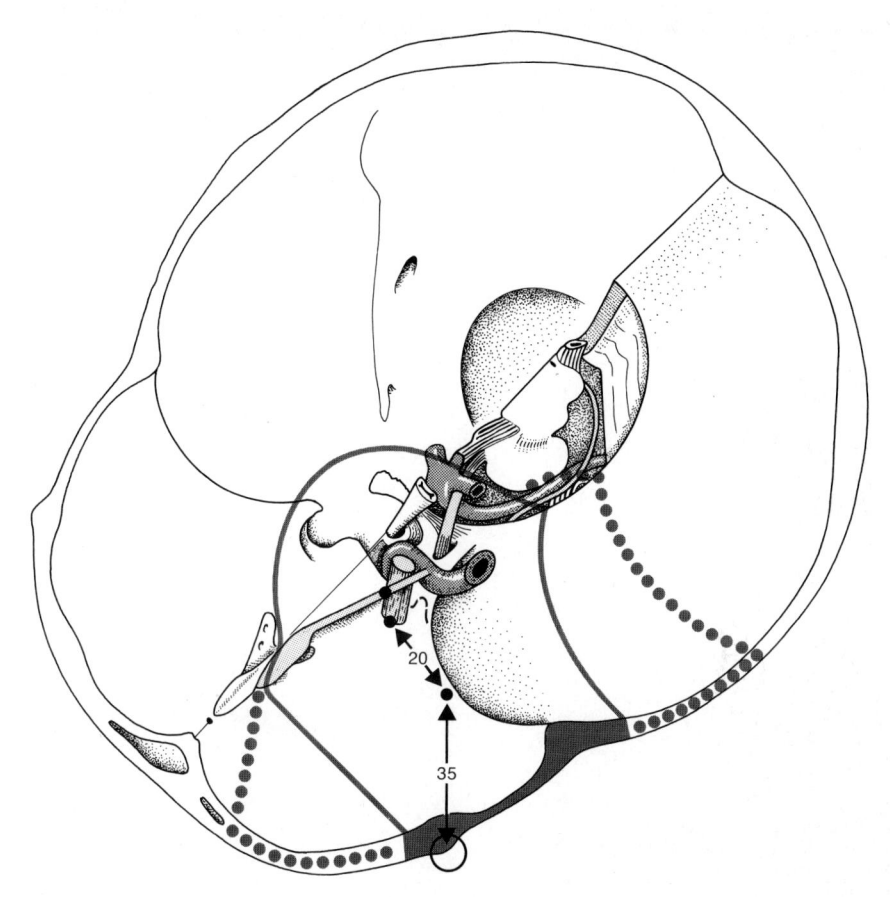

Fig. 1. Survey at the pterional trepanation with frontal and temporal enlargement

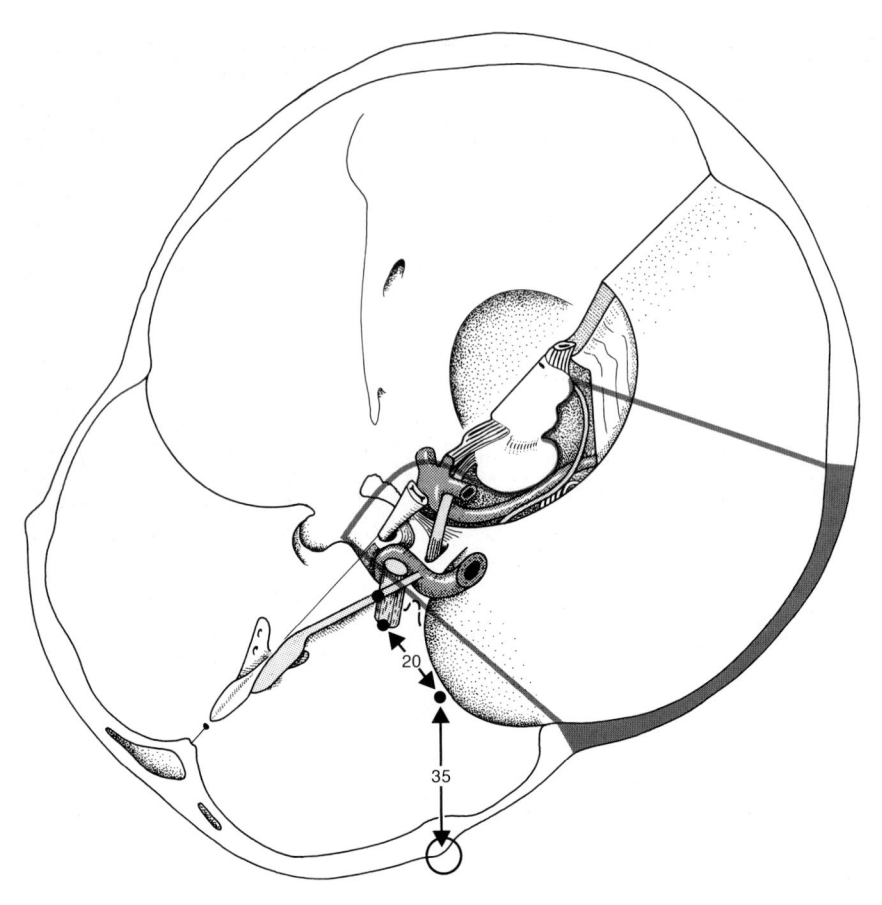

Fig. 2. View at the subtemporal approach with enlargement of the trepanation towards the temporopolar region

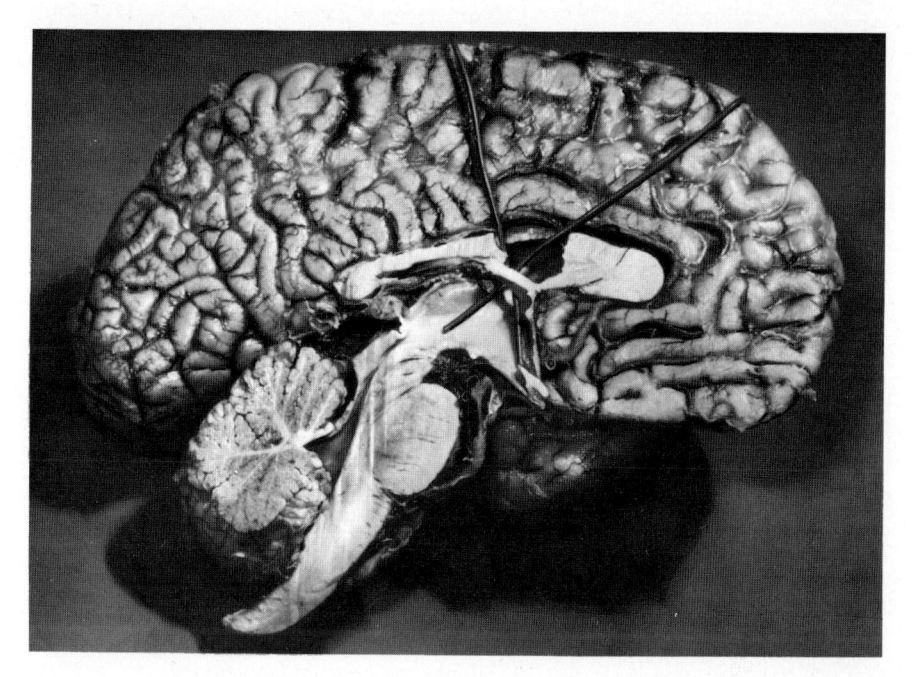

Fig. 3. View at the interhemispherical approach through the foramen of Monro

On the Extended Indication for Operation of Deep Seated Brain Tumors

W. ENTZIAN

Deep-seated and large tumors in the cerebral hemispheres (GREENWOOD, 1973) or tumors of the brain stem (LASSITER, 1971) have always presented problems as far as indications for excision are concerned. It seems worthwhile, therefore, to discuss the role of cerebral computer tomography (CT), since this diagnostic tool has, in our experience, been very instrumental in several instances in influencing the selection of the operative approach.

The successful excision of deep-seated and large tumors presumes (1) benignity (2) sufficient demarcation from normal brain tissue, and (3) exactly known, approachable localization. These concepts need to be defined: By deep-seated and large is meant, that the lateral boundaries of a tumor of the cerebral hemisphere is touching the cortex or the subcortex whereas the medial border approaches the midline beneath the falx as seen by computer tomography. Additionally, from a variety of relatively small tumors of the brain stem, two cases of intrapontomesencephalic spongioblastomas will be presented here. "Benignity" indicates primarily spongioblastomas, benign mixed gliomas and ventricular meningiomas. The meaning of "sufficient demarcation" and "approachable localization" will be discussed as the X-ray findings and postoperative results are demonstrated.

Results

A general survey of our diagnostic as well as our operative experience in children and adults of the last years is given in Table 1. It is the purpose of this paper to discuss these problems, and this will be done by demonstrating some typical cases.

Case 6 (File no. 106/78, 14 years, ♀)

History. Slightly diminished performance in high-school, writing disability and strange walking movements of 6 months duration.

Findings. Right-handed, mild hemiparesis and slightly impaired coordination on the right side.
The carotid angiogram (Fig. 1 above) shows the signs of a large hemispheric tumor sparsely vascularized, CT (Fig. 1 below) confirms the large tumor and shows good demarcation of the solid and cystic portions. After the operation the girl presented with (a) a complete homonymous hemianopsia, that vanished within weeks, (b) a hemiparalysis of the right extremities, that regressed to the preoperative stage, (c) a global aphasia, that became regressive to where she was able to continue her English and French studies with moderate results in high school at a level two years below her age and finally (d) an in-

tention dyskinesia of athetotic character of her right hand, thereafter she learned to write with her left hand.

Discussion of the Case. Angiography revealed a very large space-occupying lesion. The decision to operate was difficult to make since the tumor was of unknown type in the dominant hemisphere and in a girl with little neurological deficit. CT, however, supported the indication for operation because of sharp demarcation of cystic and solid tumor portions indicative of a spongioblastoma or an astrocytoma grade I. The late clinical result is to be considered as relatively good and justifies the dangerous procedure. Still the case underlines the problem of sparing the (phasic etc.) centers of the angular gyrus region by chosing an adequate approach through silent cortical areas.

Case 5 (File no. 837/80, 36 years, ♀)

History. Tingling sensation in her face of two years duration and double vision of 5 months duration.

Findings. Hypesthesia of the right cheek, CN-VI-paresis on the right side, slight incoordination in heel-knee-test, and early papilloedema. Angiography of the left carotid artery demonstrated an elevation of the middle cerebral artery, a shift of the anterior cerebral artery and a typical vascularization pattern of an intraventricular meningioma. CT, in addition demonstrated hydrocephalus. Postoperatively the patient presented with a severe aphasia of several weeks duration, but she started full work again as a secretary 6 months after the operation without any neurological deficits.

Discussion of the Case. CT showed partial enlargement of the temporal horn (Fig. 2). Instead of penetrating the cortex at a point where the tumor was nearest to the surface, which here was in the area of the angular gyrus, it was decided to approach the tumor anteriorly through the partially enlarged temporal horn, which was outlined in the computer tomogram. This specific information contributed to the good outcome.

Case 3 (File no. 65/81, 12 years, ♀)

History. Generalized seizures of 7 years duration, headaches 10 days prior to admission.

Findings. Left handed, papilloedema, spastic hemiparesis of the left extremities.
Angiography shows signs of a large mass in the right hemisphere, which is partially vascularized. CT revealed solid and cystic tumor portions which are well demarcated. The ventral tumor pole is located near the foramen of Monro, and the dorsal tumor pole in the occipital horn, which is still partially open. Complete tumor resection was done through an occipital, horizontal and very basal cortical incision two centimeters from the midline and 1-2 cm superior to the transverse sinus. Postoperatively, the girl presented with a complete homonymous hemianopsia to the left side probably as a result of damage to the right occipital artery which was surrounded by tumor tissue. There were no other remarkable deficits of her dominant hemisphere.

Table 1. Deep-seated tumors and CT. Among 23 patients, observed consecutively, the preoperative CT-diagnosis of a benign deep seated tumor was mostly confirmed, however was wrong or questionable in others

Patients		Histology	Follow-up		Preoperative benign CT-diagnosis

Deep seated and large tumors of a cerebral hemisphere

1	5 ♂	Benign mixed glio.	7 years	Highschool	Conf.
2	5 ♂	Benign mixed glio.	+	collaps of brain mantle	Conf.
3	8 ♂	Mal. mixed glio.	+	Recid. 10 weeks	Wrong
4	8 ♂	Spongiobl.	4 years	Highsch.	Conf.
5	9 ♀	Spongiobl.	3 months	Hemianopsia, dyspr.	Conf.
6	14 ♀	Spongiobl.	3 years	Highsch.	Conf.
7	36 ♀	Ventr. mening.	6 months	Secret. work	Conf.
8	40 ♂	Oligo., infiltr.	12 months	Severely handic.	Wrong
9	41 ♂	Oligo., delin.	2 months	Severely handic.	Conf.
10	42 ♂	Oligo., malign.	+	Infarcat. 1 week	Wrong
11	46 ♂	Ventr. mening.	9 months	Mod. handic.	Conf.

Brainstem tumors, in one level only

12	3 ♂	Medullobl., foramen of Monro	+	Second. pneum. 3 months	Wrong
13	9 ♂	Spongiobl., hypothal.	6 months	Elem. school	Question
14	13 ♀	Spongiobl., Wall 3rd ventr.	4 years	Highschool	Conf.

Brainstem tumors, along two etages

| 15 | 8 ♀ | Spongiobl., ponto-mesenc. | 3 years | Elem. sch. | Conf. |
| 16 | 10 ♀ | Spongiobl., di-mesen. | + | Subtot. res. | Conf. |

17	10 ♂	Spongiobl., med. obl.-cerv. cord.	9 years		Highsch.	Question
18	13 ♀	Spongiobl., ponto-mesenc.	4 years		Able to stand	Conf.

Brainstem tumors, along three etages or infiltr. a hemisphere

19	3 ♀	Epend.-spongiobl., bienc.-for. mag.		+	2 weeks subt. exc.	Question
20	5 ♂	Spongiobl., pons-cerv. cord.	4 years		Biopsy, handic.	Question
21	9 ♀	Spongiobl., bienc.-for. mag.		+	2 months biopsy	Question
22	9 ♂	Astrocytoma, mesenc.?- left hemisph.	4 years		Severely handic.	Question
23	12 ♀	Spongiobl., pons-cerebell.		+	4 years recid.	Question

Discussion of the Case. The topography of the occipital horn and the posterior pole of the tumor, as identified in CT, offered an occipital approach, which could not be gleaned from the angiography. The pathway was short to the posterior tumor portions, however, long to the anterior tumor portions. Nevertheless, disturbances of the typical dominant hemispheric centers could be almost completely avoided.

Case 15 (File no. 1311/78, 8 years, ♀)

Findings. CN VI-paresis left more than right, CN VII-paresis right, Parinaud-syndrome, spastic hemiparesis of the right extremities, but an acceptable gait (Fig. 3). CT revealed a solid tumor portion in the pons-region, and a cystic portion in the mesencephalon. Pneumencephalogram showed an irregular contour of the elevated floor of the 4th ventricle. A posterior fossa craniotomy and aspiration of the cystic contents was planned. On exploring the floor of the 4th ventricle it was found to be elevated laterally off the ponto-cerebellar peduncle in a small field of 2-3 mm. After perforating 1 mm into the normal tissue the smooth outlines of the solid and cystic tumor became visible and resectable. Five months after the operation there is still a spastic hemiparesis of the right extremities and a moderate CN VI-paresis on the right side. There are no clinical symptoms of tumor recurrence after 3 years of follow-up.

Discussion of the Case. CT allowed the diagnosis of the rare variant of a circumscribed intraponto-mesencephalic spongioblastoma, which could be differentiated from a glioma with its usual diffuse growth (or anlage). CT (and pneumencephalography of the 4th ventricle) and local findings finally encouraged us to undertake this operative procedure, which is generally not recommended.

Conclusions and Summary

In patients with deep seated tumors of the cerebral hemispheres, computer tomography supports the indication for an operation, which otherwise may be doubtful. It may show the probable benign character and the clear delineation as presumption of operability. Furthermore, CT may give precise information that helps in chosing an adequate approach according the topography of the tumor, ventricular system and brain mantle.
Finally, with the diagnostic aid of computer tomography, the excision of circumscribed intraponto-mesencephalic spongioblastomas via the floor of the 4th ventricle has become possible in special cases.

References

1. Greenwood, J.: Radical surgery of tumors of the thalamus, hypothalamus and third ventricle area. J. Surg. Neurol. $\underline{1}$, 29-33 (1973)
2. Lassiter, K.R.L.: Surgical treatment of brainstem gliomas. Case reports. J. Neurosurg. $\underline{34}$, 719-725 (1971)

Fig. 1 see pp.70/71

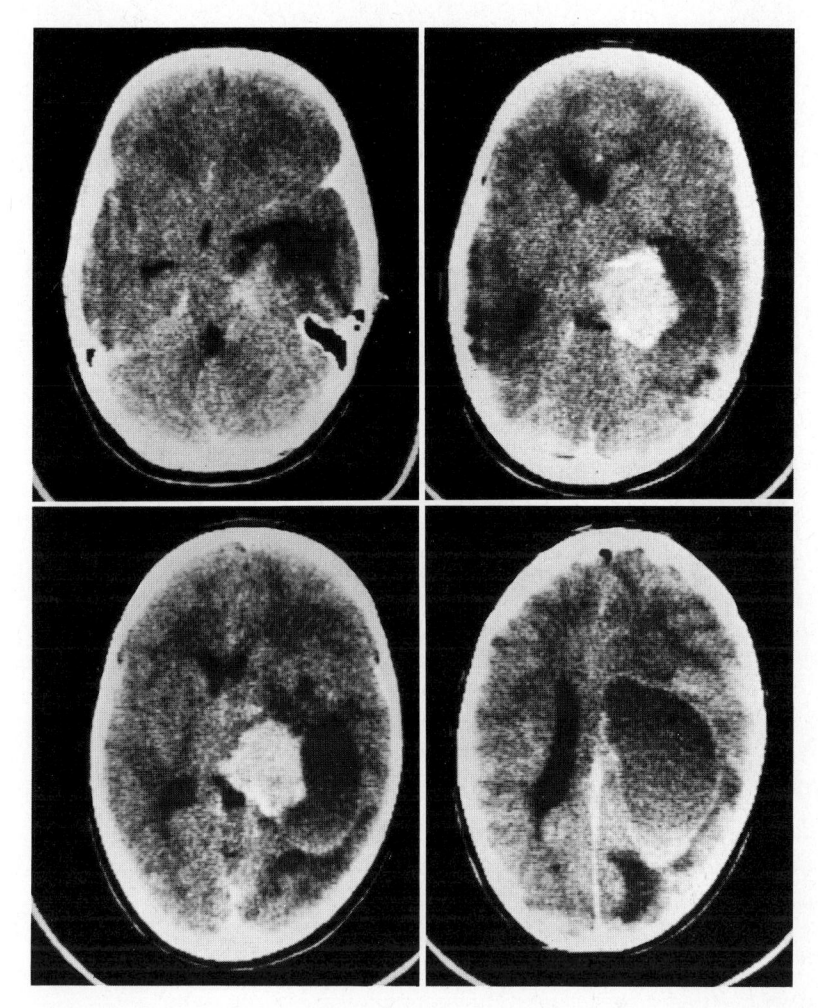

Fig. 2. Large spongioblastoma of right dominant hemisphere (case no. 5). CT suggests approach through occipital horn

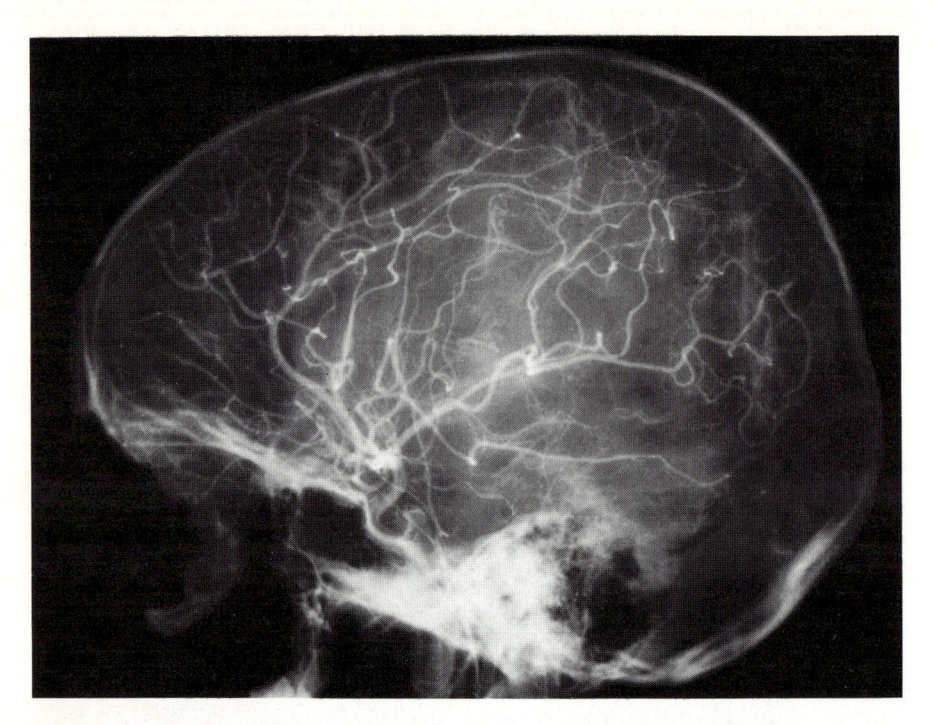

Fig. 1. Angiogram demonstrates signs of large tumor of left hemisphere (above), whereas CT reveals signs of benign glioma, supporting indication for operation see p.71 (case no. 6)

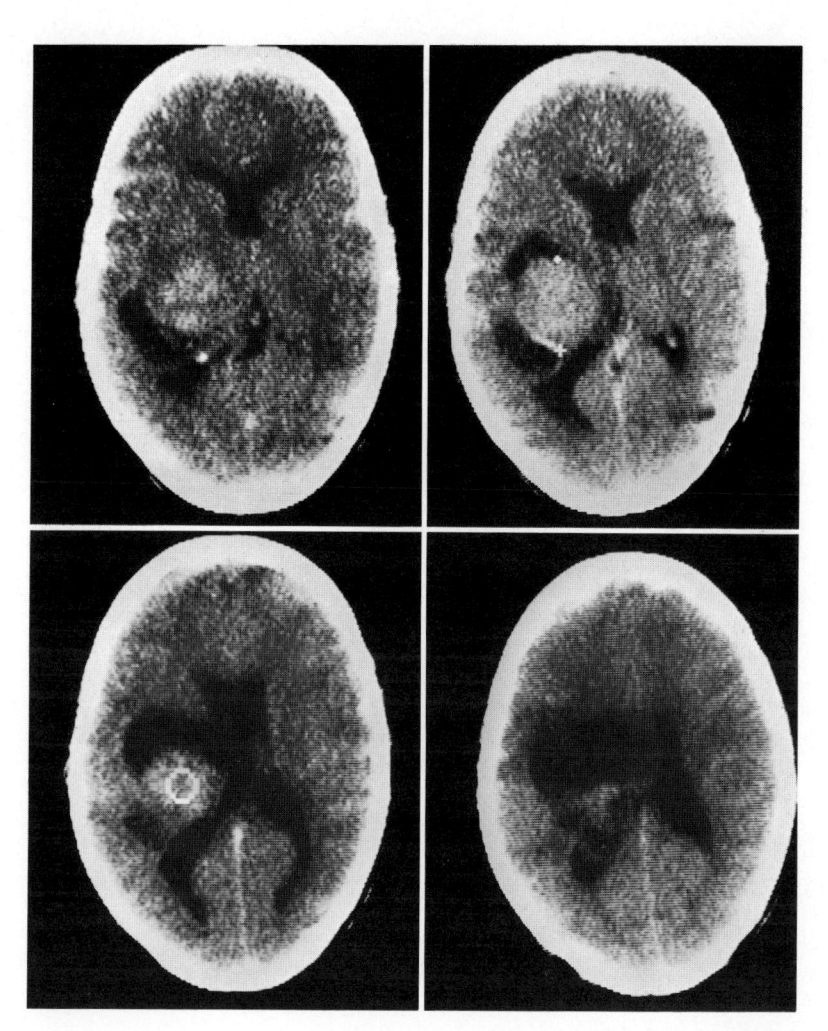

Fig. 1. Legend see p.70

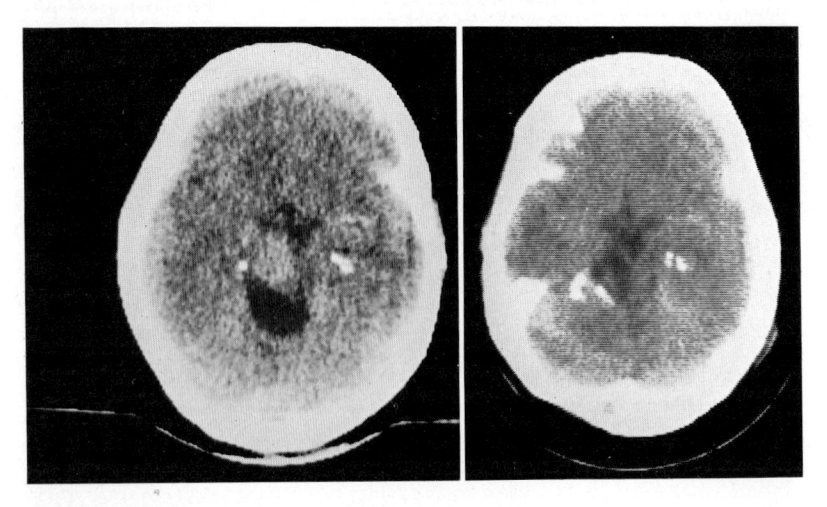

Fig. 3. Intraponto-mesencephalic spongioblastoma with solid and cystic tumor portion (*left* CT) of case no. 15 and control (*right*) 6 mo. after radical excision via the floor of the 4th ventricle

CT in Diagnosis and Treatment of 20 Cases with Brain Abscesses and Subdural Empyemas

H. KLINGE, U. MUHTAROGLU, and M. RAUTENBERG

With the aid of computer tomography, the development of cerebral abscesses and empyemas can be examined at a very early stage. Furthermore, one can differentiate clearly between the degree of liquefication and other accompanying reactions, even though it admittedly is problematic to do so in the case of a persistent oedema and a still existent encephalitic reaction. The animal experiments of WALLENFANG et al. made with cats on the development of abscesses is thus in general accordance with our observations. Therefore, the time factor plays a central role when determining the method of neurosurgical treatment. This is especially important when deciding whether the encapsulated abscess has to be removed by surgery, due to an already existent membrane, or whether to puncture, when computer tomography and clinical findings indicated this treatment to be most beneficial.

Between 1976 and 1980, 14 patients with brain abscess and 6 patients with subdural empyema were examined by means of computer tomography. The patients were treated and follow-up studies were made. Therapy varied, depending on the number and location of the abscesses and their age. Taking also into account the clinical findings, therapy consisted of four methods.

Brain Abscess

1. Puncture Alone

Seven patients with cerebral abscesses were only punctured. Neomycin-Sulfate was instilled and antibiotics were prescribed after testing. The causative agent could be traced in 5 cases. In the other two cases high dosage of antibiotics had been used previously.

Case 1 (Fig. 1). A 3-months-old infant with pneumonia was treated with antibiotics and developed meningo-encephalitis with hemiparesis and increasing disturbances of consciousness plus apathy. Rapid improvement after first puncture. The second one followed two weeks later still with distinct associated reactions. Up to now there is normal psycho-motor development with a still identifiable focal EEG-abnormality.

Case 2 (Fig. 2). An 8-year-old child with maxillary sinusitis developed headache, vomiting, fever and light somnolence. The aspirate showed pneumococcus mucosus, the progress of the patient has been unimpaired for 2 years.

Case 3. A 16-year-old boy with sinusitis frontalis suffered increasingly from headache, vomiting, and a slight hemiparesis. The first aspirate contained diplococcus pneumoniae, the second puncture after 6 weeks was sterile. Since then, the patient is symptom-free.

2. Puncture and Subsequent Surgery (2 Cases)

Case 4. A 16-year-old boy with a diagnosed vitium cordis, suffered clinical meningo-encephalitis with headache, vomiting, hemiparesis, and increasing clouding of consciousness. After antibiotic treatment, the abscess with a diameter of 1 cm was removed by surgery, after the relatively thick abscess wall had been detected by CT. The aspirate is now sterile.
Histologically, there is a lining of granulation tissue around the coarser membrane.

Case 5. After a trivial trauma, a 15-year-old boy developed nausea and headache. A week later, nuchal rigidity set in, followed by pneumonia and spreading hemiparesis with high temperature although antibiotic medication varied. 14 days after the puncture of the frontal abscess, the causative agent not having been traced, a total apocatastasis occurred. The parietal abscess, encapsulated in a distinct membrane was removed surgically.

3. Conservative Treatment Only (1 Case)

Case 6. With a 19-year-old patient a subdural hematoma was removed by surgery at another hospital. After three weeks, a discrete hemiparesis developed, antibiotics were prescribed, the causative agent could not be traced. After a week there was still a minimal impairment of the finer motor-functions, however, the patient was symptom-free. There was a continual decrease in the abscess' size. After the last check-up, a year ago, the patient has been symptom- and attack-free and neurologically without findings. The patient is now able to work again.

4. Surgery Alone

The removal of the abscess by operation was successful in 4 patients. In one case, the indication for surgery was based on the faulty assumption of a malignant glioma.

Subdural Empyema

CT proved especially helpful for the diagnosis of two empyemas in the interhemispheric fissure, for the observation of the development of an empyema above the convexity, as well as for the determination of the most beneficial date for surgery. Treatment was performed either by aspiration or by surgery.

Puncture Alone (2 Cases)

Case 7 (Figs. 3, 4). After purulent sinusitis a 16-year old boy developed headache, fever and an acute paresis of the right leg, as well as increasing somnolence. A single puncture of the empyema in the interhemispheric fissure was undertaken. The patient has been unimpaired in every sense for the last 2 years.

Case 8. A 17-year-old patient with sinusitis, osteomyelitis and pyosinus frontalis. Resection of large parts of the os frontalis by an ENT-surgeon. Two days later, the first cerebral attack occurred.

An increasing empyema development could be traced by CT. The patient was aspirated twice (in each case the aspirate was sterile). The patient has been symptom-free and without neurological deficit for the last 6 months.

Surgery Alone (4 Cases)

Four patients with subdural empyema over the convexity were operated upon; the following case under the faulty assumption of subdural effusion.

Case 9. An 8-months-old infant, who had fallen out of bed 3 months ago, showed abrasions and an apparently fractured skull left-frontal-parietal. Antibiotic medication followed. Increasing clumsiness of the right hand. Surgery on the relatively hard empyema membrane on the left side was undertaken. On the right side (low density) there was a subdural effusion without indication of a previous inflammation. The healing process was normal not only in this case, but also in 2 other cases with subdural empyema as a consequence of sinusitis. A 42-year-old patient died however, after surgery followed by encephalitis.

It can be assumed, that not only the development of encapsulated abscesses can be prevented, but also that accompanying encephalitic reactions can be controlled by means of aspiration of recent brain abscesses and instillation of Neomycin-Sulfate with simultaneous intravenous antibiotic medication.
As opposed to all previous possibilities of neuroradiological examination, atypical localisations of subdural empyema and their development can also be observed with CT.

Up to now, our results seem to prove that treatment of an empyema with aspiration only, is justifiable in those cases, where the observation of the developing empyema by CT does not lead to the assumption that solid membranes can be expected.

Case 10. A 33-year-old patient with cerebral gas gangrene caused by falling into a shrub from 2 m above. Treatment of the lacerated wound in an outpatient clinic. Two days later, the patient developed headache, swelling, reddening and secretion in the wound area, and increasing clouding of consciousness. In the first computer-tomogram, the temporal depressed fracture was identified, as well as gas in the area of the temporal cranial fossa, and brain oedema. The patient was transferred to Kiel. Tests of the secretion proved that the causative agent belonged to the clostridium group.
On admission there was a strongly indurated wound with secretion, nuchal rigidity, somnolence, and increasing confusion. Hyperbaric oxygen treatment was applied in the naval-medical institute. The intracerebral gas development receded completely.
There were renewed meningitic symptoms, despite antibiotic treatment. During surgery bone fragments, a 2 cm long splint and an abscess of about 1 cm in size were removed.
So, after primary hyperbaric oxygen treatment and subsequent surgery, the patient not only survived cerebral gas gangrene infection but could return to his native country after four weeks without neurological deficits.

Reference

Wallenfang, T., Bohl, J., Kretschmar, K.: Evolution of brain abscess in cats. Formation of capsule and resolution of brain edema. Neurosurg. Rew. 3, 101-111 (1980)

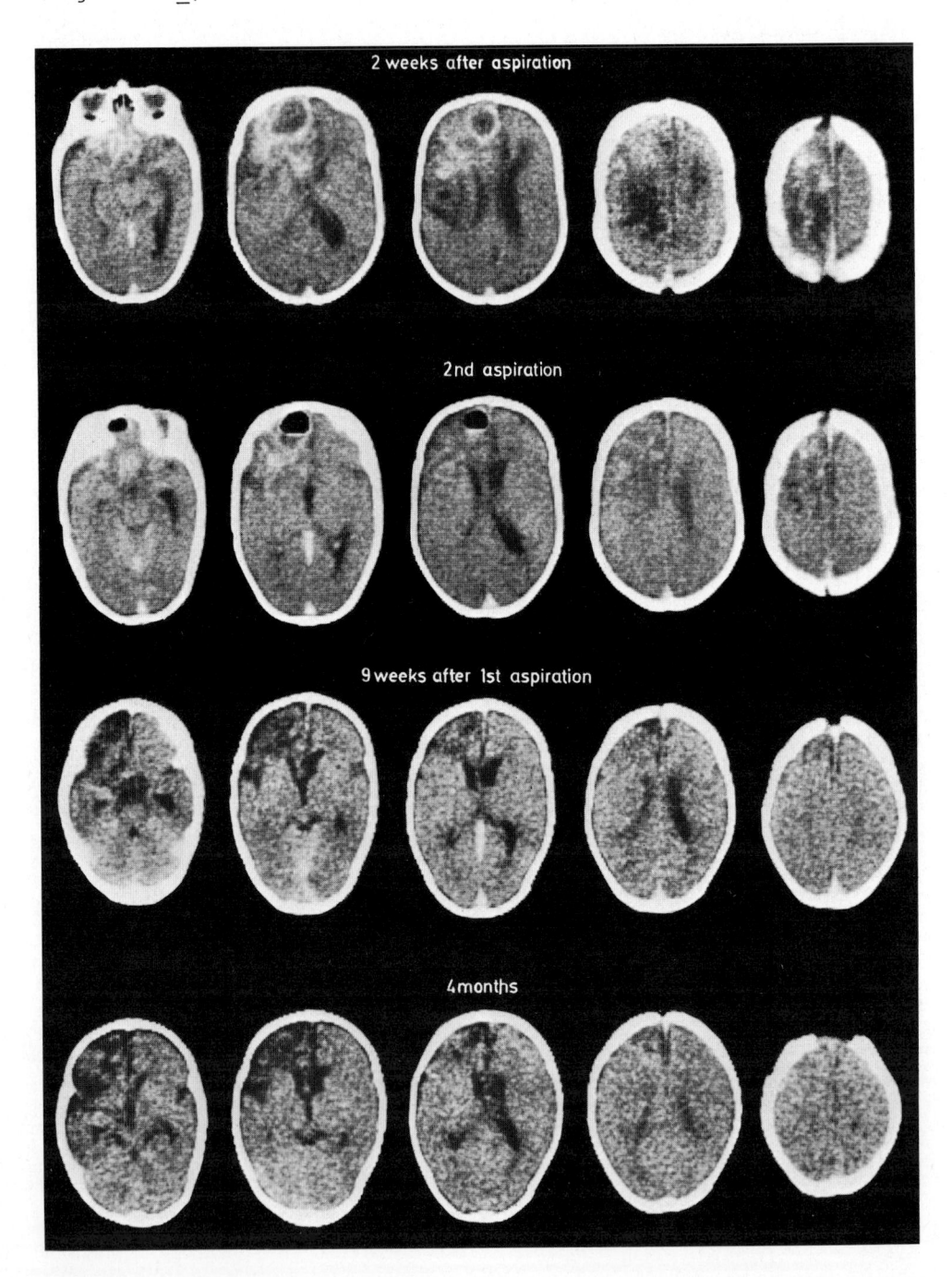

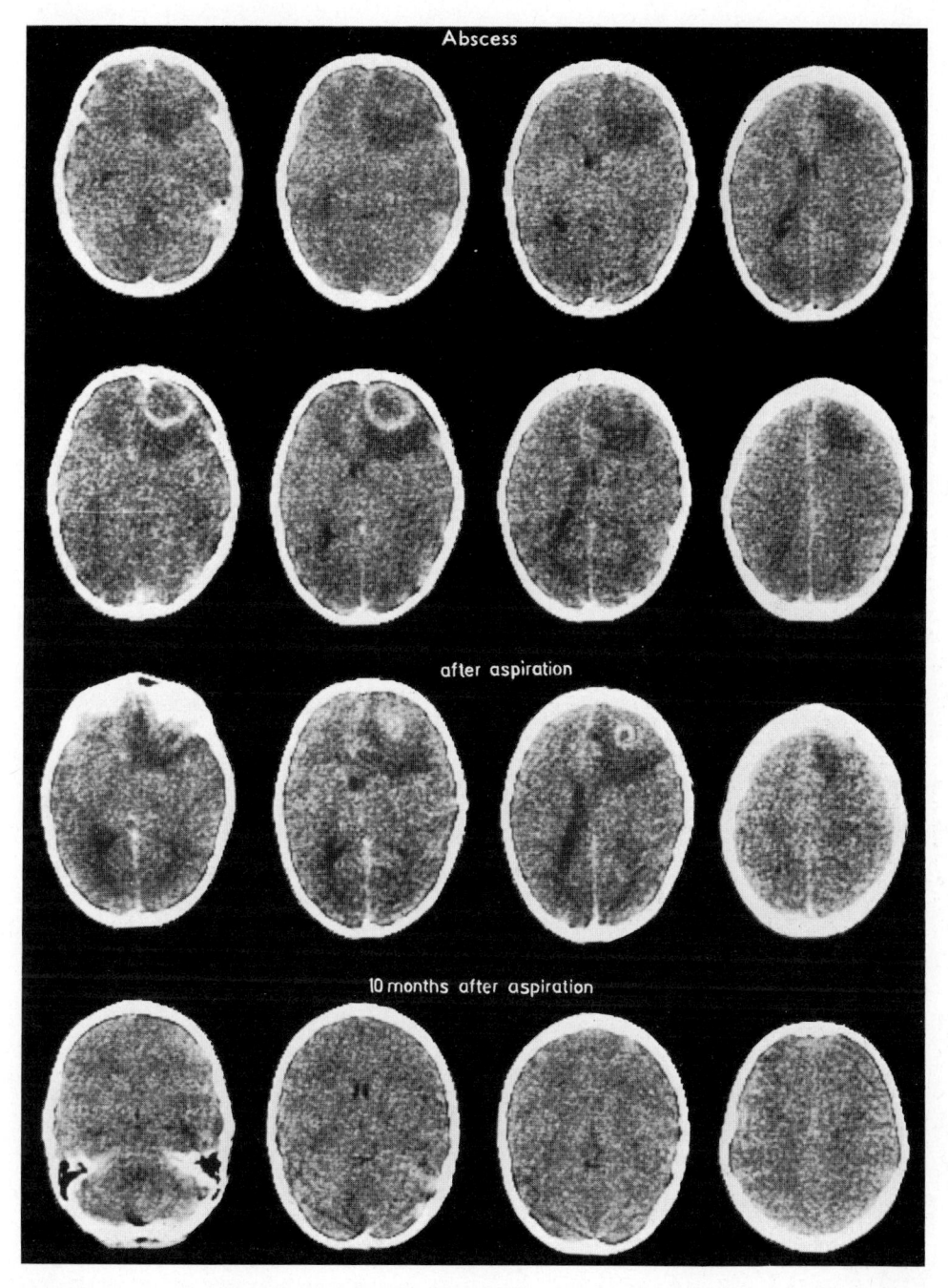

Fig. 2. 8-year-old child, right frontal cerebral abscess, follow-up study

◁ Fig. 1. 3-months-old infant. *Note:* Encephalitic reaction 2 weeks after first aspiration

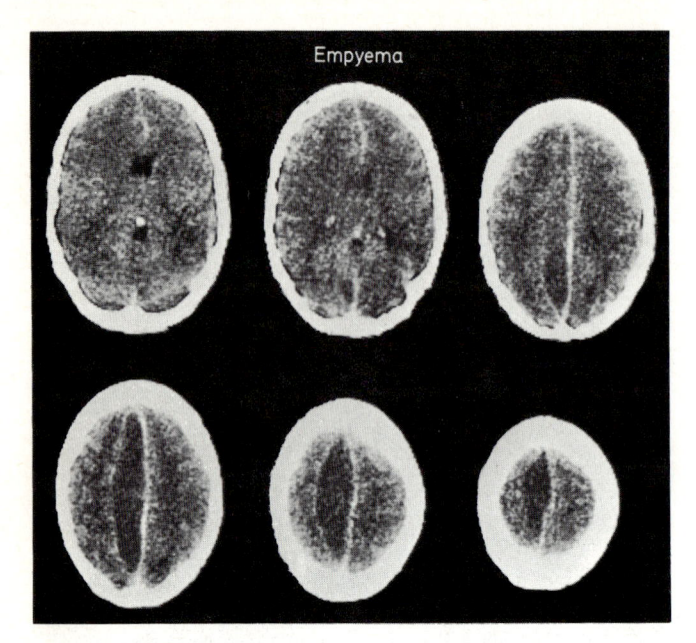

Fig. 3. 16-year-old boy with empyema of the interhemispheric fissure

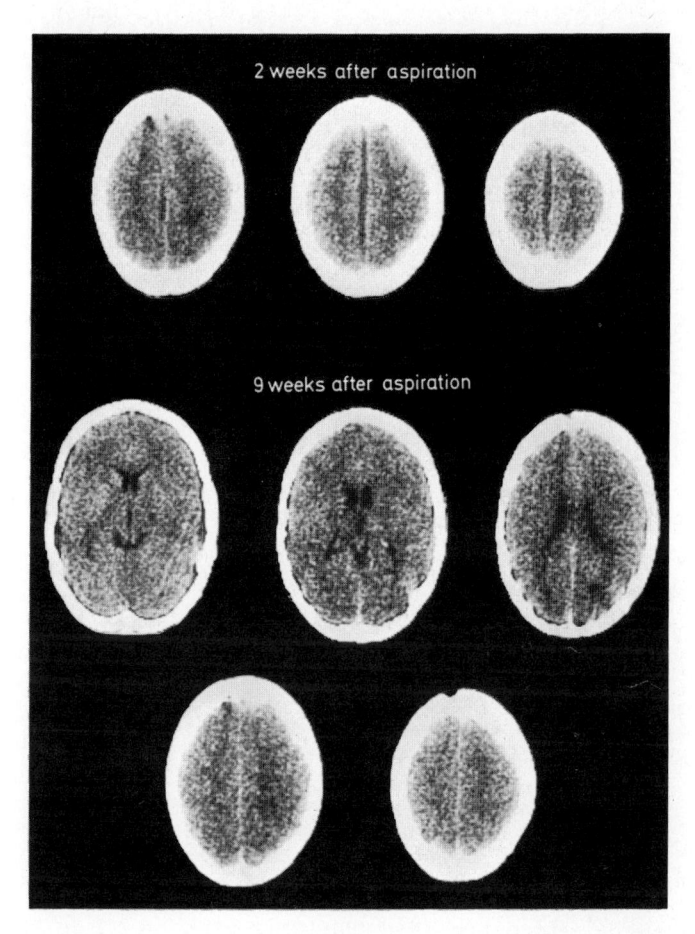

Fig. 4. Same patient as in Fig. 3 after aspiration

Diagnosis and Two-Dimensional Localization of Intracranial Metastases with Computerized Tomography

F. BRANDT, H. C. NAHSER, H.-E. CLAR, and H. M. MEHDORN

Introduction

In comparison with scintigraphy (5) and angiography computerized tomography (CT) offers a greater security in diagnosing cerebral metastases. On the other hand difficulties remain in the topographical determination of minor lesions and the operative approach based on these informations.

Preferring a localization near the border of the subcortex, brain metastases cannot be readily recognized by the inspection of the brain surface. Anti-oedematous therapy is an additional factor for these difficulties.

Material and Approach

The precise topographical reference of CT findings on the analogous pictures to the gyral structure involved is impossible. Only the stereotactic apparatus permits exact three-dimensional localization (3). Stereotactic methods for this purpose are limited to specialized neurosurgical centers. For localization of small brain metastases in routine clinical use this method is not useful. To minimize the risk of exstirpation of intracerebral metastases in strategic brain areas we therefore preceded the operation by CT-guided localization and scalp marking.

Scans were performed by a Siemens Siretom 2.000-scanner, which has a 256 x 256 matrix.

After CT-scanning without and with contrast media for diagnostic investigation, a preoperative scalp marking was done by the neurosurgeon if the following criteria were fulfilled:

1. Patient's good physical condition
2. No fatal prognosis of the underlying disease
3. No other systemic metastases
4. Presence of solitary metastases and situated near to cortical structures.

Occasionally an indication was accepted if the primary tumour was unknown.

Results

Basically two methods of localization were applied.

1. Marking by Meridians. After visualization of the metastasis in 5 mm thick axial CT-sclices with contrast enhancement, the X-ray path of the slice in question was marked on the shaved scalp (Figs. 1a, b). This procedure was repeated in the coronal plane (Figs. 1c, d). The crossing point indicated the area of craniotomy and the cortical point which was to be incised.

2. Marking by Point. Alternatively a radiopaque material was fixed on the scalp in the meridian of the detected lesion and the exact position was controlled by repetition of the axial scan (Fig. 2).

Discussion

To localize metastases in deeper brain structures we applied the method of visualization in axial and coronal scanning, i.e. marking by meridians. This procedure gives information about the level of cut and the resulting angle for incision.

Metastases of the cerebral convexity and close to vertex structures are better marked by method 2, because only in this way the shortest approach for removal can be determined.

The suggested method permits a reduction of the operation to straight exstirpation of the metastasis and diminishes possible damage to the surrounding brain tissue. By means of angiography and scintigraphy this was not yet possible. We could at the same time reduce the size of the craniotomy defect. The described method of localization is suitable, too for a reduction of operative risks in multiloculated intracerebral lesions in which biopsy is needed.

Two propositions for simple CT localizations have recently been described: O'LEARY and LAVYNE (1978) construct a baseline on the patient's lateral skull film corresponding to identical landmarks of prominent bony structures found on CT scan. All other sections obtained by CT examination are parallel to this baseline. The height of the lesion above the baseline can thus be calculated. The method of CAIL and MORRIS (1979) uses plain radiographs for localization, too. HINCK and CLIFTON (1981) use radipaque material in defined graduated lengths which is fixed extracranially during CT-scanning to detect the height of the lesion.

Essential for the accuracy of our method of localization are the following criteria:

1. The position of the patient may not be changed during examination.
2. Coronal scanning must be practicable in regard of constitutional factors and neurological circumstances for marking by meridians.
3. Any movements resulting from flapping have to be taken into account.

If these criteria are fulfilled an exact position according to the orbito-meatal line is not compulsory. For our way of localization a reference line is not necessary since the marking is only referred to the lesion itself in CT. Anatomical variants are therefore without importance.

References

1. Cail, W.S., Morris, J.J.: Localization of intracranial lesions from CT scans. Surg. Neurol. 11, 35-37 (1979)
2. Hinck, V.C., Clifton, G.L.: A precise technique for craniotomy localization using computerized tomography. J. Neurosurg. 54, 416-418 (1981)
3. Jacques, S., Shelden, C.H., McCann, G.D., Freshwater, D.B., Rand, R.: Computerized three-dimensional stereotaxic removal of small nervous system lesions in patients. J. Neurosurg. 53, 816-820 (1980)
4. O'Leary, D.H., Lavyne, M.H.: Localization of vertex lesions seen on CT scan. J. Neurosurg. 49, 71-74 (1978)
5. Zeidler, U.: Hirnszintigraphie. In: Handbuch der Medizinischen Radiologie. Diethelm, L. et al. (eds.) Vol. 15 (2). Berlin 1978

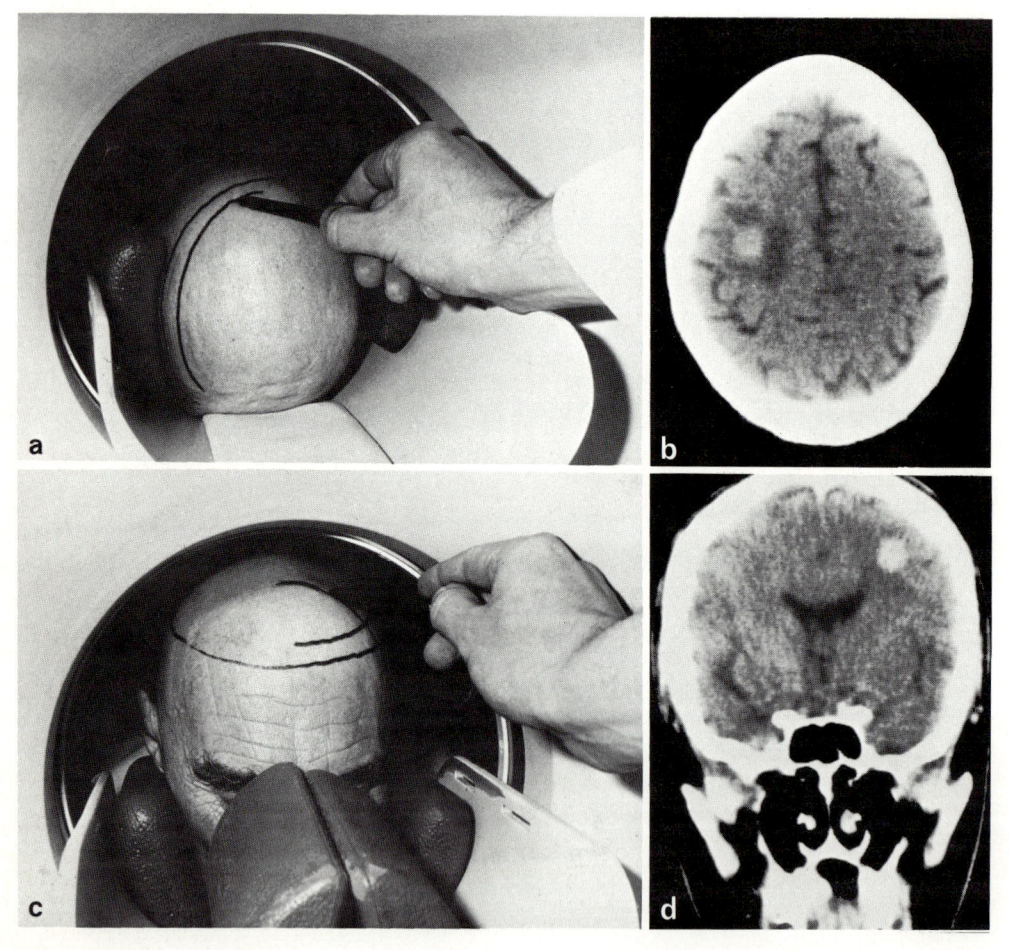

Fig. 1a-d. Marking by meridians for localization of a left parietal metastasis (a,b) and in coronal plane (c,d)

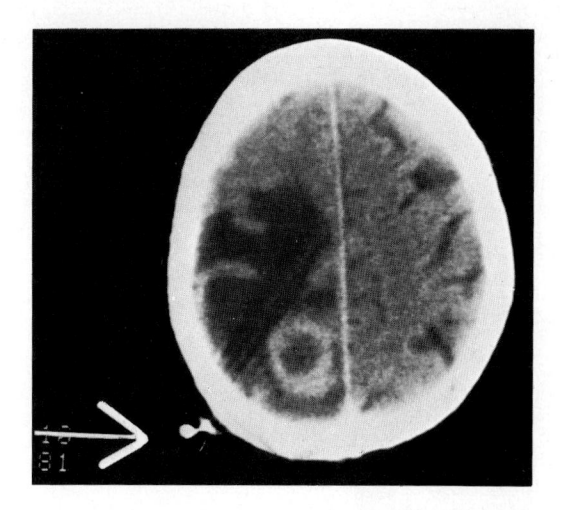

Fig. 2. Marking by point. The arrow points to the extracranially fixed radiopaque material

The Influence of Computerized Tomography on Treatment of Spontaneous Intracerebral Hematoma

TH. GRUMME, W. LANKSCH, and D. KOLODZIEJCZYK

The conservative and operative treatment of patients with spontaneous intracerebral hematoma has always caused problems to any neurosurgeon. The results of operative treatment vary considerably - as can be noted from a survey of the last thirty years' literature, which is mainly due to the difference in patients and to the non-uniformity of indications for operation (Tables 1, 2). In this survey it has been distinguished as far as possible between typical hypertensive hematoma involving the basal ganglia and the atypical hematoma, situated in the white matter or the lobes.

The introduction of computer tomography has considerably improved diagnosis and treatment of various neurosurgical diseases by enabling a more exact indication to be worked out and more precise planning of surgical methods. With regard to this we have tried to find out whether the results of operative treatment of spontaneous intercerebral hematoma have been changed by computer tomography.

From the beginning of 1975 until the end of 1980 74 patients with spontaneous intracerebral hematoma have been operated on in the neurosurgical departments of the university Munich (Klinikum Großhadern) and Berlin (Klinikum Charlottenburg). 7 hematomas were situated infratentorially. For interpretation of results we have coordinated the neurological findings into four stages (Table 3). Special attention was focussed on the development of the neurologic situation between the beginning of the disease until the moment of surgical intervention. We considered computertomographically only size and position of the hematoma. Displacement of midline structure has intentionally been disregarded because the degree of midline shift could not be correlated with the neurological signs.

Out of our 67 patients with supratentorial hematoma 28 died, i.e. 42%. Out of 7 patients with cerebellar hematoma only 2 survived. For reasons of vital urgency and for lack of undoubted prognostic criteria, 9 patients in stage 4 were operated upon immediately; all of them died within the first week after operation without having recovered consciousness (Table 4). Out of 20 patients who were operated upon because of an imminent and/or an advanced stage of midbrain compression within 24 hours after the acute event, only 9 survived. 4 out of these 9 patients suffered either from a relatively small temporal basal ganglia hematoma and 4 from frontal hematoma. One patient suffered from a most extensive hematoma of basal ganglia with severe postoperative neurological deficit. Out of this group, 5 patients recovered without neurological deficit. Out of 30 patients who were operated upon during the acute phase of the first day, 20 died, i.e. 67%. The mortality among those patients who were - with the same indication - operated upon only in the second day was 25%. All but one of the surviving patients of the group who

Table 1. Survey of the literature on spontaneous intracerebral hematoma during the pre-CT-era

Author	Year	No. of patients (n)	Mortality (total) (%)	Typical hematomas mortality (n)	(%)	Atypical hematomas mortality (n)	(%)
DAVID et al.	1953	287	27				
LAZORTHES	1956	481	27				
TÖNNIS, FROWEIN	1958	588	31				
McKISSOCK et al.	1961	189	65	20	75	60	62
CUATICO et al.	1965	102	8	55	13	47	0
PASZTOR et al.	1980	156	17	70	27	86	9
Total		1803	28,3	145	29	202	26

Table 2. Survey of literature on spontaneous intracerebral hematoma in the CT-era

Author	Year	No. of patients (n)	Mortality (total) (%)	Typical hematomas mortality (n)	(%)	Atypical hematomas mortality (N)	(%)
KANAYA et al.	1980	145	19	145	19		
SCHÜRMANN et al.	1980	61	36	29	41	32	31
MÜKE	1980	42	48				
KARIMI, HAMEL	1980	104	61	47	69	57	54
MATSUKADO, SAKURAMA	1980	25	20	25	20		
ZIERSKI	1980	102	54	57	67	45	38
Total		479	40,3	303	38	134	43

Table 3. Classification of the neurological status

Stage 1: Neurologically normal

Stage 2: Alert, but with focal neurological signs (hemiparesis, dysphasia, hemianopsia)

Stage 3: Unconsciousness, focal neurological signs with pupillary signs (imminent midbrain compression)

Stage 4: Unconsciousness, rigidity, fixed dilated pupils on one or both sides (advanced midbrain compression)

Table 4. Results of operative treatment dependent on the neurologic stage of the patient and on the time of operation

Operation days	Stage 2 n	(+)	Stage 3 n	(+)	Stage 4 n	(+)	Total n	(+)	=	%
1.	1	(−)	20	(11)	9	(9)	30	20		67
2.	−	(−)	9	(2)	3	(1)	12	3		25
3. − 7.	4	(−)	7	(2)	1	(−)	12	2		17
> 8.	8	(1)	5	(2)	−	(−)	13	3		23
							67	28		42

were operated on during the second day showed no development of the focal-neurological deficit. Both of the surviving patients, who were operated upon in stage 4 are totally disabled. Among the group of patients who were operated upon after the second day but within the first week, two died because of extracerebral and one for neurological reasons. Most tragic is the death of a 33-year-old patient who had been operated upon after 3 weeks in stage 2 and who had several postoperative hematomas.

Beyond the age of 50, prognosis clearly deteriorates (Fig. 1). A volume of hematoma of more than 40 ml as well as a hematoma of basal ganglia and/or rupture into the ventricles diminishes the survival rate considerably; on the other hand the position of the hematoma in atypical regions influences the focal-neurological deficit more.

An analysis of the results of the surviving patients who were operated upon after the second day shows that all except two of those patients who were submitted to an operation during stage 3 had no alteration in their distinct neurologic deficit. Out of 11 patients who had been operated upon during the more favourable stage 2 because of non-existent or not progressing recovery, 7 came to total remission, 2 to progressing recovery, whilst the status of 2 patients remained unchanged. Only 18% of our patients were nearly completely cured by neurosurgical intervention.

The CT-follow up's in conservatively treated cases show that under strict neurological status-control there is a legitimate reason to postpone surgical treatment. The rate of resorption depends on the size of the hematoma. Small hematoma with an average diameter of between 1,5 and 3 cm are often reabsorbed leaving within 4 to 5 weeks hypodense defects; larger hematoma, however, need usually up to 9 weeks before complete resorption takes place.

Intraventricular haemorrhages are not seen in CT scan between 14 and 20 days after bleeding. The return of midline structures does not occur simultaneously with the diminishing or density decrease of the hematoma, and is seen at the earliest after a period of 3 weeks. According to CT-follow-up-examinations there is no hard and fast rule governing the rate of resorption in intracerebral bleedings. It appears that the size and the location of the hematoma, penetration of the ventricles, perifocal edema, extent of displacement of cerebral structures, preexistent brain atrophy, age, general physical condition and previous illness may all cause great variation in these processes of haematoma absorption. Before the CT-era we would most certainly have operated on some patients from this group, because of the space occupying lesion.

Summary

1. The operative mortality amounts to 42%; 40% of patients survived with neurologic deficit; only 18% came up to an almost complete recovery.
2. Our experience proves that operations during the first day on patients suffering from a typical midbrain compression lead to a mortality rate of 100%. Therefore an operation seems to be senseless.
3. A comparison with former results clearly demonstrated that the results of operative treatment have not changed in spite of improved diagnosis by computerized tomography (Table 5).
4. An exact demonstration of hematoma and its correlation to adjacent cerebral structures by computerized tomography permits one nowadays to reject operations which in former times would have been carried out in case of doubt only on indirect proof of an intracerebral hematoma.
5. The indication for operation still depends in each particular case on the neurologic symptomatology and mainly on its speed.

Table 5. Comparison between results of operative treatment of spontaneous intracerebral hematoma (pre-CT-era, CT-era, own results)

	n	Mortality Total (%)	Typical hematoma (%)	Atypical hematoma (%)
Survey of literature pre-CT-era	1703	28,3	29	26
Survey of literature CT-era	479	40,3	38	43
Own results CT-era	67	42	63	24

References

1. Cuatico, W., Adib, S., Gaston, P.: Spontaneous intracerebral hematomas. J. Neurosurg. 22, 569-575 (1965)
2. David, M., Hecaen, H., Frowein, R.A.: Revue critique sur le traitment chirurgical de l'hématome intracerebrale spontane. Sem. Hôp. Paris 29, 500-510 (1953)
3. Grumme, Th., Kretzschmar, K., Lanksch, W.: Natural history and follow-up of spontaneous intracerebral hematomas. In: Spontaneous intracerebral hematomas. Advances in diagnosis and therapy. Pia, H.W., Langmaid, C., Zierski, J. (eds.), pp. 216-221. Berlin, Heidelberg, New York: Springer 1980
4. Kanaya, H., Yukawa, H., Itoh, Z., Kutsuzawa, H., Kagawa, M., Kanno, T., Kuwabara, T., Mizukami, K., Araki, G., Irino, T.: Grading and the indications for treatment in ICH of the basal ganglia (Cooperative study in Japan). In: Spontaneous intracerebral hematomas. Advances in diagnosis and therapy. Pia, H.W., Langmaid, C., Zierski, J. (eds.), pp. 268-274. Berlin, Heidelberg, New York: Springer 1980
5. Karimi-Nejad, A., Hamel, E.: Comparative study of the results in spontaneous and traumatic ICH. In: Spontaneous intracerebral hematomas. Advances in diagnosis and therapy. Pia, H.W., Langmaid, D., Zierski, J. (eds.), pp. 310-316. Berlin, Heidelberg, New York: Springer 1980
6. Lazorthes, G.: L'hémorrhagie cérébrale. Vue par le Neurochirurgien. Paris: Masson 1956
7. Matsukado, Y., Sakurama, N.: Putaminal ICH with regard to its size in CT scanning. In: Spontaneous intracerebral hematomas. Advances in diagnosis and therapy. Pia, H.W., Langmaid, C., Zierski, J. (eds.), pp. 341-345. Berlin, Heidelberg, New York: Springer 1980
8. McKissock, W., Richardson, A., Taylor, J.: Primary intracerebral haemorrhage. Controlled trial of surgical and conservative treatment in 180 unselected cases. Lancet II, 221-226 (1961)
9. Müke, R.: Burr-hole evacuation. In: Spontaneous intracerebral hematomas. Advances in diagnosis and therapy. Pia, H.W., Langmaid, C., Zierski, J. (eds.), pp. 379-382. Berlin, Heidelberg, New York: Springer 1980
10. Pasztor, E., Afra, D., Orosz, E.: Experiences with the surgical treatment of 156 ICH (1955-1977). In: Spontaneous intracerebral hematomas. Advances in diagnosis and therapy. Pia, H.W., Langmaid, C., Zierski, J. (eds.), pp. 251-257. Berlin, Heidelberg, New York: Springer 1980
11. Schürmann, K., Dei Anang, K.: Indication and contraindication for surgery of spontaneous intracerebral hematomas. Neurosurg. Rev. 3, 17-22 (1980)
12. Stender, A.: Operative Therapie der Massenblutungen. Acta neurochir. (Wien) Suppl. 7, 283-290 (1961)
13. Zierski, J.: Hematomas in hemispheric lobes. In: Spontaneous intracerebral hematomas. Advances in diagnosis and therapy. Pia, H.W., Langmaid, C., Zierski, J. (eds.), pp. 322-326. Berlin, Heidelberg, New York: Springer 1980

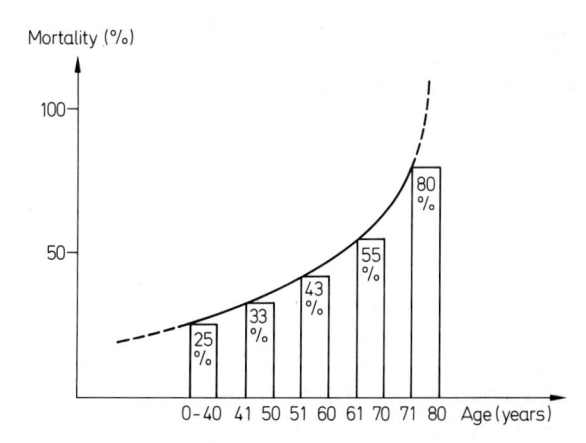

Fig. 1. Dependency of mortality on age

The Prognosis of Traumatic Intracranial Hematomas Before and After the Introduction of Computerized Tomography

E. HEISS, F. ALBERT, and H. WEILAND

The localization and expansion of an intracranial hemorrhage can be detected by CT within a few minutes. Therefore, the advantages of this exact identification and time-saving diagnostic method may be assumed to influence the results of surgical treatment of traumatic intracranial hematomas.

For this purpose we have compared the clinical courses of acute epidural (EDH) and subdural (SDH) hematomas, as well as of traumatic intracerebral blood clots (ICH), which were operated on between 1971 and 1979 in the Neurochirurgische Universitätsklinik Erlangen. During this period 468 patients were treated for these 3 types of hematomas (EDH: 213 cases; SDH: 168 cases; ICH: 87 cases). The diagnosis was made by CT in 51.9%, by other methods (angiography, echoencephalography = AE) in 48.1%.

It is worth mentioning that the frequency of operative treatment of CT-diagnosed intracerebral hematomas was more than one-third higher than in the pre-CT era, whereas subdural hematomas were operated on about one third less frequently (Fig. 1).
In 338 cases we were able to determine the time interval between the accident and the surgical procedure. The 24 hour-time-limit for acute subdural hematoma (FROWEIN and KEILA, 1972) was drawn into consideration in these cases.
Owing to the use of CT, the time interval between accident and operation could be reduced for all types of hematomas (Fig. 2). On the average, EDH were operated on 4 hours earlier than in the pre-CT era, SDH 2.3 hours earlier, and ICH 0.3 hours earlier.

With regard to the postoperative outcome, the different types of hematomas were classified into 3 groups: *good* (cured or eligible for rehabilitation), *poor* (persisting unconsciousness or apallic syndrome), and *death*. The tendency towards a more rapid diagnosis with the help of CT was observed in all these 3 subdivisions for all types of hematomas (Fig. 3).

Comparing the two different diagnostic methods (CT, AE), the patients of the CT group revealed a better survival rate and an improved postoperative state (good condition in 60.9%, in contrast to 57.6% in the AE group), and a corresponding decrease in the mortality rate (4.3%).

The evaluation of the outcome in the various types of hematomas showed some remarkable differences in the postoperative conditions (Fig. 4):

Epidural hematomas (n = 213)

	CT (123 cases)	AE (90 cases)
Good	73.2%	73.3%
Poor	8.9%	13.3%
Death	17.9%	13.3%

Subdural hematomas (n = 168)

	CT (66 cases)	AE (102 cases)
Good	42.4%	49.0%
Poor	22.7%	13.5%
Death	34.9%	37.5%

Intracerebral hematomas (n = 87)

	CT (54 cases)	AE (33 cases)
Good	55.6%	40.6%
Poor	13.0%	9.4%
Death	31.4%	50.5%

In spite of the use of the CT, the mortality of epidural hematomas in our series increased by 4.6%, that of subdural hematomas on the other hand, decreased by 2.6%. At the same time a rise (9%) in the number of patients with a poor outcome after SDH was seen. Intracerebral hematomas were not only operated on more frequently, but the results of their treatment also improved considerably, the decrease in the mortality being nearly 20%.

The following factors are thought to influence the result of therapy of traumatic intracranial hematomas: the time interval between accident and operation, the age and the condition of the injured person, additional injuries, and the occurrence of unfavourable clinical signs (primary or secondary unconsciousness, dilatation of the pupils, pyramidal tract signs, extensor spasms of the extremities).

No significant age differences were observed between the CT and the AE groups of the various hematoma types. The survival chances of cases with acute traumatic hemorrhages declined rapidly in patients over 60 years of age. Furthermore, investigations in patients with prolonged unconsciousness or apallic syndrome indicated that younger people tend to recover in the course of time, while older people die.

With regard to the determining factors mentioned above, the patients who died of *epidural hematomas* had exhibited an unfavourable clinical condition at an early stage, despite the time-saving diagnostic CT procedure: 33.3% of these had a primary unconsciousness persisting since the accident. Out of these, 71.4% had additional severe injuries, and 95.5% exhibited dilated pupils. A primary unconsciousness was seen in only 8.3% of the patients in the AE group. These, moreover, had no substantial secondary injuries. Dilatation of the pupils was found in 91.6% of these latter patients.

Patients with *subdural hematomas* were found to have a decrease in the mortality rate by 2.6% in the CT group. Furthermore, a conspicuous increase of survivors in a poor clinical condition (+9%) was observed in this group.

A primary unconsciousness and multiple injuries were seen equally often in the deceased of both diagnostic groups. Compared to the CT-diagnosed group, the operation in the AE group was not only delayed in time, but also took place under more unfavourable clinical conditions: dilatation of the pupils in 89.5% (CT group: 86.7%), extensor spasms in 44.7% (CT group: 31.3%).
The survivors of SDH in a poor postoperative condition had likewise been primarily unconscious in both diagnostic groups. The CT-diagnosed survivors, however, had multiple injuries in a higher percentage of cases (CT group: 37.5%; AE group: 0%), and more often exhibited dilated pupils (CT group: 75.0%; AE group: 71.4%). It must therefore be assumed that they had been in a more unfavourable condition immediately after the accident, a further loss of time resulting in death.

The most remarkable observation in our series was the decrease in the mortality rate - almost 20% - of the traumatic *intracerebral hematomas* since the introduction of CT. In respect to their survival, the patients of the AE group were already in a less favourable condition at the time of operation, surgery being performed approximately 5 hours later on the average. In these patients we found higher rates of primary unconsciousness (+15%), of dilated pupils (+6%), of a tendency to extensor spasms of the extremities (+12%), and of pyramidal tract signs (+24%). The incidence of multiple injuries was about the same.

In summary, we conclude that the diagnosis of a traumatic intracranial hemorrhage is unquestionably facilitated and accelerated by CT, but more patients come to surgery in a primarily adverse clinical condition. Especially the diagnosis of ICH has been improved by the localizing abilities of the CT, which has positive effects on the number and the outcome of surgical interventions, and which results in a substantial decrease of the mortality.

Despite the unquestionable benefit of the CT, the fate of patients with traumatic intracranial hematomas remains dependent on the rapidity of hemorrhage development, and on the alertness of the admitting physician.

Reference

Frowein, R.A., Keila, M.: Einteilung der traumatischen subduralen Hämatome. Acta traumat. 2, 205-213 (1972)

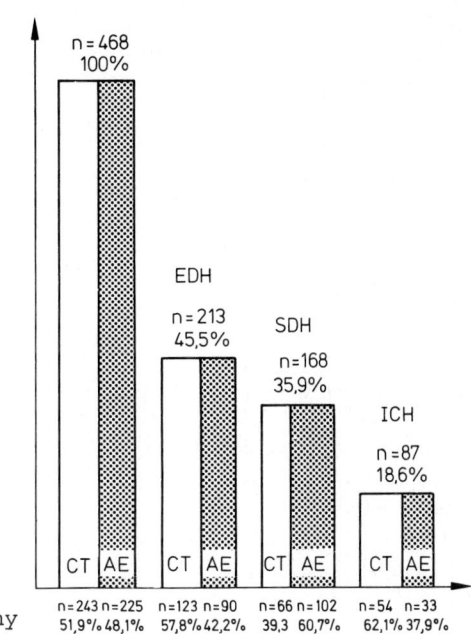

Fig. 1. Frequency of diagnostic methods
CT, computer tomography;
AE, angiography, echoencephalography

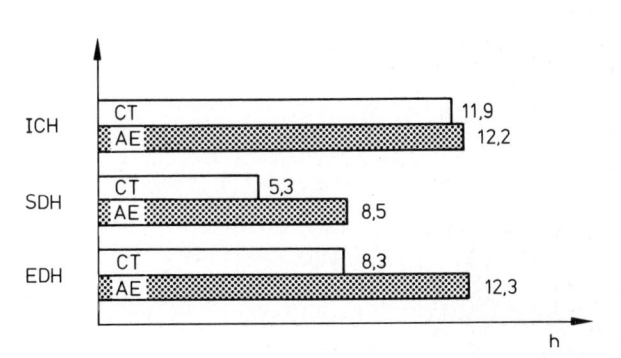

Fig. 2. Time differences between CT- and AE-diagnosed hematomas

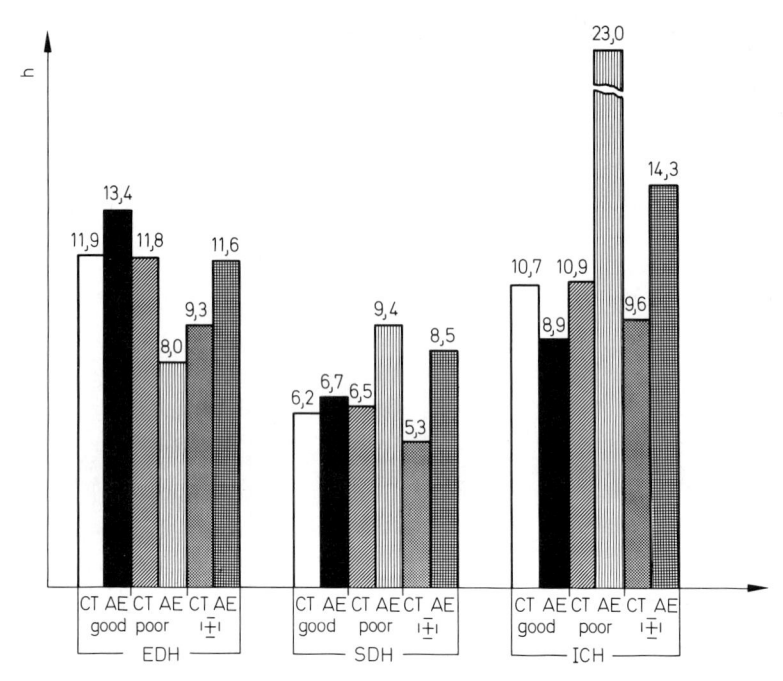

Fig. 3. Time differences of the results depending on the diagnostic method

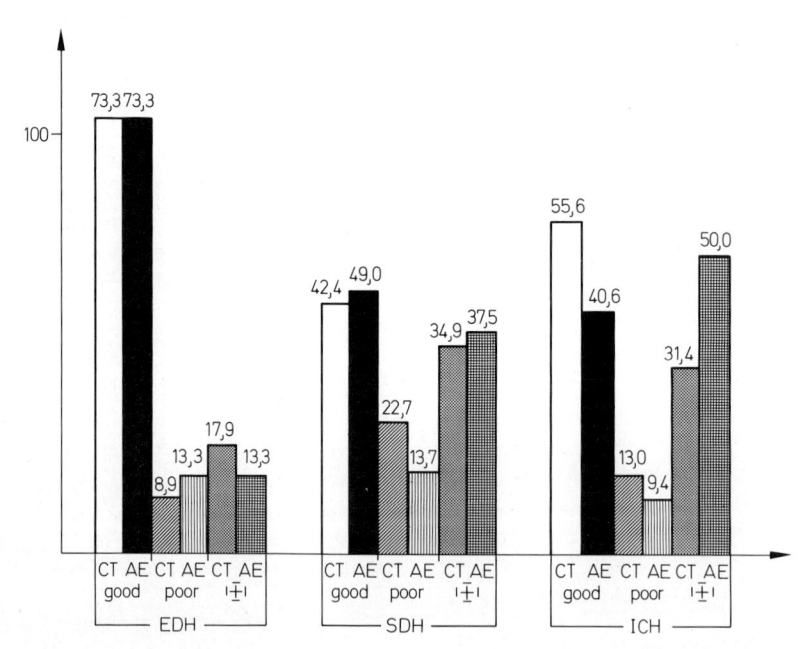

Fig. 4. Results of the individual hematoma-groups depending on the diagnostic method

Postoperative CT-Follow-Up of Chronic Subdural Hematoma

J. R. Moringlane, M. Samii, and K. D. Lerch

Introduction

Chronic subdural hematomas show not only during the preoperative examination characteristic computertomographic changes of the subdural space and cortex, signs of compression of the basal cisterns and ventricular system, rabbit-ear-phenomenon etc. (1, 2, 3). In the postoperative period repeated CT-examinations show important peculiarities - depending on the surgical technique - which give essential information of the healing process. Neurosurgeons and neuroradiologists should undertake the analysis of postoperative CT findings, always taking into consideration the operative technique employed in each case and the clinical situation in order to avoid false interpretations which could lead to superfluous reinterventions.

Material and Method

Since 1977, 55 patients with chronic subdural hematomas between 12 and 87 years of age were treated at the Neurosurgical Clinic of the City of Hannover (FRG). Depending on the extent of the subdural fluid collection, evacuation was performed via 2 or 3 seldom enlarged burr holes. The membranes were resected in the visible area of the burr holes. After irrigation of the subdural space with saline solution a JACKSON-PRATT drain was introduced into the subdural space between the cortex and the inner membrane. This drain was withdrawn as soon as the cortex had reached the inner table of the skull bone, otherwise it was left in place till the drained liquid became clear.

The following 3 cases demonstrate exemplary CT findings in the postoperative course of chronic subdural hematomas.

Case 1

A 50-year-old male patient with psychic disorders and headache, later followed by deterioration of state of consciousness (Fig. 1 a-e):

a) Preoperative finding: Chronic mixed hypo-isodense subdural hematoma over the right hemisphere, fronto-temporo-parietal. Compression of the right lateral ventricle, shifting of the midline structures to the left.

b) 7th postoperative day: Drain is still in place. Rest of hematoma and air. Beginning of widening of ventricle.

c) 11 days after surgery. The drain has been removed. Residuum of air.

d) 17th postoperative day. Rest of air and level of liquid. The condition of the patient has definitively improved.

e) 4th postoperative week. No residual hematoma. No air. Normal configuration of the ventricular system. The surface of the brain has reached the inner table of the skull.

Case 2

A 66-year-old male patient. Admission in the hospital after a fall on the street with short loss of consciousness. No neurologic deficit, no (subjective) complaint. Routine CT-examination (Fig. 2 a-e):

a) Preoperative CT-finding showing a hypodense bilateral subdural hematomas with depressed (flattened) gyri, rabbit-ear-phenomenon on the right side and compression of the right lateral ventricle.

b) 8th postoperative day with drainage on both sides. Rest of liquid and of air over both frontal lobes (patient is in the supine position.

c) 3 weeks after surgery. The drains have been removed. Rest of air and liquid. Collapse of ventricles and hemispheres. Patient clinically well.

d) 4 weeks after surgery. Rest of liquid. Persisting collapse of the hemispheres. The patient is clinically in excellent condition.

This patient had check-ups at regular intervals of 3 months. Despite the very good condition of the patient CT finding was unchanged 8 months after the operation.

e) Final result 1 year after surgery. Complete expansion of the hemispheres. Complete resorption of subdural fluid. Normal appearance of the pattern of the cortex, cisterns and ventricles, corresponding to the age of the patient.

Case 3

A 66-year-old female patient. Admission into hospital because of psychic disorder. CT-examination was performed because of impairment of the state of consciousness.

a) Preoperative finding: bilateral isodense chronic subdural hematomas with rabbit-ear-phenomenon, flattened relief of cortex.

b) 11th postoperative day. CT showing the drain on both sides. Beginning decompression of the ventricles.

c) 15 days after surgery. Drains removed. Brain mass still collapsed. Tent-like moulded frontal lobes. Rest of air over the frontal lobes (supine position). Clinical improvement.

d) 3 weeks after surgery. No subdural liquid. No air. Persisting signs of compression with rabbit-ear-phenomenon. Patient clinically improved. No indication for a new surgical intervention.

In this patient normalization of the ventricular system and of the cisterns required a period of 6 months.

e) 7 months after surgery. Enlargement of lateral ventricles. Normalization of cortex, sulci open, no rabbit-ear-phenomenon. Ventricular system and surface of the brain corresponding to the age of the patient.

Conclusion

After evacuation of chronic subdural hematomas via 2 or 3 enlarged burr holes with subsequent postoperative drainage of the subdural space, CT examinations show well defined peculiarities as demonstrated by the 3 representative cases described above.

In the 1st postoperative week, the CT picture shows the drains as well as a residuum of air and fluid and persistance of signs of compression. After removal of the drains the space is occupied by a residuum of air and fluid. In a few cases the surface of the brain reaches the inner table of the skull and the ventricular system gets normal in a short time. In spite of the improvement of the clinical situation of the patient, signs of compression of the basal cisterns and of the ventricles can still be present. Normalization of the ventricles, of the cortical pattern, of the subdural space and basal cisterns is not a result obtained immediately after surgery, but a more or less slow process over a few weeks to several months. There is no parallelism between the clinical recovery and the normalization of the CT finding. A residuum of air and of fluid in the subdural space as well as the persistence of preoperative signs of compression should not be taken for a recurrence of the chronic subdural hematoma. The length of time required for the disappearance of pathologic signs depends not only on the age of the chronic subdural hematoma, but also greatly on the general condition of the patient and on his biological age.

References

1. Lanksch, W., Grumme, Th., Kazner, E.: Schädelhirnverletzungen im Computertomogramm. Berlin, Heidelberg, New York: Springer 1978
2. Nadjmi, M., Piepgras, U., Vogelsang, H.: Kranielle Computertomographie. Stuttgart, New York: Thieme 1981
3. Marcu, H., BEcker, H.: Computed-Tomography of bilateral isodense chronic subdural hematomas. Neuroradiology 14, 81-83 (1977)

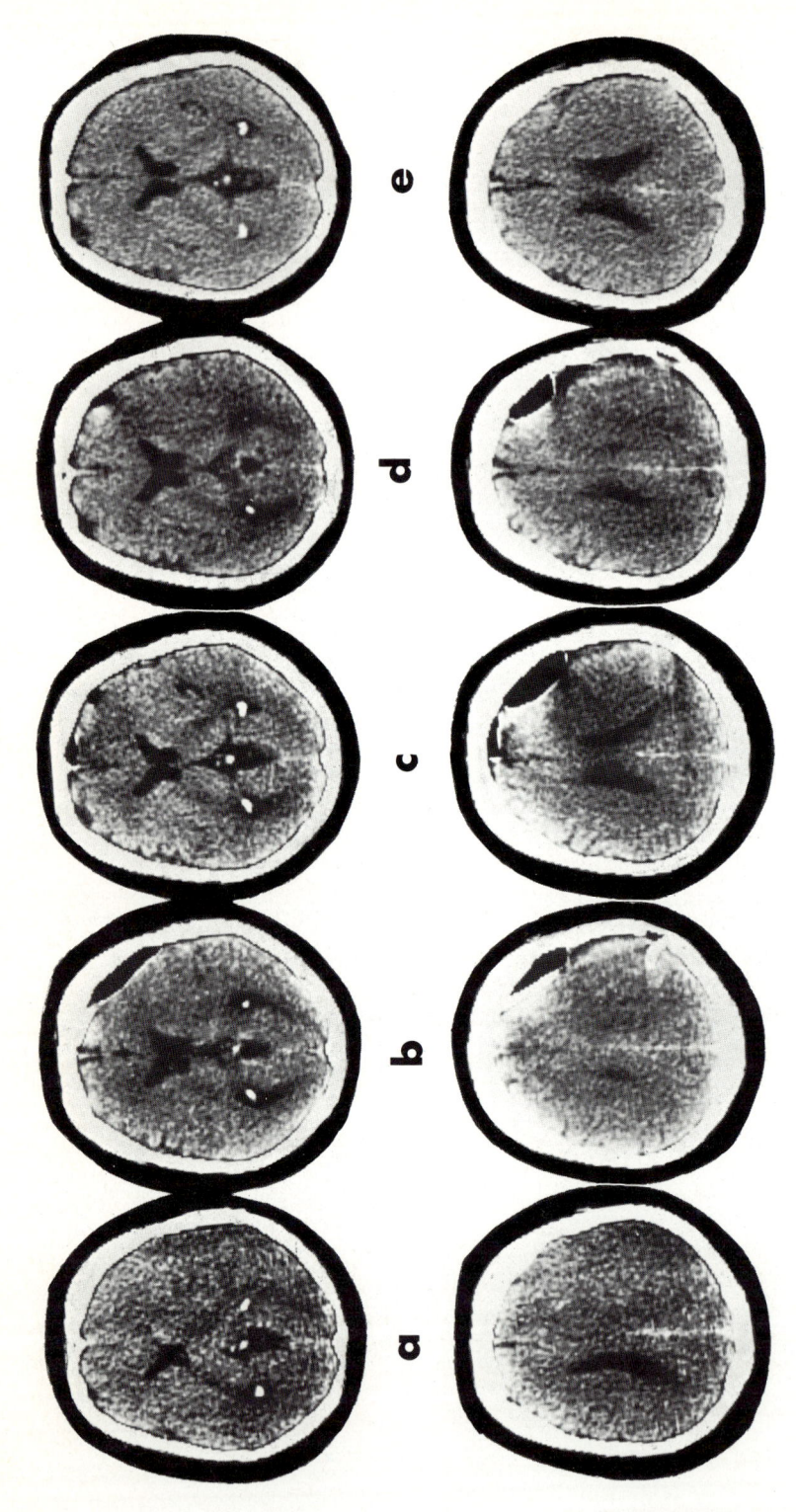

Fig. 1 a-e. Chronic iso-hypodense subdural hematoma over the right hemisphere in a 50-year-old patient. a Preoperative CT; b 7th postoperative day; c 11th postoperative day; d 17th postoperative day; e 4 weeks after surgery

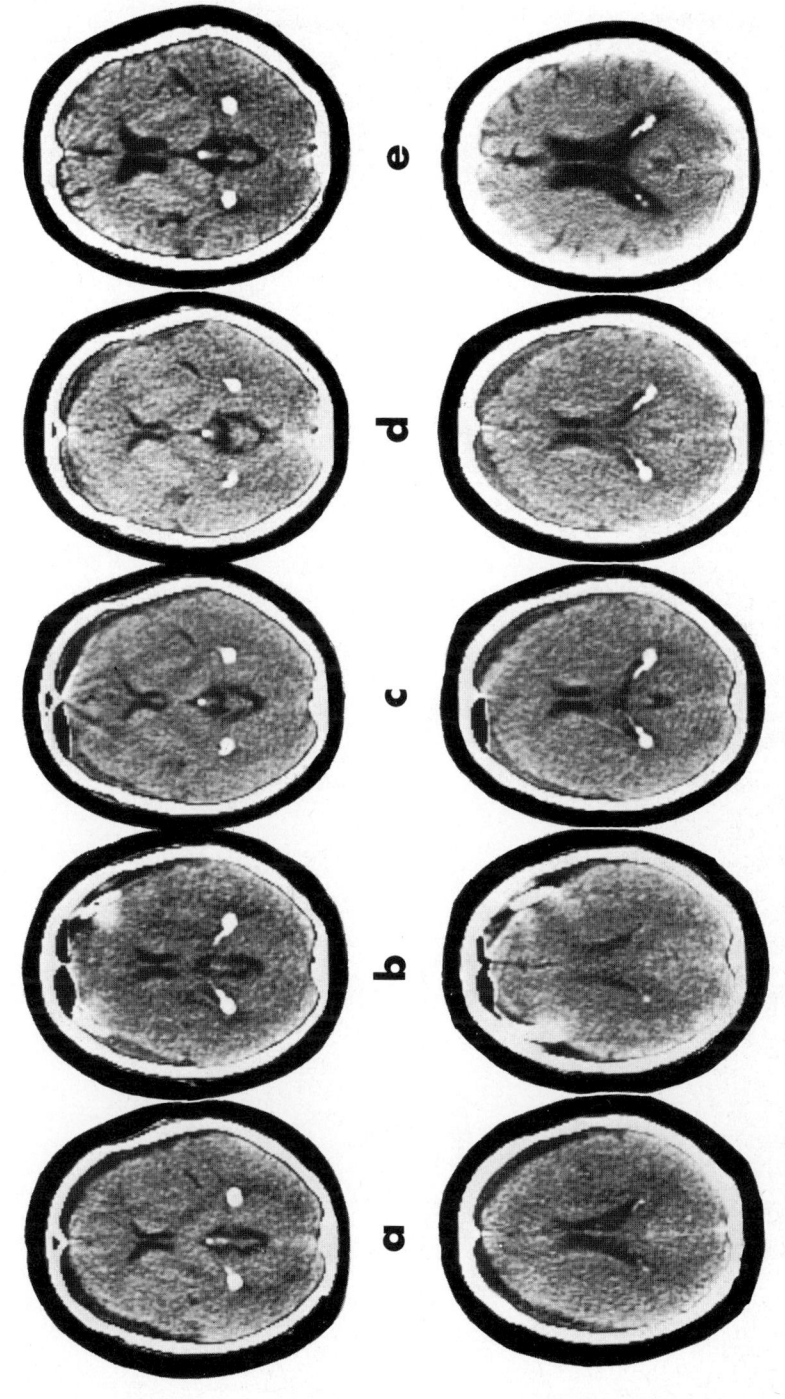

Fig. 2 a-e. Chronic hypodense bilateral subdural hematoma in a 66-year-old patient. a Preoperative CT; b 8th postoperative day; c 3 weeks after surgery; d 4 weeks after surgery; e 1 year after surgery

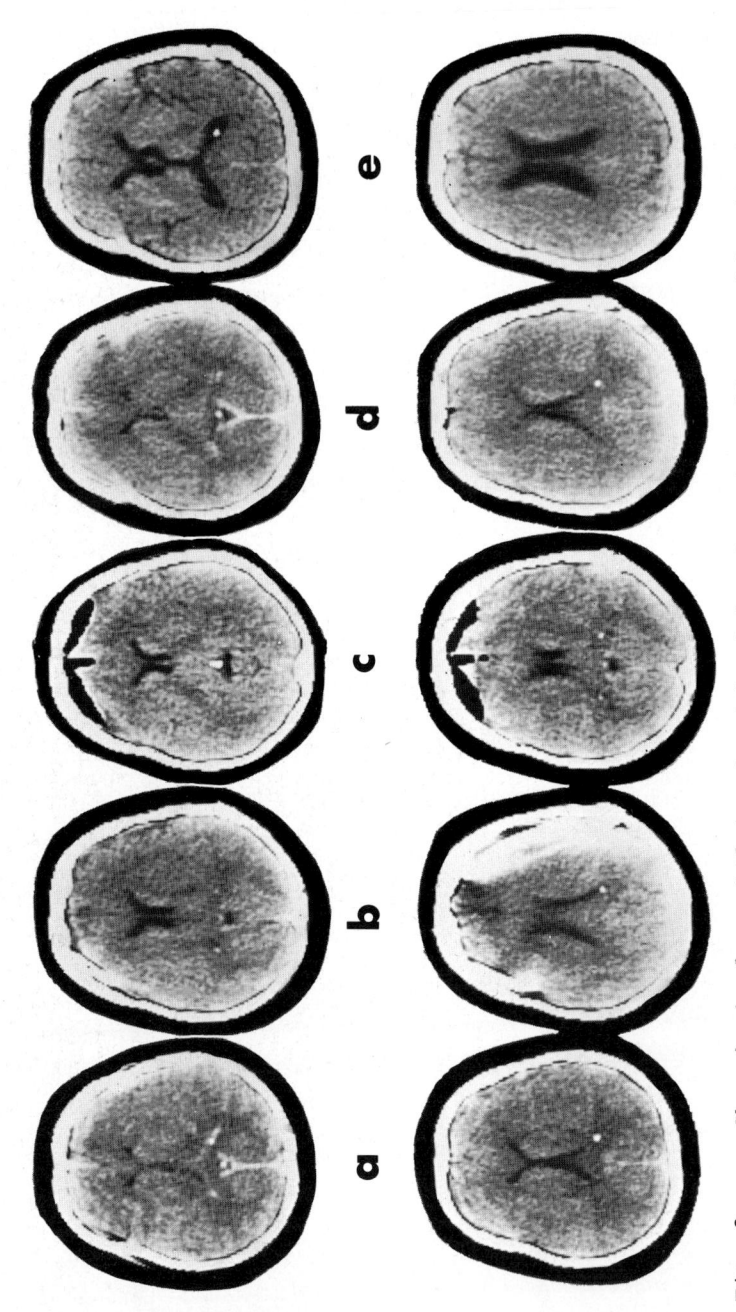

Fig. 3 a-e. Chronic isodense bilateral subdural hematoma in a 66-year-old patient. a Preoperative CT; b 11th postoperative day; c 15th postoperative day; d 3 weeks after surgery; e 7 months after surgery

Cranial Computed Tomography: Its Influence on Results of Treating Traumatic Intracranial Extradural Hematomas

H. M. MEHDORN, W. GROTE, H. C. WEICHERT, A. BUCH, and S. BERGNER

Introduction

Computed tomography (CT) has become a major adjunct in the treatment of intracranial lesions, including those caused by head trauma (1-3, 8, 11, 13-16, 18, 20). In order to find out to which degree it has influenced management and outcome of patients presenting with intracranial extradural hematomas (EDH), we reviewed a series of 139 consecutive patients admitted to the Department of Neurosurgery at the University of Essen, between 1973 and 1980.

Material

The majority of the 139 patients was referred to us from various local hospitals located at a distance of up to seventy kilometers and were brought to us via ambulance or helicopter. Only a few patients were admitted primarily to our department. The exact number of patients admitted for each year is listed in Fig. 1. We used the Glasgow-Coma Scale (GCS) (6, 7, 17, 19), to identify a patient's initial clinical status, his status upon arrival in our department and at consecutive intervals, although it was sometimes difficult to identify precisely the initial status due to a lack of information in the admitting notes. Whenever possible, patients were examined after follow-up intervals ranging from 1 to 7 years. If patients were not available for follow-up examinations, they were interviewed by telephone or their clinical status at any later examination was used to identify the outcome.

Sixty-four patients were treated in our department before a CT became available for clinical applications in early 1977, and seventy-five patients were treated after this date. Among the 64 patients treated prior to 1977, 44 patients underwent angiography; between 1977 and 1980, 9 patients underwent angiography, usually in an outside hospital. Furthermore, 42 patients received a late follow-up CT-scan; among them, 30 patients had received one or more previous CT-scans.

Results

The patient's age ranged from less than a year to 76 years, with a first peak between 11 and 20 years and a second in the group aged 41 to 50 years. The extradural hematomas were located predominantly (1/3) over the temporal region, the remaining regions accounting for the other two-thirds. Among the 139 patients, 109 had only an EDH at surgery, 10 patients presented with EDH and brain contusion, 8 patients with an EDH and a subdural hematoma and 5 patients with a combination of EDH + subdural hematoma + contusion. Seven patients with an EDH diagnosed on CT did not undergo surgery. Most patients were referred to our department within 24 hours after a trauma, approximately 5% of the patients had a chronic EDH and were admitted a few days or later after the initial trauma.

A summary of the 139 patients' initial status and their status upon admission to our department is given in Fig. 1. In the lower part of this figure, the respective mortality rates are given in per cent. There was an overall mortality of 25,9% at time of discharge and 30,2% at time of the follow-up examination. The mortality rate for the years 1973 to 1976 was 34,4%, from 1978 to 1980 20%. It was exceedingly high in 1977: 53%. Thirty-three patients presented with neurological defects at the follow-up examen (38% morbidity): 18 patients were able to work as well as they had done prior to the trauma; 8 patients showed such a neurological deficit that they were not able to work, but were able to care for themselves and 7 patients were disabled and required daily care.

Discussion

The value of computed tomography in the management of patients presenting with head injuries has been shown previously (1-3, 8, 11, 13-16, 18, 20). It allows for rapid, non-invasive detection of intracranial lesions in critically ill patients who often required rapid (neuro-)surgical treatment. The ease with which one can perform the CT-scan had led us to obtain an initial CT-scan on practically every patient presenting with a major head injury. This also includes the management of patients with the initial diagnosis of EDH. JAMIESON and YELLAND (5), have emphasized the importance of precise and "intelligent observation" of the patient's level of consciousness and did not usually rely on radiological procedures in order to define the extent of head trauma. In our series, approximately half of the patients presented with initial localizing signs. From 1973 until 1976, when only angiography was available to identify intracranial lesions, it was performed only in two-thirds of those patients presenting with primary localizing signs; however, since the advent of CT-scan, 28 patients presenting with localizing signs still underwent CT examination, and only 5 patients were taken directly to the operating theatre. The emergency situation in those cases is reflected by the high mortality rates: among those patients undergoing an initial CT examination, mortality was 21% compared to 67% in those patients who were taken immediately to the operating theatre. There is a smaller difference when comparing the patients who did or did not undergo initial angiography in 1973 to 1976: the mortality rate of 27% for those undergoing initial angiography compared to 45% mortality in those who did not undergo initial angiography.

Prior to the introduction of CT, mortality rates were around 34%; since then, they have been reduced to 27,6% for the period 1988-80, with a high of 53% in 1977 and 0% in 1980. 1977 seemed to have been an uncommon year: there was a high number of older patients admitted for surgery, and 20% of all patients presented with GCS grades 1-3. A similar situation was only reached in 1979 when 6% of the patients were clinically dead at time of admission and another 10% were GCS grades 1-3. Whether this could be due to an effort in the referring hospitals to obtain a maximum of diagnostic information and treatment performed on their critically ill patients remains an open question.

When one tries to identify any possible influence of the CT-scan on the outcome, one has to consider first the patient's clinical status. The percentage of patients presenting with GCS grades 1-6 upon admission varied markedly from one year to another. Mortality rates seem to correlate best with the percentage of patients presenting, upon arrival in our department, with GCS grades 1-6; this has been reported by other authors, as well (6, 7, 12, 17, 19). The data presented here do not support the opinion (2) that CT alone has significantly reduced mortality after EDH. This difference may be due to differences in the referral systems, since the large majority of our patients was referred to us from other hospitals; an analysis of 16 case histories of patients who had died in the period 1977-80 revealed that 4 had died because of inadequate time delay from the onset of clinical warning signs until the decision was taken to transfer the patient into a neurosurgical centre. A similar experience was noted by other previously (5, 10). CT-scan therefore is not, in our experience, of exclusive value to reduce mortality rates in patients with EDH, because the initial clinical situation and acuteness of evolution of an EDH are the major factors influencing outcome. However, it has become a major diagnostic tool in the management of EDH:

1. With CT, intracranial lesions can be localized better than with conventional diagnostic methods; this has led us to practically always perform an osteoplastic craniotomy instead of an exploratory burrhole

2. Associated intracranial lesions can be detected easily and therefore adequately dealt with (Fig. 2); 16% of our patients presented with this problem. Often, the second lesion may be fatal (8, 15, 16). In 5 instances we observed a lesion on CT that was considered to be fatal, and in conjunction with the patients' poor clinical status it was decided not to perform surgery for the EDH

3. Occasionally, CT shows an EDH without major mass effect in patients who are in stable clinical conditions. In 2 such cases our decision to postpone surgery, was eventually followed by the patient's spontaneous complete recovery and resolution of the EDH (Fig. 3)

4. After evacuation of an EDH, other lesions may become visible or more pronounced which may require further therapy (Fig. 4).

Summary

Nowadays, CT is an important neuroradiological tool. Physicians caring for patients with head traumas in peripheral hospitals should be more aware of its possibilities and decide earlier to transfer a patient for diagnostic workup and possible treatment. This should help to establish the full benefit of this method in order to reduce the mortality rate towards the 10% target set by HOOPER (4) and aimed at by others, as well (2, 5, 9, 10).

References

1. Clifton, G.L., Grossmann, R.G., Makela, M.E., Miner, M.E.: Neurological course and correlated computerized tomography findings after severe closed head injury. J. Neurosurg. 52, 611-624 (1980)

2. Cordobes, F., Lobato, R.D., Rivas, J.J., Munoz, M.J., Chillon, D., Portillo, K.M., Lamas, E.: Observations on 82 patients with extradural hematoma. Comparison of results before and after the advent of computerized tomography. J. Neurosurg. 54, 179-186 (1981)

3. French, B.N., Dublin, A.B.: The value of computerized tomography in the management of 1000 consecutive head injuries. Surg. Neurol. 7, 171-183 (1977)

4. Hooper, R.: Observations on extradural haemorrhage. Br. J. Surg. 47, 71-87 (1959)

5. Jamieson, K.G., Yelland, J.D.N.: Extradural hematoma. Report of 167 cases. J. Neurosurg. 29, 13-23 (1968)

6. Jennett, B., Teasdale, G.: Assessment of coma after severe brain damage: A practical scale. Lancet 1, 480-484 (1975)

7. Jennett, B., Teasdale, G., Braakman, R., Minderhoud, J., Heiden, J., Kurze, T.: Prognosis of patients with severe head injury. Neurosurgery 4, 283-288 (1979)

8. Koulouris, S., Rizzoli, H.V.: Acute bilateral extradural hematoma: case report. Neurosurgery 7, 608-610 (1980)

9. Kvarnes, T.L., Trumpy, J.H.: Extradural haematoma. Report of 132 cases. Acta Neurochirurg. 41, 223-231 (1978)

10. McKissock, W., Taylor, J.C., Bloom, W.H., Till, K.: Extradural haematoma. Observations on 125 cases. Lancet 2, 167-172 (1960)

11. Merino de Villasante, J., Taveras, J.M.: Computerized tomography (CT) in acute head trauma. Am. J. Roentgenol. 126, 765-778 (1976)

12. Miller, J.D., Butterworth, J.F., Gudeman, S.K., Faulkner, J.E., Choi, S.C., Selhorst, J.B., Harbison, J.W., Lutzm H.A., Young, H.F., Becker, D.P.: Further experience in the management of severe head injury. J. Neurosurg. 54, 289-299 (1981)

13. Omar, M.M., Binet, E.F.: Peripheral contrast enhancement in chronic epidural hematoma. J. Comp. Ass. Tomogr. 2, 332-335 (1978)

14. Svendsen, P.: Computer tomography of traumatic extracerebral lesions. Br. J. Radiol. 49, 1004-1012 (1976)

15. Sweet, R.C., Miller, J.D., Lipper, M. et al.: The significance of bilateral abnormalities on the CT scan in patients with severe head injury. Neurosurgery 3, 16-21 (1978)

16. Taneda, M., Irino, T.: Enlargement of intracerebral haematomas following surgical removal of epidural haematomas. Acta Neurochirurg. 51, 73-82 (1979)

17. Teasdale, G., Jennet, B.: Assessment of coma and impaired consciousness: A practical scale. Lancet 2, 81-84 (1974)

18. Tsai, F.Y., Huprich, J.E., Gardner, E.C., Segall, H.D., Teal, J.S.: Diagnostic and prognostic implications of computed tomography of head trauma. J. Comp. Assist Tomography 2, 323-331 (1978)

19. Young, B., Rapp, R.P., Norton, J.A., Haack, D., Tibbs, P.A., Bean, J.R.: Early prediction of outcome in head-injured patients. J. Neurosurg. 54, 300-303 (1981)

20. Zimmerman, R.A., Bilaniuk, L.T., Gennarelli, T., Bruce, D., Dolinskas, C., Uzzell, B.: Cranial computed tomography in diagnosis and management of acute head trauma. Am. J. Roentgenol. 131, 27-34 (1978)

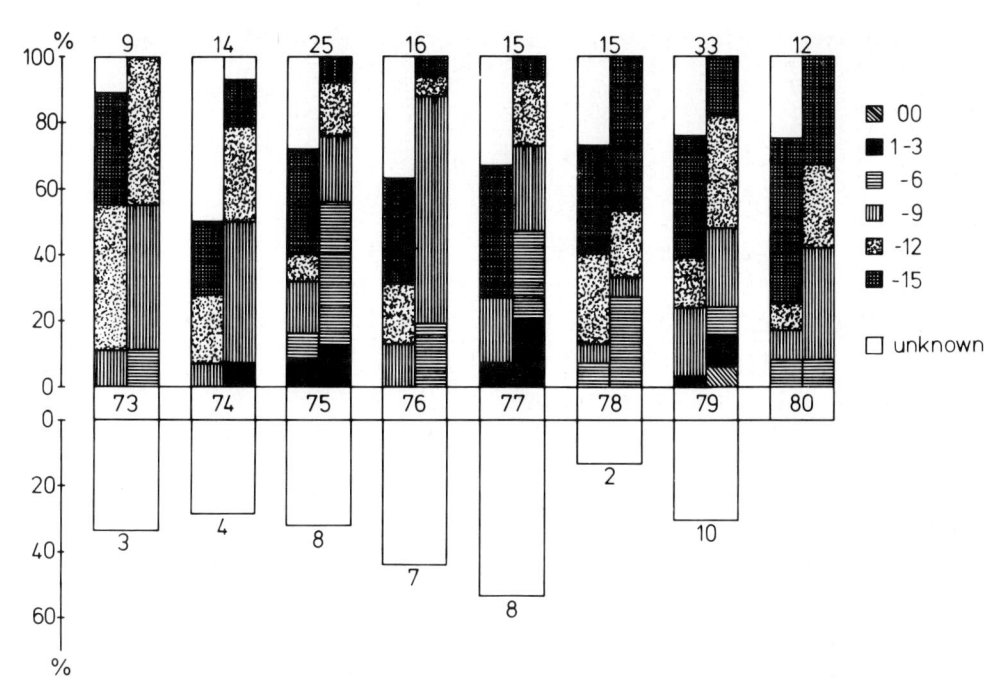

Fig. 1. Extradural hematomas, 1973 - 1980: Mortality related to patient's clinical status according to the Glasgow Coma Scale

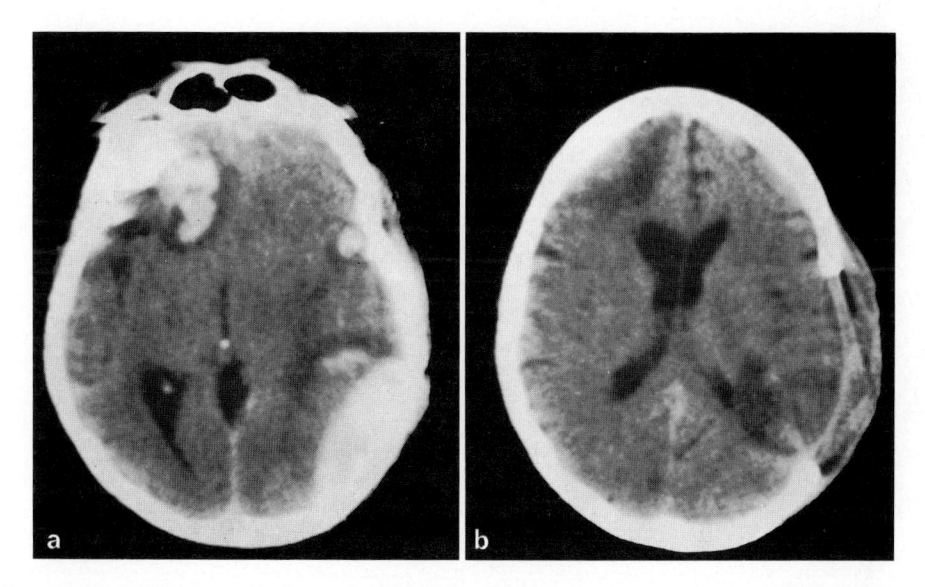

Fig. 2. Combined EDH and frontal brain contusion requiring decompressive craniotomy; preoperative *(left)* and postoperative *(right)* CT scans

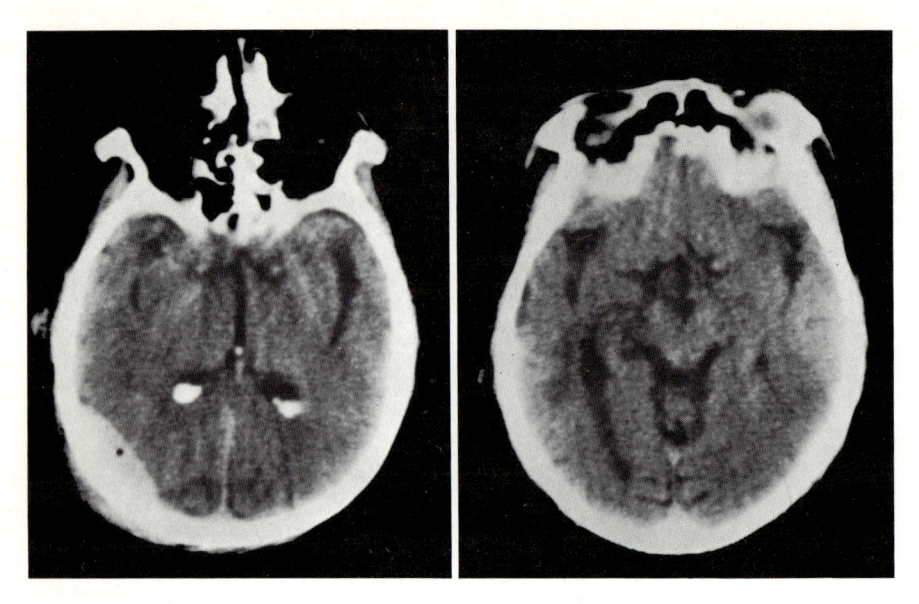

Fig. 3. Conservatively treated and completely resolved EDH

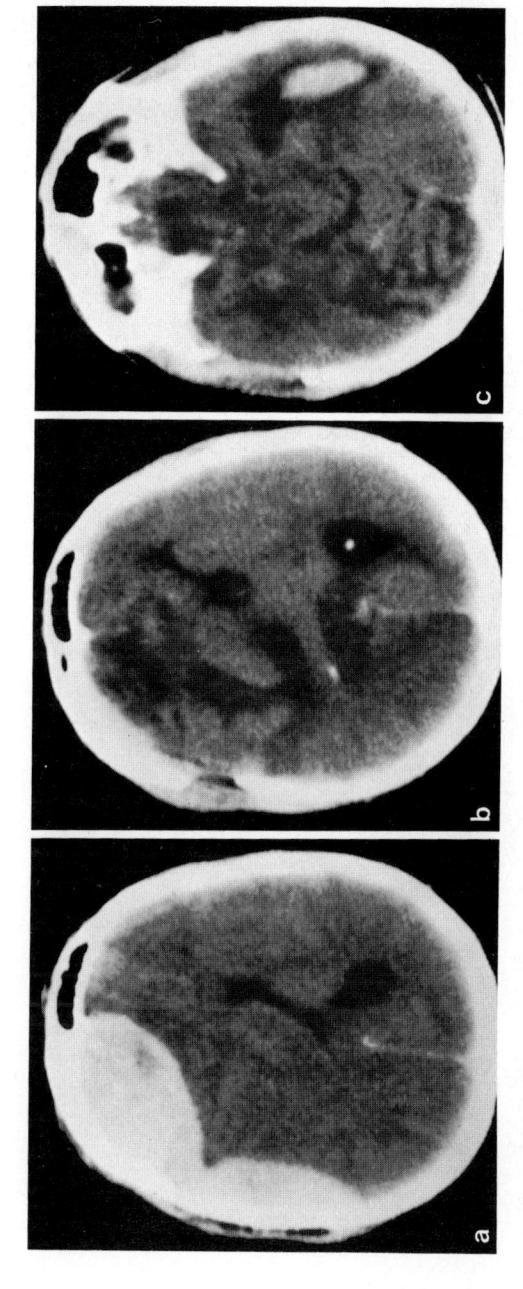

Fig. 4 a-c. Large EDH (a); after decompression a massive brain swelling of the ipsilateral hemisphere was observed (b); the initially present brain contusion (c) in the contralateral hemisphere remained unchanged

Value of Computerized Tomography in Setting the Indication for Surgical Treatment of Extradural Hematomas with a Delayed Course

U. DIETRICH, N. NICOLA, and H. K. SEIBERT

The value of the computerized tomography (CT) in recognizing epidural hematomas is unquestionable. The same is true for epidural hematomas the development of which is delayed, since their symptomatology may be atypical (3, 5). On the other hand, the computerized tomography reveals sometimes beneath a fracture of the skull, an epidural accumulation of blood that does not account for the clinical symptoms. In those cases, surgical intervention would be inappropriate.

At our clinic, 159 patients have undergone surgical interventions in the course of 11 years, on account of epidural hematomas (Fig. 1). In 25 cases, the intervention took place 3 days or even more, after the accident. In 14 cases of this group of patients, the diagnosis had been confirmed by computerized tomography (Fig. 2). We compared the clinical development with the indications for a CT-investigation. This comparison has shown that in 11 cases, a progressive symptomatology had called for a neuroradiological elucidation and led to operation.

A computer tomogram was performed in 5 cases because a deterioration of the patients' condition had occurred some days after the accident. In 4 other cases, a primary CT had already been performed, but it had revealed no hematoma. The further course of the patients' conditions prompted us to repeat the CT that now visualized epidural hematomas (Fig. 3). Finally, in 2 cases, a primary CT had been made, but the epidural hematoma it had revealed had not been recognized as such. In an one-year-old child, a subdural hematoma was assumed, but the surgical intervention was postponed for two weeks, until tapping of the fontanelle performed elsewhere, had failed. In the other case, the picture of a hematoma of the vertex revealed by CT could not be safely interpreted. However, radiographies of the skull displayed a biparietal circular fracture, and the angiogram showed that the sinus sagittalis had been pushed away from the tabula interna.

The clinical symptoms of three patients were rather inconspicuous. Two patients complained of headache and vomiting some days after the trauma had occurred, while the third patient had a local pain with a subgaleal swelling above the temporal bone together with trismus. These complaints persisted several days, and showed no clear tendency to regress. The surgical intervention had been decided upon because in the CT, the hematoma below the fracture of the skull had attained a certain volume, and thus contributed to the displacement of tissues.

In 4 other patients, no operation was carried out. They had suffered minor cranial and cerebral injuries which had caused fractures of their skulls. In each case, the CT revealed a small, biconvex zone located beneath the site of the fracture. Epidural accumulations of blood must be reckoned with although no objective evidence could be produced by surgical intervention. In the first case, the symptomatology consisted of somnolence and slight unrest. As the clinical signs subsided, and since the hematoma was a small one in the CT and hardly displaced the neighbouring tissues, the further development could be watched (Fig. 4) without intervening. In the course of the following days, the hematoma disappeared spontaneously, as could be proved by clinical examination and CT (Fig. 5). The symptomatology of the three other patients had been even less pronounced, and the accumulation of blood visualized by CT had been smaller. These patients complained of slight headache, but informative neurological findings could not be registered. In these cases, too, clinical follow-up examinations and CT-controls proved to be sufficient measures.

The computerized tomography has proved that epidural hematomas may appear with a certain delay, after a head injury. However, they are not always revealed, by a primary CT (1). If hematomas of that kind become more voluminous, they must generally be removed by surgical intervention (2, 4). On the other hand, the computerized tomography reveals sometimes, epidural accumulations of blood below a fracture of the skull, but the clinical symptomatology cannot be ascribed fairly, to such a little hematoma. If the hematoma does not surpass a certain volume in CT, and does not displace the neighbouring tissues, it is good practice to watch its further development clinically, and by CT. In several cases of that kind, surgical intervention can be avoided (6).

References

1. Cordobes, F., Lobato, R.D., Amor, T., Lamas, E.: Epidural haematomas of the posterior fossa with delayed operation. Acta Neurochirurgica 53, 275-281 (1980)
2. Iwakuma, T., Brunngraber, C.V.: Chronic extradural hematomas. J. Neurosurg. 38, 488-493 (1973)
3. Jackson, I.J., Speakman, T.J.: Chronic extradural hematoma. J. Neurosurg. 7, 444-447 (1950)
4. Sparacio, R.R., Khatib, R., Chiu, J., Cook, A.W.: Chronic epidural hematoma. J. Trauma 12, 435-439 (1954)
5. Trowerbridge, W.V., Porter, R.W., French, J.D.: Chronic extradural hematomas. Arch. Surg. Chicago 69, 824-830 (1954)
6. Weaver, D., Pobereskin, L., Jane, J.A.: Spontaneous resolution of epidural hematomas. J. Neurosurg. 54, 248-251 (1981)

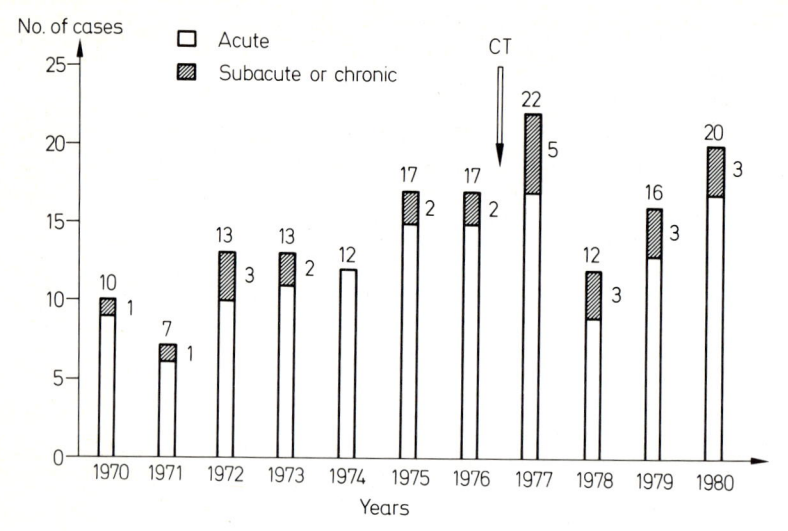

Fig. 1. Surgically treated extradural hematomas

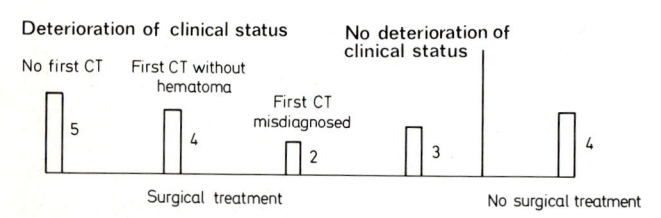

Fig. 2. CT-diagnosis of 14 delayed extradural hematomas

Fig. 4 (left). Computerized tomography scan on the day of admission showing an extradural hematoma in the right parieto-occipital region

Fig. 5 (right). Repeat computerized tomography demonstration spontaneous resolution of the right extradural hematoma (scan on the 10th postoperative day)

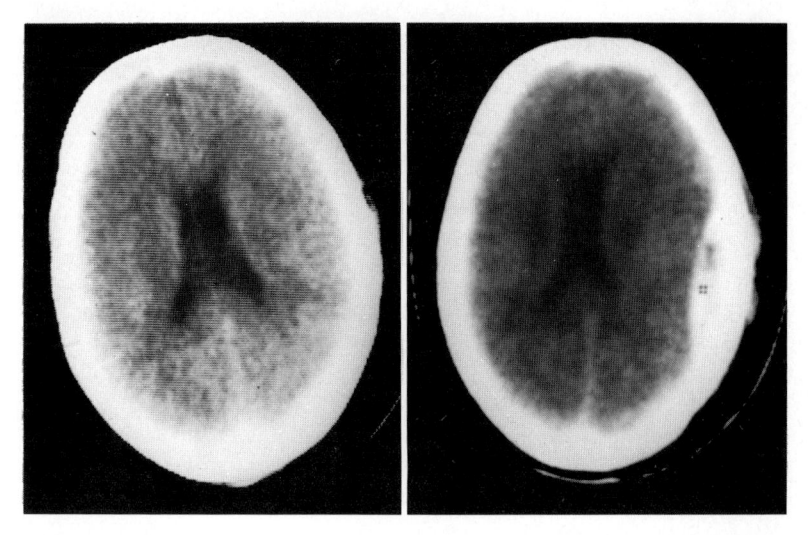

Fig. 3. Computerized tomography scan on the day of admission *(left)* and 48 hours after injury *(right)* showing the development of a right-sided extradural hematoma

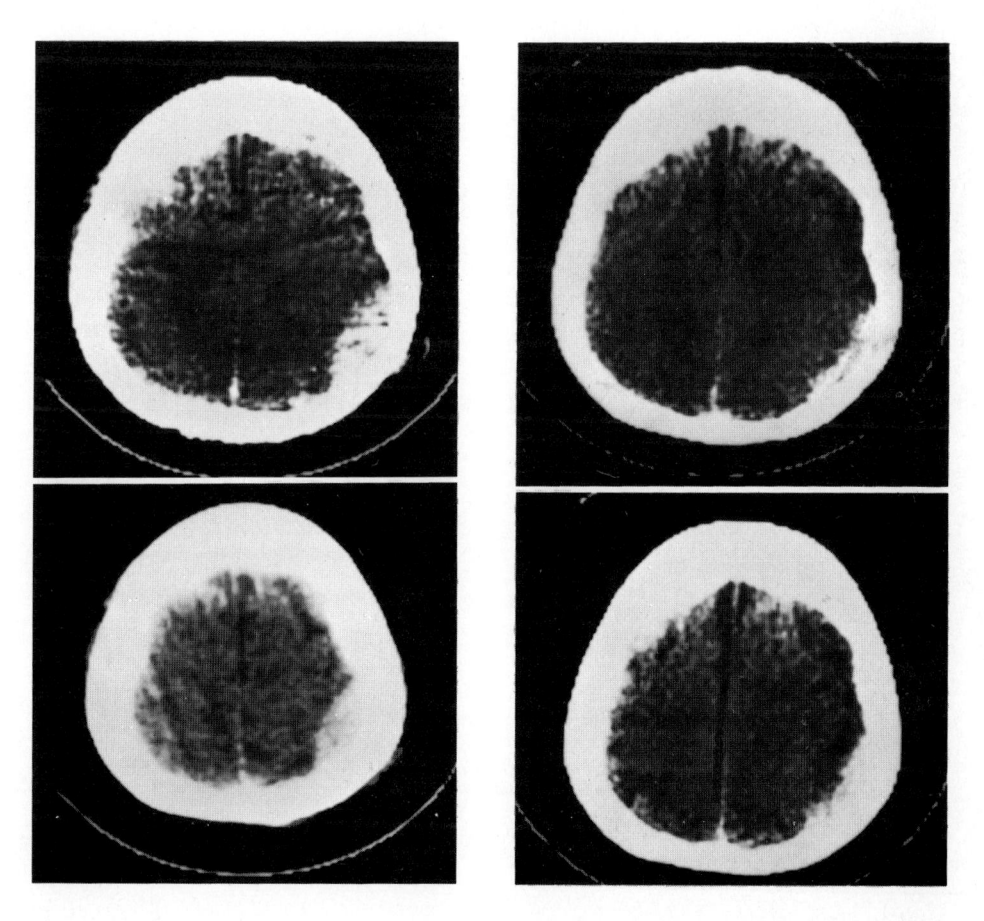

Surgery in Traumatic Intracerebral Bleeding Based on Computerized Tomographical Findings

H. KRETSCHMER, P. TZONOS, and R. GUSTORF

Introduction

Routine use of axial computerized tomography in neurotraumatology has very much facilitated rapid diagnosis and exact classification of traumatic intracranial hemorrhages. As a result, it has also become possible to distinguish intracerebral hematomas from so-called space-occupying contusions. This was hardly possible using earlier, conventional methods (echoencephalography, carotid angiography) which were associated with a high rate of error. It is, however, necessary to examine our former attitude toward surgical indications.

Material

Within a three-year period, 316 patients were operated on for traumatic intracranial bleeding; 79 had epidural, 181 subdural, and 56 intracerebral hematomas, as opposed to approximately the same number of patients with severe brain contusions not requiring surgery. Without exception, the intracerebral hematomas were caused by severe craniocerebral traumas, half of which resulted from traffic accidents and half from falls. The sex distribution was male : female, 4 : 1. The average age was 44.7 years. The location was: frontal and temporal, 44,6% each; fronto-temporal, 10,8%.

Results

Skull fractures (2/3 on the hematoma side, 1/3 on the opposite side) were found in 71.4% of the 56 patients later operated upon. Leading *neurological symptoms* were disturbances of consciousness of various degrees. 1/3 of the patients were unconscious upon admission (coma I - IV); in 2/3 of the cases, consciousness was clouded. The disturbance of consciousness followed various courses: primary, lasting (41.1%) or secondary, increasing (53.6%); a free interval could be detected in only a few cases (5.3%). Further neurological symptoms we found were: pupil irregularities (in 48.2%), a contralateral hemiparesis (in 35.7%), and extensor spasms caused by compression of the midbrain (in 12.5%).

Axial computerized tomography provided a wide spectrum of different findings: extensive, space-occupying hematomas (Fig. 1), multiple hematomas of different sizes (Fig. 2), deep-lying bleeding with connection to the brain stem and basal ganglia (Fig. 3), and giant hematomas with ventricular collapse (Fig. 4).

In cases where surgery was indicated, we always performed an extensive osteoplastic craniotomy in order to completely evacuate the hematoma and treat still-bleeding vessels. Aspiration via drill-hole is, in our opinion, not sufficient. All in all, mortality rate in our cases was 62.5% and compares with the results of other authors (1, 2, 4, 6).

Discussion

Based on our experience, indication for surgery in traumatic intracerebral hematomas should depend on a number of criteria:

Course. Acute and subacute hematomas are to be distinguished from each other on the basis of speed of development until manifestation of neurological signs (1, 3), although there is a disagreement upon the time intervals (12 to 48 hours). We classified according to the 12-hour limit and found 62.5% acute and 37.5% subacute hematomas. The two forms differ markedly as far as prognosis is concerned: Mortality rate in acute cases, 80%; in subacute, 33.3%.

State of Consciousness. The severity of the disturbance of consciousness is a dependable indicator of the extent of brain damage, as can be seen by the surgical results. Mortality rate was 12.5% in somnolent patients, 53.3% in suporous, and 100% in comatous.

Age. Age also clearly influences survival chances. In general, the prognosis for patients over 50 years is poor (1, 3).

Computerized Tomographical Findings. Based on computerized tomographical (5, 7-10) and clinical findings, we recommend the following approach.

Surgery Indicated
- In cases of isolated, large hemorrhages of a space-occupying nature, manifesting clinical symptoms of brain pressure.
- In hemorrhages where, under conservative treatment and computerized tomography supervision, the patient's clinical condition worsens or secondary symptoms of brain pressure appear.

Surgery Contraindicated
- In cases of multiple, minor contusional bleeding, independent of the clinical state.
- In hemorrhage anywhere, without neurological signs and symptoms of brain pressure.
- In hemorrhage of any size and location in comatous patients with bilaterally dilated and fixed pupils.

Conclusion

In deciding for or against surgery in traumatic intracerebral hematomas, not only computerized tomographical findings but also course (acute or subacute), severity of disturbance of consciousness, and the age of the patient should be taken into account. Despite taking consideration of these factors, the mortality rate is very high (over 60%) and also, in part, a result of constantly severe primary traumatic brain damage. No comatous patient over 50 years of age having extensive hematomas with ventricular collapse survived.

References

1. Hamel, E., Karimi-Nejad, A.: Traumatic intracerebral hematomas. Adv. Neurosurg. 5, 56-61 (1978)
2. Jamieson, K.G., Yelland, J.D.N.: Traumatic intracerebral hematoma - Report of 63 surgically treated cases. J. Neurosurg. 37, 528-532 (1972)
3. Karimi-Nejad, A., Hamel, E., Frowein, R.A.: Verlauf der traumatischen intrazerebralen Hämatome. Nervenarzt 50, 432-435 (1969)
4. Kretschmer, H.: Traumatische intrazerebrale Hämatome - Analyse von 88 operativ behandelten Fällen. Neurochirurgia 22, 35-41 (1979)
5. Lanksch, W., Grumme, Th., Kazner, E.: Schädelhirnverletzungen im Computertomogramm. Berlin, Heidelberg, New York: Springer 1978
6. Levinthal, R., Stern, W.E.: Traumatic intracerebral hematoma with stable neurologic deficit. Surg. Neurol. 7, 269-273 (1977)
7. Messina, A.V., Chernik, N.: Computed tomography: the "resolving" intracerebral hemorrhage. Radiology 118, 609-613 ( )
8. Pineda, A.: Computed tomography in intracerebral haemorrhage. Surg. Neurol. 8, 55-58 (1977)
9. Weigel, K., Ostertag, C.B., Mundinger, F.: CT-follow-up control of traumatic intracerebral hemorrhage. Adv. Neurosurg. 5, 62-67 (1978)
10. Wüllenweber, R., Zum Winkel, K., Grumme, Th., Lange, S., Meese, M.: Differentialdiagnose des Schlaganfalls im Computertomogramm. Neurochirurgia 19, 1-9 (1976)

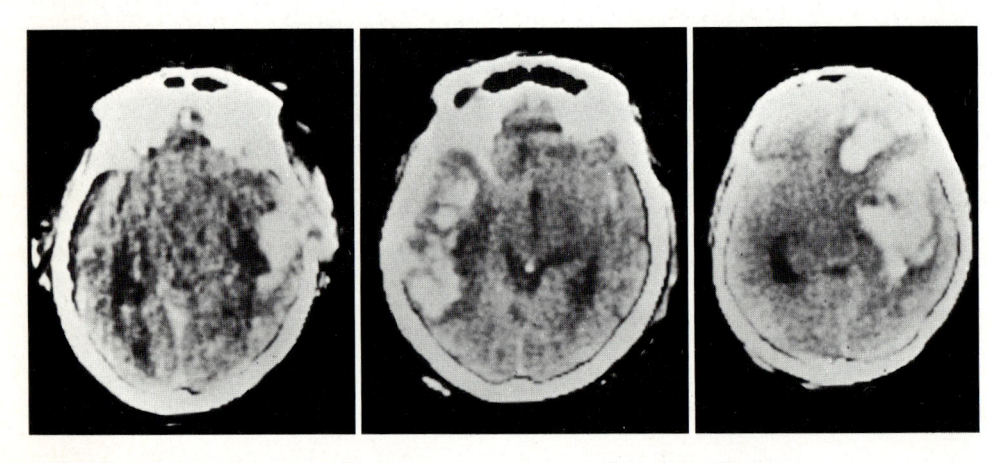

Fig. 1. Extensive, solitary, space-occupying hematomas

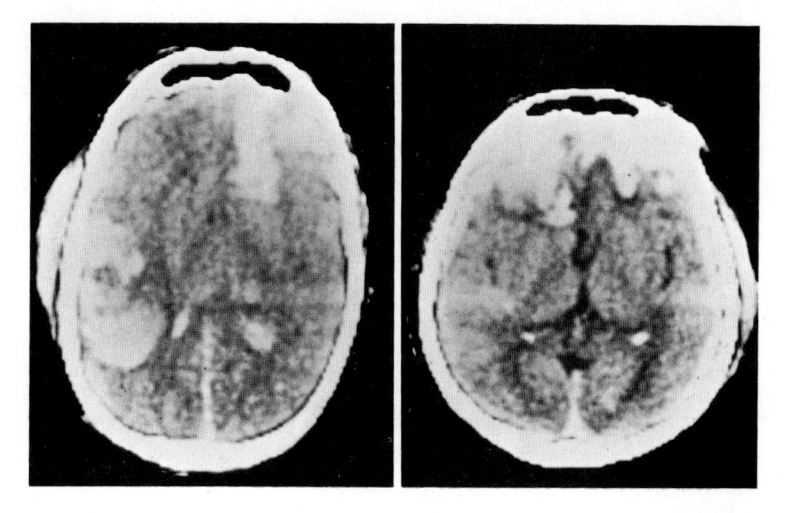

Fig. 2. Extensive, multiple hematomas

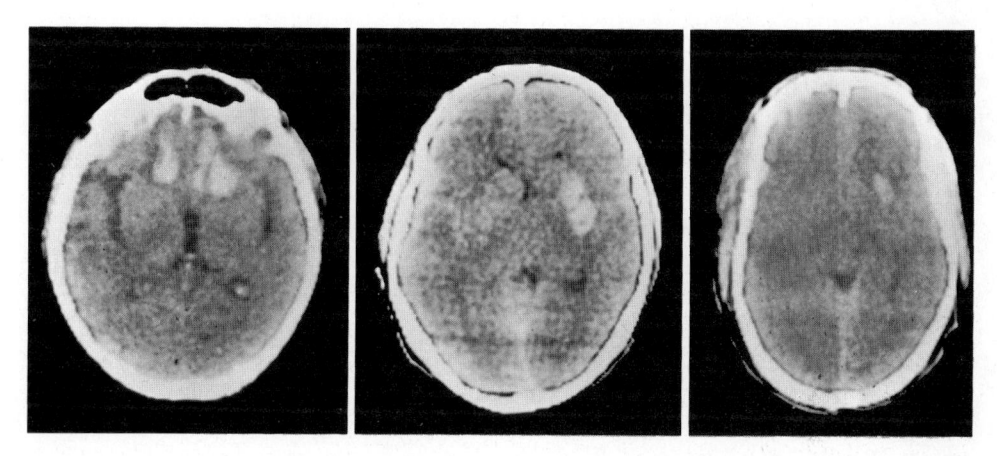

Fig. 3. Small, deep-lying hematomas without space-occupation

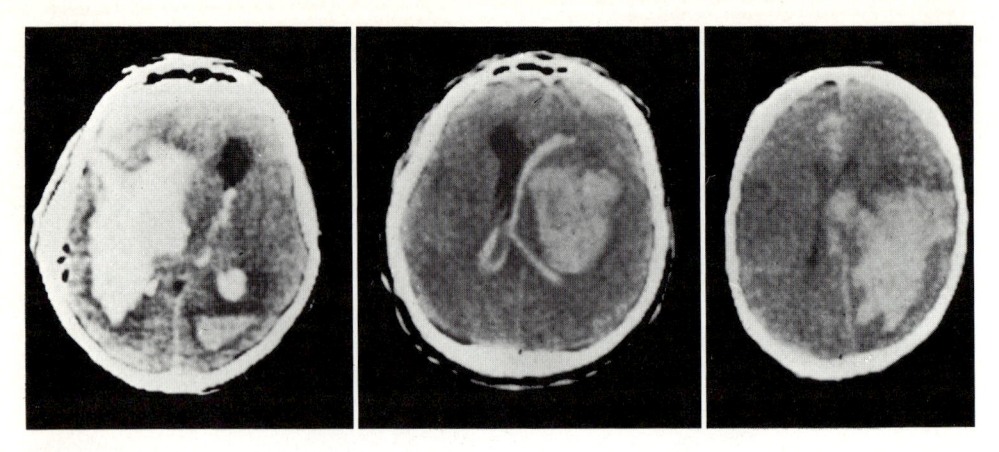

Fig. 4. Giant hematomas with or without ventricular collapse

Detection of the Angiographically Cryptic Cerebrovascular Malformations by Computerized Tomography

S. Tiyaworabun, U. Pasch, N. Nicola, M. Schirmer, and H. K. Seibert

Since HAWKIN and REWELL (2) in 1946 called attention to the role of small angiomatous malformations in the production of fatal intracerebral hemorrhage and RUSSELL (12) in 1954 described the clinically "cryptic" nature for this entity, many investigations have been done on analysis of the clinical manifestation, improvement of neuroradiological technique, equipment and modality, as well as precise definition in neuropathology of this "cryptic" cerebro-vascular malformation (CVM).

However, some of these CVM, due to hemodynamic or pathological changes, failed to be opacified on cerebral angiography. Recently, with the aid of computerized tomography (CT), many of these angiographically cryptic CVM can be promptly and accurately suggested or diagnosed preoperatively.

The purpose of this communication is to attempt to review and analyse the usefulness and limitation of CT in the identification of this subgroup of CVM.

Case Material

During the past 15 years, i.e. from 1965 to 1980, 240 cases of CVM have been seen and treated in the neurosurgical department of the University Hospital Düsseldorf. Among these, 10 cases of histologically proved CVM with the absence of definitive angiographic evidence were detected. Seven patients received CT examination while the other 3 did not. Isotope scanning had been done in 2 cases. The pertinent clinical information is summarized in Table 1. Four examples of cases, which showed various clinical manifestations and provided different CT-patterns, are briefly described as follows:

Case 2 (Table 1). A 10-year-old boy had done well until 6 months ago when he complained of frontal headache and malaise. 1 month before admission, he had 2 grand mal seizures. Neurological examination was unremarkable. EEG showed slow waves with spike waves in the left temporo-parietal region. Plain CT showed a mottled and tubular oval mass in left middle fossa (Fig. 1a). Slight contrast enhancement was observed (Fig. 1b). Left carotid angiography revealed an avascular mass of the middle fossa (Fig. 1c). A 4x2x2 cm calcified multicystic mass filled with old blood was totally evacuated. Histology confirmed cavernous haemangioma with calcification and old hemorrhage (Fig. 1d). He was followed up 1 year later, where he was in good condition, free of seizures on anticonvulsants.

Table 1. Summary of clinical, neuroradiological and pathological findings of 10 patients with CVM

Case No.	Age (years)	Sex	Chief complaints	Skull X-ray	Isotope Scan	Angiography	Location
1. K.T.	10	M	Choreoathetotic movements of right extremities and hemiparesis for 1 month	Calcified lesion	Not performed	Normal	Left fronto-parietal
2. K.B.	10	M	Headache for 6 months, seizure for 1 month	Normal	Not performed	Mass	Left tempral
3. S.R.	54	F	Episodic faintings for 5 months	Normal	Not performed	Mass	Left frontal
4. S.B.	38	F	Episodic faintings for 25 years	Calcified lesion	Not performed	Mass	Right frontal
5. K.G.	47	M	Disorientation for 1 month	Normal	Positive	Normal	Right frontal
6. W.R.	25	M	Aphasia and right hemiparesis for 4 weeks	Normal	Not performed	Mass	Left parietal
7. S.D.	2	M	Seizure, papilledema, meningism for 10 days	Normal	Not performed	Mass with abnorm. Vascularity	Right fronto-parieto-temporal
8. F.I.	56	F	Headache for 4 years, coma, left hemiparesis, decerebrate rigidity	Normal	Positive	Mass	Right basal ganglia
9. S.E.	47	F	Subarachnoid haemorrhage, left hemiparesis, right mydriasis for 8 days	Normal	Not performed	Mass	Right temporal
10. K.H.	52	M	Headache, vertigo and vomiting for 1 month	Normal	Not performed	Mass	Left basal ganglia

Table 1 (continued)

Case No.	Computerized tomography					Pathology	Follow-Up	
	Morphology	Calcification	Mass effect	Enhancement			Interval (year)	Result
1. K.T.	Irregular mottled	Yes	Minimal	Minimal	Cavernous haemangioma	1	Hemiparesis improved
2. K.B.	Oval, tubular mottled	Yes	No	Minimal	Cavernous haemangioma	1	Seizure-free with drugs
3. S.R.	Oval finely, uneven	Yes	Minimal	Minimal	Arteriovenous angioma	1	Normal
4. S.B.	Oval, vermiform, mottled	Yes	Minimal	Minimal	Arteriovenous angioma	3	Decreased in frequency
5. K.G.	Hypodense focus	No	No	Well defined ring-shaped	Capillary haemangioma	2	Normal
6. W.R.	Haemorrhage	?	Minimal	Not performed	Arteriovenous angioma	3	Hemiparesis improved
7. S.D.	Hypodense focus	No	Extensive	Irregular polylobulated	Cavernous haemangioma and malignant haemangioendothelioma	2/12	Seizure-free with drugs
8. F.I.		Not existing			Arteriovenous angioma		Died 72 hours thereafter
9. S.E.		Not existing			Arteriovenous angioma		Died 72 hours thereafter
10. K.H.		Not existing			Arteriovenous angioma		Died 8 days after posterior fossa exploration

Case 5 (Table 1). A 47-year-old man was admitted with a one month's history of disorientation, loss of concentration and ambition. Neurological examination was unremarkable. EEG was read as normal. Plain CT revealed a right frontal hypodense focus (Fig. 2a). After contrast administration a well defined ring-shaped enhancement was detected, with perifocal edema but no mass effect (Fig. 2b). Isotope scanning showed a similar finding (Fig. 2c). Selective right internal carotid angiography was unremarkable (Fig. 2d). At surgery, a 5x5x4 cm encapsulated intracerebral haematoma with surrounding gliotic tissue was evacuated. Microscopy revealed an intracerebral capillary microhaemangioma with old hemorrhage (Fig. 2e). He was in good condition at the follow-up examination 2 years later.

Case 6 (Table 1). A 25-year-old male was admitted with a one month's history of aphasia, right hemiparesis and meningism. Left carotid angiography revealed an avascular lesion fronto-parietal without abnormal vascularity (Fig. 3a). Plain CT showed left parietal haematoma (Fig. 3b) with ventricular bleeding. At surgery, the haematoma and the surrounding gliotic tissue were totally evacuated. Histology confirmed an arterio-venous angioma with fresh haematoma (Fig. 3c). He was followed up 2 years later with improved right hemiparesis.

Case 7 (Table 1). A 2-year-old boy was transferred to us because of grand mal seizures, papilloedema and meningismus for 10 days. In addition to this, multiple cafe-au-lait spots over the whole body were detected. CSF was normal. EEG showed mixed foci of slow and sharp waves in the right fronto-temporo-parietal region. Plain CT defined a large hypodense focus right fronto-parietal. After contrast administration, an irregular, multilobulated mass with extensive perifocal edema was detected (Fig. 4a). Right carotid angiography revealed a space-occupying lesion in the same region (Fig. 4b, c). At surgery, a 8x5x4 cm large cystic mass with surrounding gliotic brain tissue was totally removed. Histology confirmed a mixed tumor of cavernous haemangioma and malignant haemangioendothelioma (Fig. 4d).

Discussion

The clinical manifestations of CVMs show a broad spectrum. They may be dominant, deserving the nomer "cryptic" and found incidentally at autopsy, or lead to catastrophic fatal hemorrhage (2, 3, 9, 10, 12). The clinical symptoms and signs were chiefly effected by the severity of mass effect, ischemic deficiency of surrounding brain, episodic hemorrhages and subsequent complications. The true incidence of clinically cryptic CVM is unknown. However, many reports on angiographically cryptic CVM have been made. During the past 15 years, 10 cases (4%) of this subgroup of patients have been detected in our department. The ages ranged from 2 to 56 years. There was no significant sex preponderance, although males showed a slight prevalence. The neurological findings of the patients are summarized in Table 1. Surprisingly, there was no antecedent history suggestive of hemorrhage in these cases but clinically manifested as those of tumors (case 1, 2, 5, 6, 8, 10), cardio-vascular disorders (case 3, 4), sudden hemorrhage (case 9) and brain abscess (case 7).

Although CVMs are seen equally in the supra- and infratentorial regions (3, 9, 10, 13) they have just been observed supratentorially in this subgroup, mostly closely corresponding with the middle cerebral artery distribution, and there was no side predominance.

Skull X-ray revealed 10% (5) to 30% (11) of calcified lesions in CVM, which were also detected in 2 cases of this series. In all cases, there were no symptoms and signs of cardiac decompensation or cardiomegaly on physical examination as well as in chest X-ray.

Prior to the introduction of isotope scanning, patients with the clinical course suggestive of space occupying lesion were investigated with angiography and pneumoencephalography. In cases with angiographically "cryptic" CVM with minimal mass effect, it is impossible for a surgeon to recognise the nature of the lesion and hence would hesitate to initiate a course of treatment as seen in case 8, 9 and 10. Although isotope scans were found to be positive in nearly all cases of CVMs, some did escape enhancement (8, 15). All 2 patients who had received this examination revealed positive findings.

Nearly all clinically significant CVMs are readily diagnosed by good quality cerebral angiography; such as, rapid serial angiography, prolonged injection angiogram, magnification angiography, angiotomography and film-subtraction (1, 4, 14). However, some of these lesions may evade these examinations. They are usually present (normal) or are seen as an avascular mass after previous episodic hemorrhages. Although some angiographic features of this subgroup of lesions have been reported (1, 7), they may be confused with those of glioma especially in cases without clinical past history of hemorrhage. Eight cases (80%) presented as avascular masses in our series while the others had unremarkable angiograms. It still remain unresolved, why they remain angiographically "cryptic". There are several hypotheses suggesting the explanation of the mechanism of this partially or complete angiographic disappearance of CVM as summarized in Fig. 5. In addition to these presumptive factors, we feel that it may be possible that some of these "cryptic" CVM, have remained in the state comparable to those during embryonal life and hence fail to be opacified at angiography. At operations, most of these lesions (case 2, 3, 4, 6) were discovered to have large patent vessels in spite of unremarkable angiography. Moreover, why these lesions bleed profusely when their blood supply seems to have been obliterated remains unanswered.

KENDALL (5) reported the correct diagnosis of over 90% of angiographically proven CVM by CT. In typical cases the enlarged vessels may appear tubular or of serpigious pattern when they lie in the axis of the tomogram-section or rounded or oval with a mottled appearance when transected by it. The filling artery or draining vein of the lesion may occasionally be identified. Moreover, CT also offers supplementary information regarding mass effect, calcifications, associated hemorrhage and oedema, focal atrophy or infarct, anatomical relationship as well as ventricular configuration. Furthermore, CT provided neurosurgeons in some cases with a crucial aid in deciding on the operability and route of approach. It is also valuable for the elucidation of the cause of clinical deterioration (5, 6, 15, 16, 17).

In this subgroup, CT suggestive of CVM was made in 4 cases (case 1-4), 2 cases of gliomas (case 5, 7), 2 cases of intracerebral haematoma (case 5, 6) and 2 cases of abscess (case 5, 7). In cases suggestive of CVM (case 1-4), histology confirmed 2 cases of cavernous haemangioma and 2 cases of arterio-venous angioma. Case 5 had a presumptive CT diagnosis of glioma, metastatic tumor, old hemorrhage or abscess. Histology was found to be a capillary micro-haemangioma. As was proposed by HAWKINS (2), this small lesion, which may be inapparent to the naked eye, could be revealed microscopically if careful sectioning of the margins of haematoma was made. CT pattern of case 6 was that of intracerebral haematoma and this made the interpretation of various structures within this haematoma difficult and impossible. The presumptive CT diagnosis of case 7 was that of glioma or abscess. Surprisingly, histology revealed a rare mixed tumor of cavernous haemangioma and malignant haemangioendothelioma. There was no case of obstructive hydrocephalus, which is usually encountered in cases of vein of Galen malformation in our series.

In conclusion, there is no doubt that CT is the most valuable neuroradiological modality in diagnosis of "cryptic" CVM but its efficiency is still limited in cases of small-size CVMs, where destruction of the malformation by hemorrhage as well as by associated with haematoma occurs.

References

1. Bogren, H., Svalander, C., Wickbom, I.: Angiography in intracranial cavernous haemangioma. Acta Radiologica 10, 81-89 (1970)

2. Hawkins, C.F., Rewell, R.E.: Unheralded, fatal hemorrhages in haemangiomata of the brain. Guy's Hosp. Rep. 95, 88 (1946)

3. Hoök, O., Johanson, C.: Intracranial arterio-venous aneurysma: A follow-up study with particular attention to their growth. Archs. Neurol. Psychiat., Chicago 80, 39-54 (1958)

4. Huber, P., Krayenbühl, H., Yasargil, G.: Zerebrale Angiographie für Klinik und Praxis. 3. Aufl., S. 383-395. Stuttgart: Thieme 1978

5. Kendall, B.E., Claveria, L.E.: The use of computed axial tomography (CAT) for the diagnosis and management of intracranial angiomas. Neuroradiology 12, 141-160 (1976)

6. Kramer, R.A., Wing, S.D.: Computed tomography of angiographically occult cerebro-vascular malformations. Radiology 123, 649-652 (1977)

7. Leo, J.S., Lin, J.P., Kricheff, I.I.: Pseudoaneurysms formation secondary to spontaneous thrombosis of a massive cerebral anterior-venous malformation. Neuroradiology 17, 115-119 (1979)

8. Landman, S., Ross, P.: Radionuclides in the diagnosis of arteriovenous malformations of the brain. Radiology 108, 635-639 (1973)

9. McCormick, W.F., Nofzinger, J.D.: "Cryptic" vascular malformations of the central nervous system. J. Neurosurgery 24, 865-875 (1966)

10. Pool, J.L., Potts, D.G.: Aneurysms and arteriovenous anomalies of the brain, diagnosis and treatment. New York: Herper and Row 1965

11. Rumbaugh, C.L., Potts, D.G.: Skull changes associated with intracranial arterio-venous malformation. Amer. J. Roentgenol. 98, 525-534 (1966)

12. Russell, D.S.: The pathology of spontaneous intracranial hemorrhage. Proc. R. Soc. Med. 47, 689-693 (1954)

13. Russell, D.S., Rubinstein, L.J.: Pathology of tumors of the nervous system. 4th ed. Arnold 1977

14. Sartor, K., Nadjmi, M.: Angiotomography for aneurysms and arteriovenous malformations. Neuroradiology 17, 89-100 (1979)

15. Savoiardo, M., Passerini, A.: CT, angiography and rn scans in intracranial cavernous haemangioma. Neuroradiology 16, 256-260 (1978)

16. Shuey, H.M., Day, A.L., Quisling, R.G. et al.: Angiographically cryptic cerebrovascular malformations. Neurosurgery 5, 476-479 (1978)
17. Weisberg, L.A.: Computed tomography in the diagnosis of intracranial vascular malformations. Computed Tomography 3, 125-132 (1979)

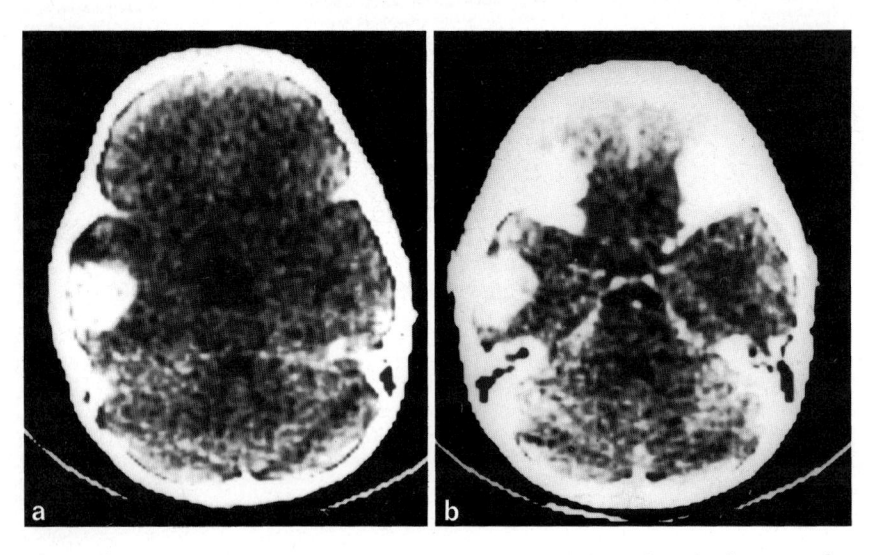

Fig. 1. a Plain CT demonstrates a mottled and tubular oval mass in left middle fossa and b with slight contrast enhancement

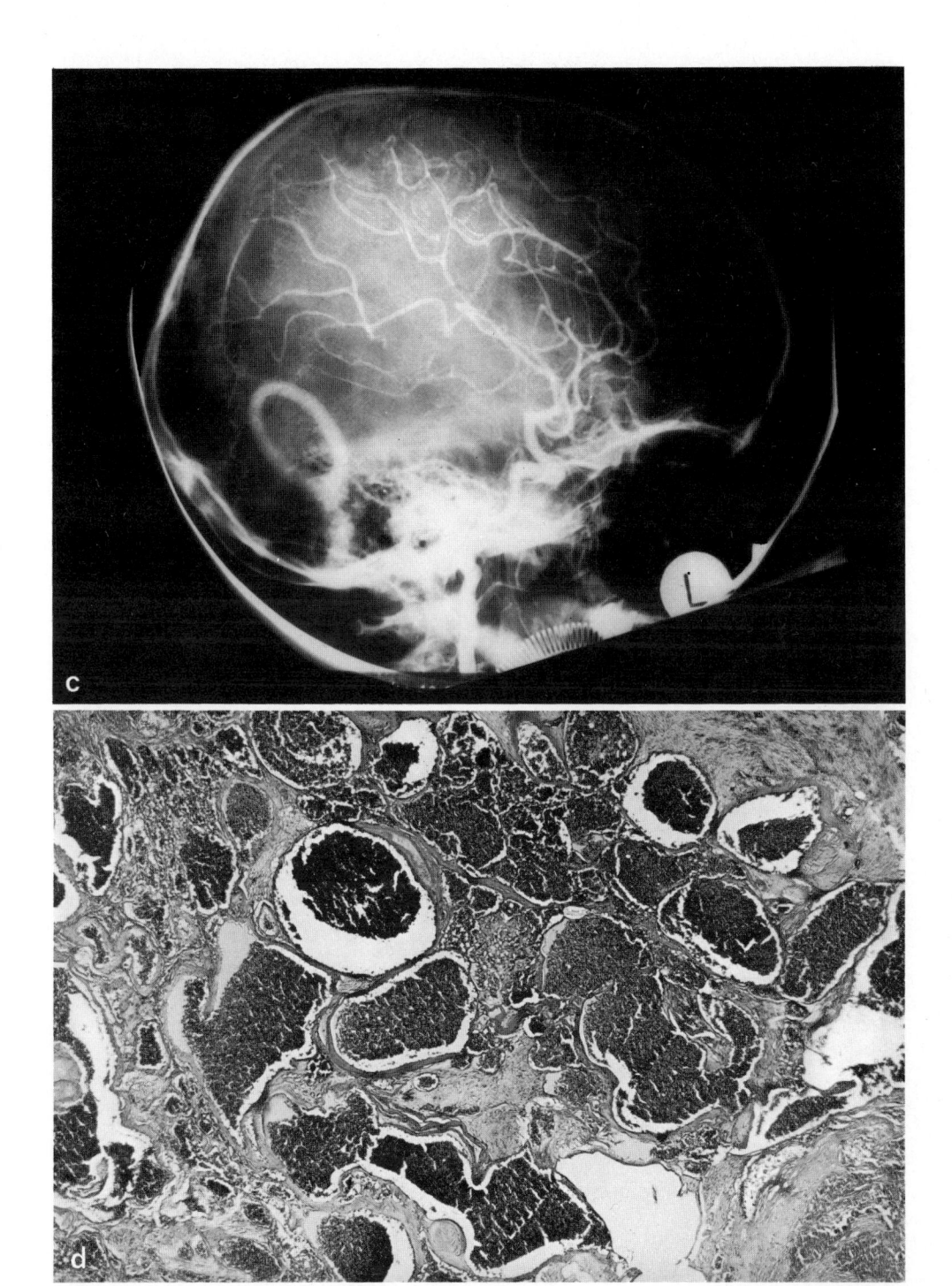

Fig. 1. c Left carotid angiography reveals an avascular mass of the middle fossa. d Histology confirms cavernous haemangioma, x 35

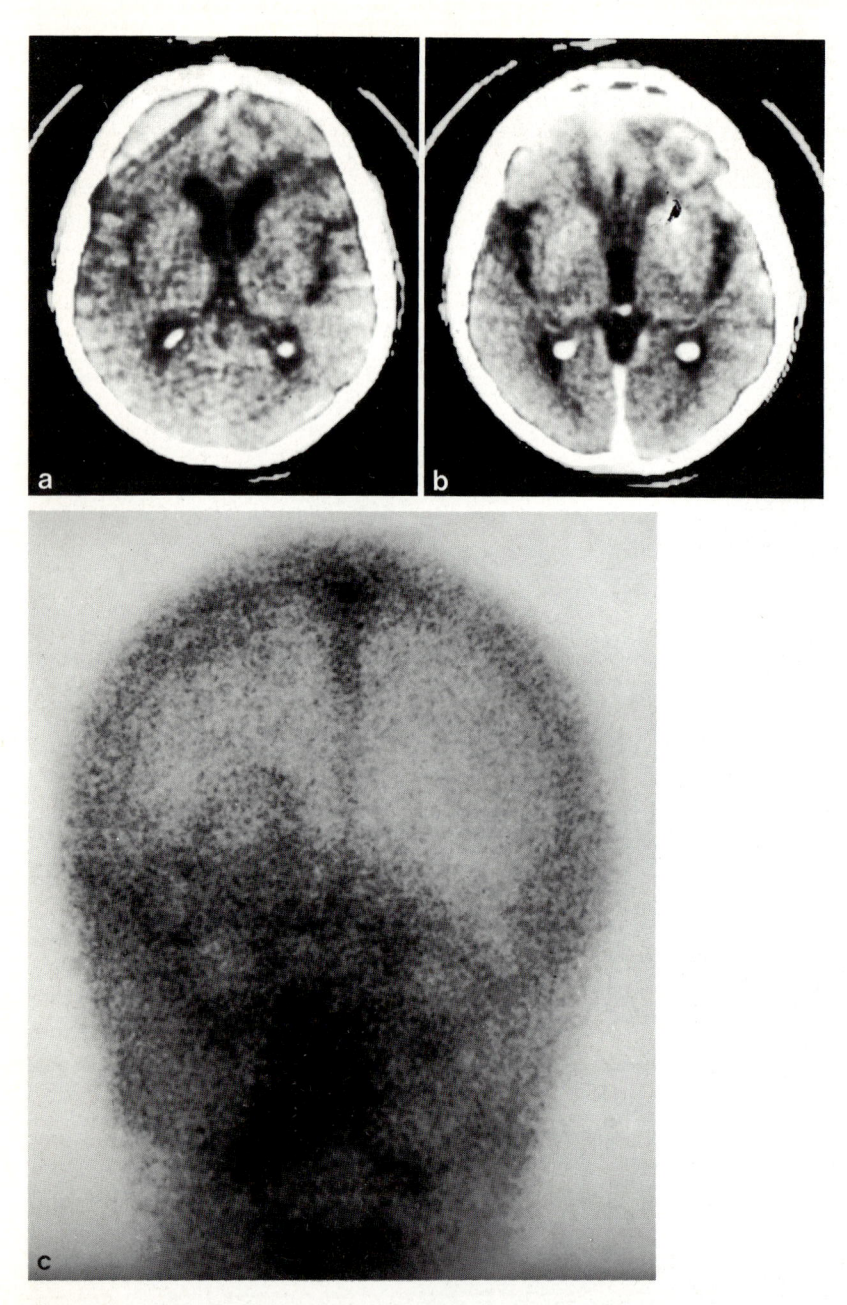

Fig. 2. a Plain CT shows a right frontal hypodense focus. b A well defined ring-shaped enhancement after contrast administration. c Scintigram using 99 m Tc pertechnetate showing a ring-shaped intense uptake, right fronto-basal.

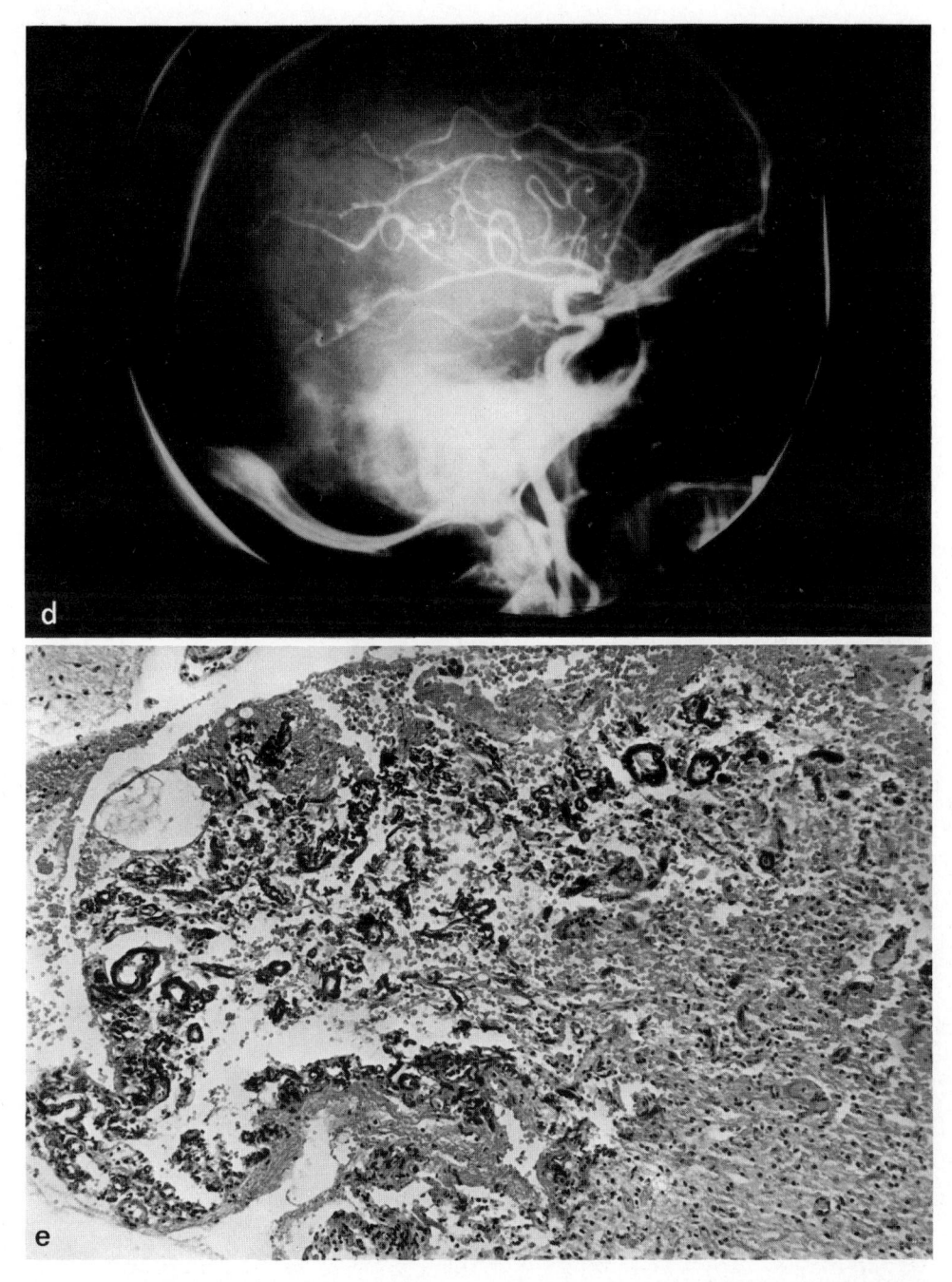

Fig. 2. d Right internal carotid angiography demonstrates no CVM.
e Histology confirms intracerebral capillary microhaemangioma with
old hemorrhage (134 x)

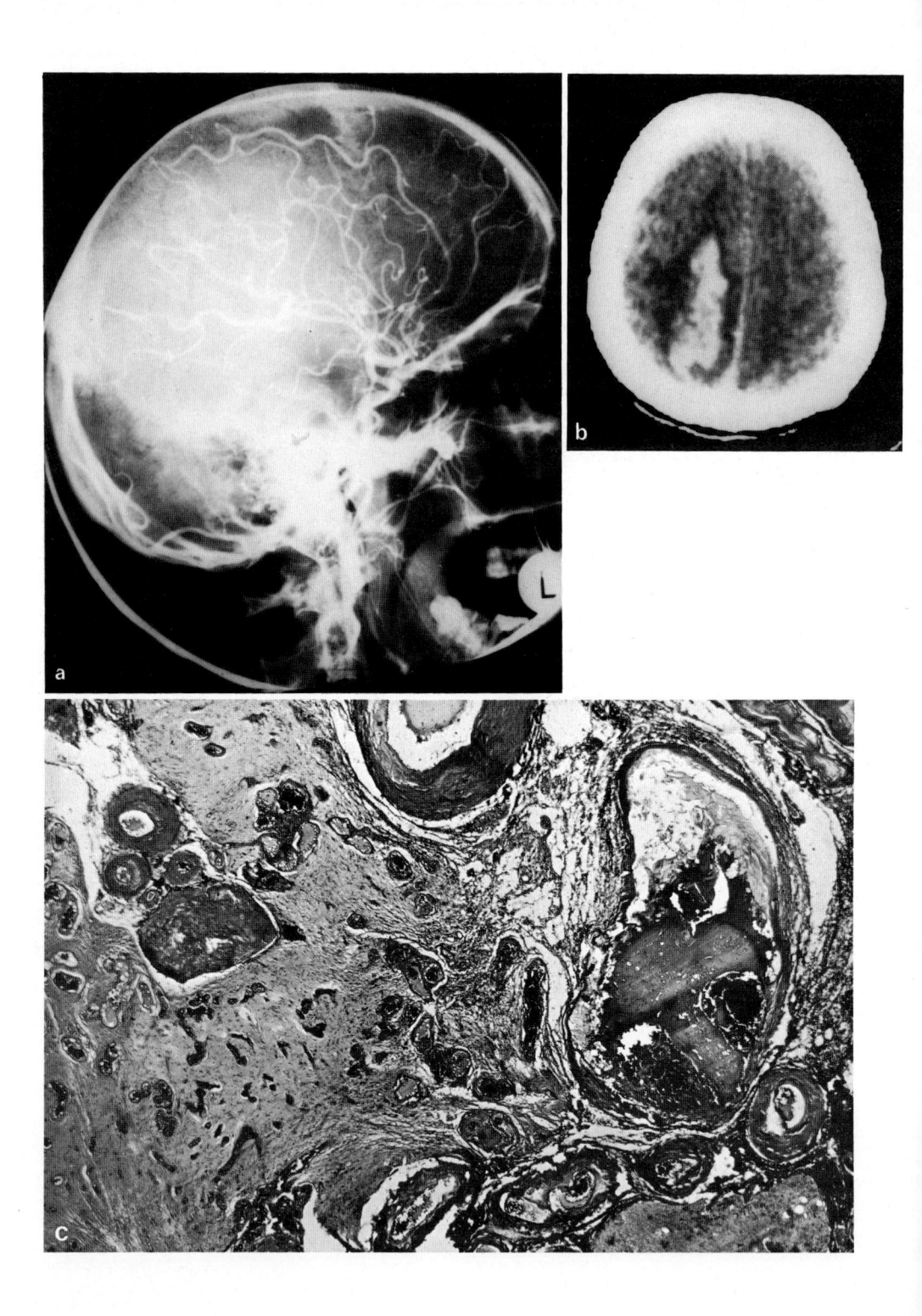
a
L
b
c

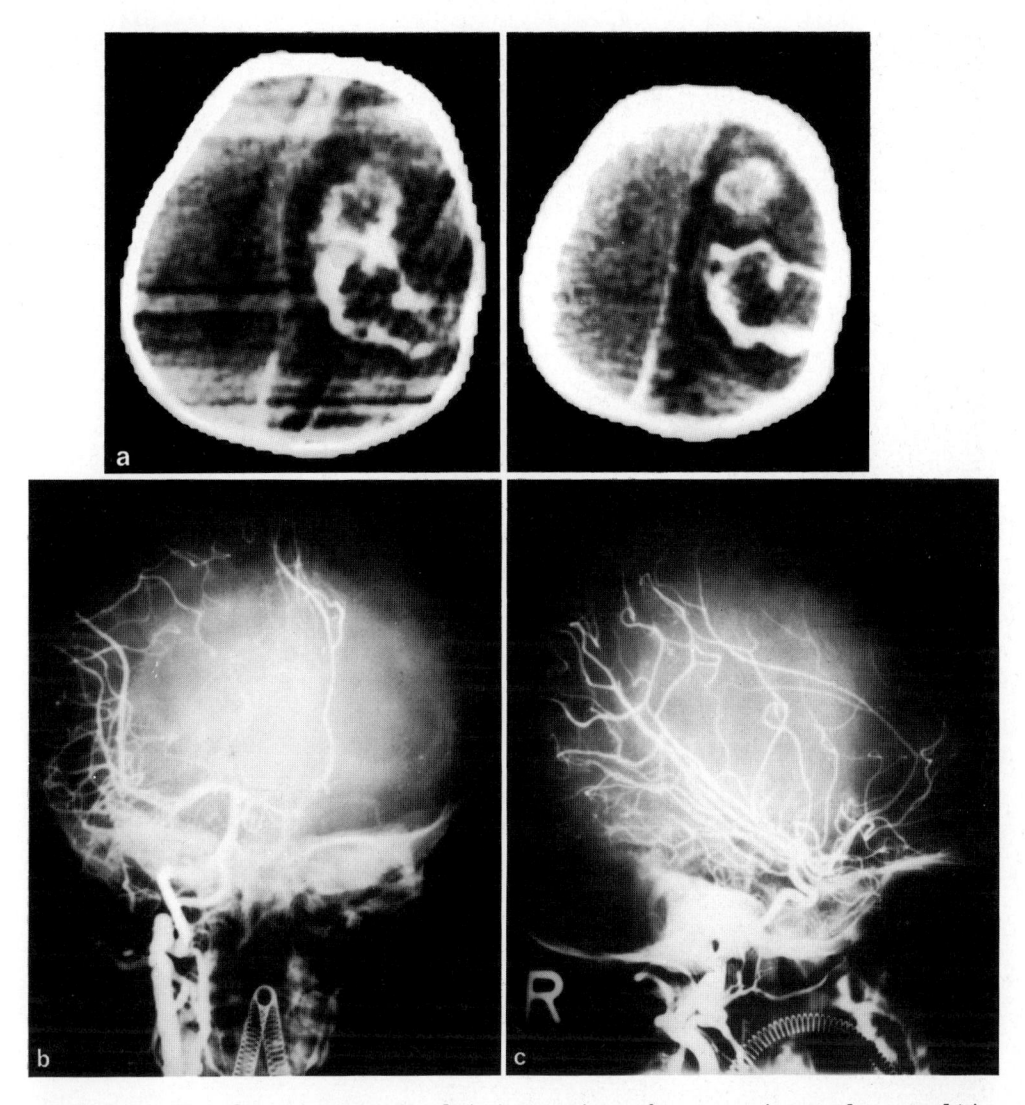

Fig. 4. a CT after contrast administration shows an irregular, multi-lobulated masses with extensive perifocal edema right fronto-parietal. Right carotid angiography reveals space-occupying lesion at the same region b A-P and c lateral view

Fig. 3. a Left carotid angiography reveals an avascular lesion fronto-parietal. b Plain CT shows left parietal haematoma. c Histology confirms an arteriovenous angioma with fresh hematoma (35 x)

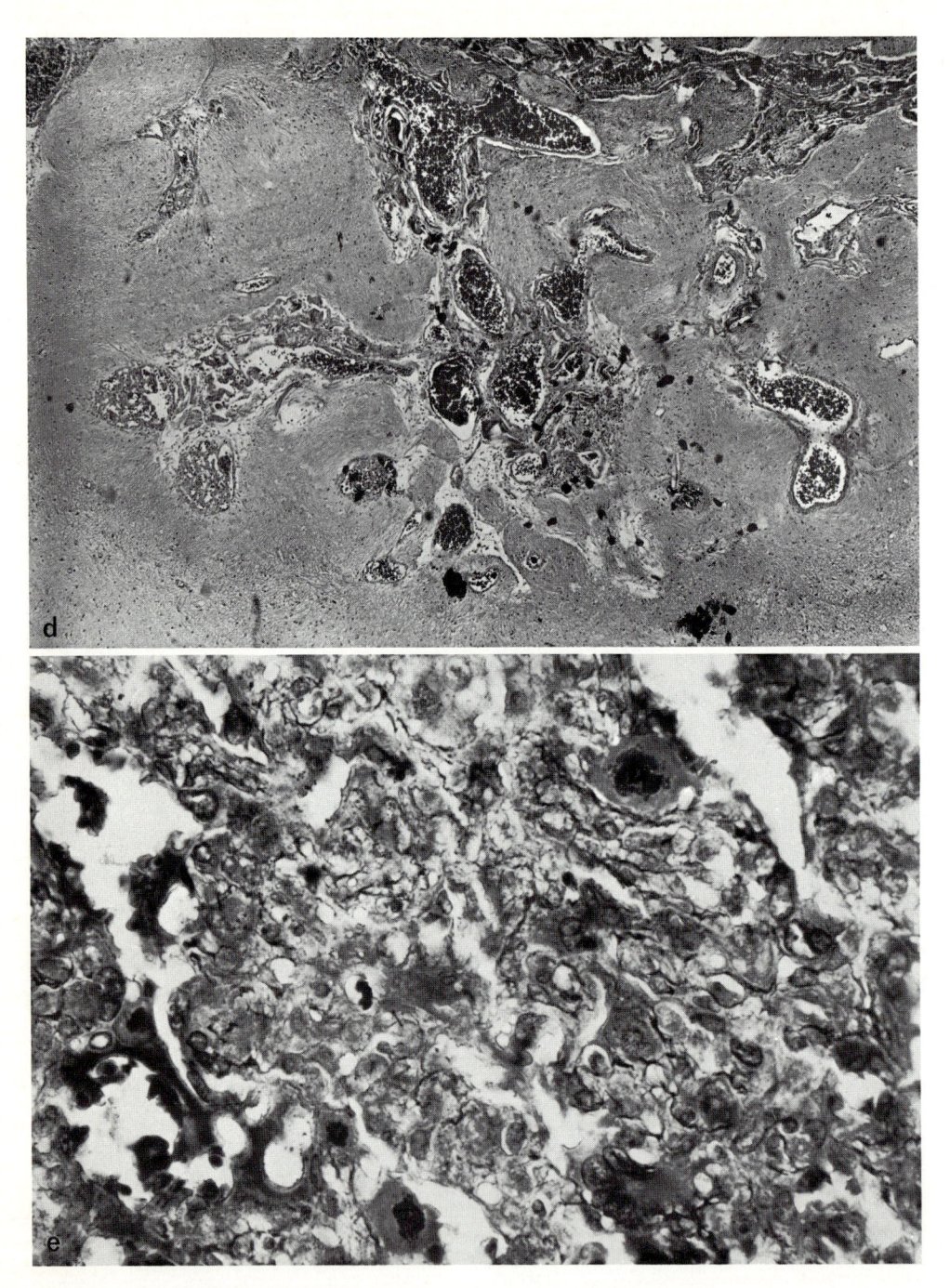

Fig. 4. Histology confirms (d) cavernous haemangioma and (e) malignant haemangioendothelioma

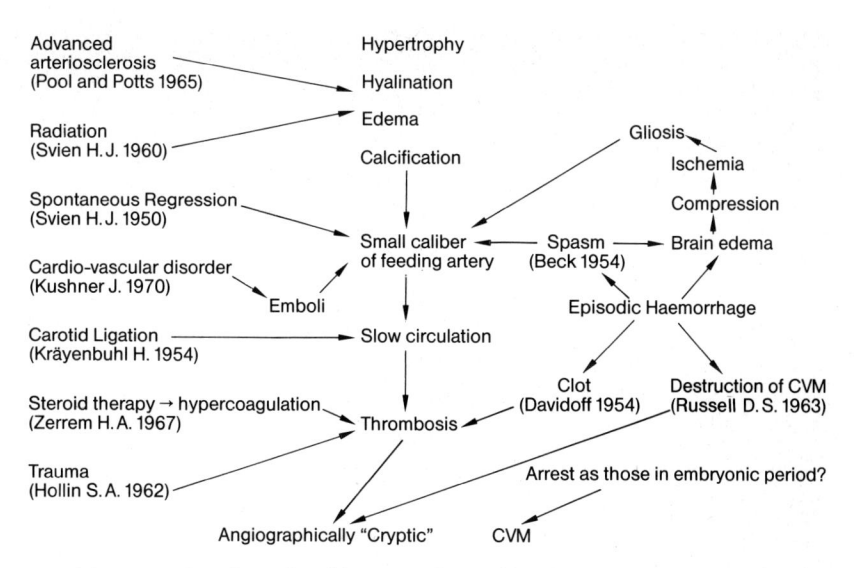

Fig. 5. Presumptive mechanism leading to haemodynamic and pathological changes with subsequent partial or complete angiographic disappearance of cerebro-vascular malformations

The Use of Computer Tomography in the Diagnosis and Postoperative Observation of Cerebral Aneurysms

W. Mauersberger and E. Lins

Coagulated blood is represented by a mean density value between 56 and 68 Hounsfield-Units (H.U.) (2, 5, 12). It thus lies clearly above the density values of normal brain tissue, 24 H.U. (white matter) and 36 H.U. (gray matter). With a density difference of nearly 30 H.U., it is possible to demonstrate lesions up to 4 mm diameter. It is thus possible to evaluate even smaller intracranial hemorrhages with computer tomography. If one takes into account the minimal burden to which this procedure subjects the patient, it becomes understandable that the computer tomogram, even in cases of spontaneous intracranial hemorrhage, represents a valuable diagnostic tool.

In respect to spontaneous intracranial hemorrhages due to aneurysms, two important questions arise.

1. How often is it possible to demonstrate an intracranial hemorrhage?
2. Is it possible to localize the aneurysm by computer tomograph?

In 71 patients with a ruptured aneurysm it was possible to demonstrate, by computer tomograph, a hemorrhage in 69. This represents a true positive quota of 97.2%.
In two cases, where a lumbar puncture confirmed a subarachnoid hemorrhage, the computer tomogram was unable to demonstrate a lesion. The false negative results thus represented 2.8%. These values correlate with those in the literature (3, 6, 7, 9, 10, 15), which lie between 97 and 100% true positives within the first 5 days following a subarachnoid hemorrhage.

Following a hemorrhage, there is a quick fall in density due to the breakdown and dilution with CSF of the clot. A rise in false negative results, after the 5th day, is thus understandable. Our false negative results were in those cases where the hemorrhage occurred 10 to 18 days prior to study.

In contrast to these patients, there is a case in which an aneurysm of the anterior communicating artery was diagnosed by computer tomography, not found on arteriography but confirmed at autopsy.

Important in the localization of an aneurysm is an exact analysis of the affected areas of the subarachnoid space and cerebral structures (3).

A hemorrhage in the area of the suprasellar cisterns, the frontal portions of the intrahemispheric space, the third ventricle, the paramedian and basal portions of the frontal lobe or in a pre-existing cyst of the septum pellucidum is indicative of an aneurysm of the anterior communicating artery (Fig. 1a).

Aneurysms of the supraclinoid portion of the carotid artery are revealed by blood in the parasellar cisterns and medial basal portion of the temporal lobe (Fig. 1b).

Hemorrhage into the Sylvian fissure and the temporal lobe is primarily indicative of an aneurysm of the middle cerebral artery (Fig. 2a), whereas aneurysms of the rostral portion of the basilar fork lead to hemorrhage into the interpeduncular cisterns and the peripontine cisterns (Fig. 2b).

Using these criteria, it was possible in 55 patients (76%) to exactly locate the aneurysm. Of course, this does not preclude the use of a carefully performed preoperative diagnostic angiogram, since a direct demonstration of an aneurysm is seldom possible by CT.

In any case, localization is made difficult if blood fully fills the basal cisterns and the subarachnoid space over the convexity or if only a small amount of blood is present.

Due to the communications which the parasellar cisterns have with the basal segments of the frontal interhemispheric space and with the Sylvian fissure, supraclinoid aneurysms may bleed into these CSF-spaces. A topographic false diagnosis, in our patient population, occurred most often with this aneurysm, which in most cases, was misdiagnosed as an aneurysm of the anterior communicating artery.

The topographic diagnosis is also important in respect of the cerebral angiogram and also in those cases in which the angiogram revealed multiple aneurysms and it must be decided which caused the hemorrhage.

If the clinical progress of the patient worsens, this is most often due to either a re-bleed or vasospasm. In these cases one is able to demonstrate either an increase in the size of the hemorrhage or the development of a hyperdense area of the brain supplied by a major brain vessel (Fig. 3).

In patients where there is a delay or lack of improvement, one must think of the development of a mal-resorptive hydrocephalus. Here the CT can easily demonstrate ventricular size. The diagnosis of a shunt dependent hydrocephalus depends upon the demonstration of a periventricular drop in density, as result of transependymal CSF diffusion (1, 4, 11, 14) (Fig. 4).

The computer tomogram is thus able to indicate the most probable localization of a bleeding aneurysm in most cases, to demonstrate the extent of the subarachnoid and intracerebral hemorrhage, to reveal possible complications and thus give guidance to any further diagnostic and therapeutic measures.

References

1. Asada, M., Tamaki, N., Kanazawa, Y., Matsumoto, S., Matsumoto, M., Kimura, S., Fujii, S., Kandey, Y.: Computer analysis of periventricular lucency on the CT scan. Neuroradiol. 16, 207-211 (1978)
2. Bergström, M., Ericson, K., Levander, B., Svendsen, P., Larson, S.: Variation with time of the attenuation values of intracranial hematomas. J. Comput. Ass. Tomogr. 3, 234-240 (1979)

3. Van Gijn, J., van Dongen, K.J.: Computed tomography in the diagnosis of subarachnoid hemorrhage and ruptured aneurysm. Clin. Neurol. Neurosurg. 82, 11-24 (1980)

4. Hopkins, L.N., Bakay, L., Kinkel, W.R., Grand, W.: Demonstration of transventricular CSF absorption by computerized tomography. Acta Neurochir. 39, 151-157 (1977)

5. Hübner, K.-H., Schmitt, W.G.H.: Computertomographische Densitometrie des menschlichen Blutes. Einfluß auf das Absorptionsverhalten von parenchymatösen Organen und Ergußbildungen. Fortschr. Röntenstr. 130, 185-188 (1979)

6. Kendall, B.E., Lee, B.C.P., Claveria, E.: Computerized tomography and angiography in subarachnoid hemorrhage. Br. J. Radiology 49, 483-501 (1976)

7. Liliequist, B., Lindquist, M., Valdemarsson, E.: Computed tomography and subarachnoid hemorrhage. Neuroradiol. 14, 21-26 (1977)

8. Marvilla, K.R., Pastel, M.S., Kirkpatrick, J.B.: White matter of the cerebellum demonstrated by computed tomography: Normal anatomy and physical principles. J. Comput. Ass. Tomogr. 2, 156-161 (1978)

9. Modesti, L.M., Binet, E.F.: Value of computed tomography in the diagnosis and management of subarachnoid hemorrhage. Neurosurg. 3, 151-157 (1978)

10. Moran, C.J., Naidich, T.P., Gado, M.H., Holloman, W.G., Shalen, P.R.: Leptomeningeal findings in CT of subarachnoid hemorrhage. J. Comput. Ass. Tomogr. 2, 520-521 (1978)

11. Mori, K., Murata, T., Nakano, Y., Handa, H.: Periventricular lucency in hydrocephalus on computerized tomography. Surg. Neurol. 8, 337-340 (1977)

12. New, P.F.J., Aronow, S.: Attenuation measurements of control blood and blood fractions in computed tomography. Radiology 121, 635-640 (1976)

13. Schultz, E., Felix, R., Lackner, K., Bergeder, H.-D., Thurn, P.: Abbildungseigenschaften der Computertomographie. II. Räumliches Auflösungsvermögen. Dichteauflösungen und Partial-Volume-Effekt bei kugelförmigen Objekten verschiedenen Durchmessers. Fortschr. Röntgenstr. 130, 479-486 (1979)

14. Sprung, C., Grumme, Th.: CT images of periventricular lucency (PVL) in various forms of hydrocephalus. In: Advances in neurosurgery, Vol. 8. Grote, W., Brock, M., Clar, H.E., Klinger, M., Nau, H.-E. (eds.), pp. 172-182. Berlin, Heidelberg, New York: Springer 1980

15. Weisberg, L.A.: Computed tomography in aneurysmal subarachnoid hemorrhage. Neurology 29, 802-808 (1979)

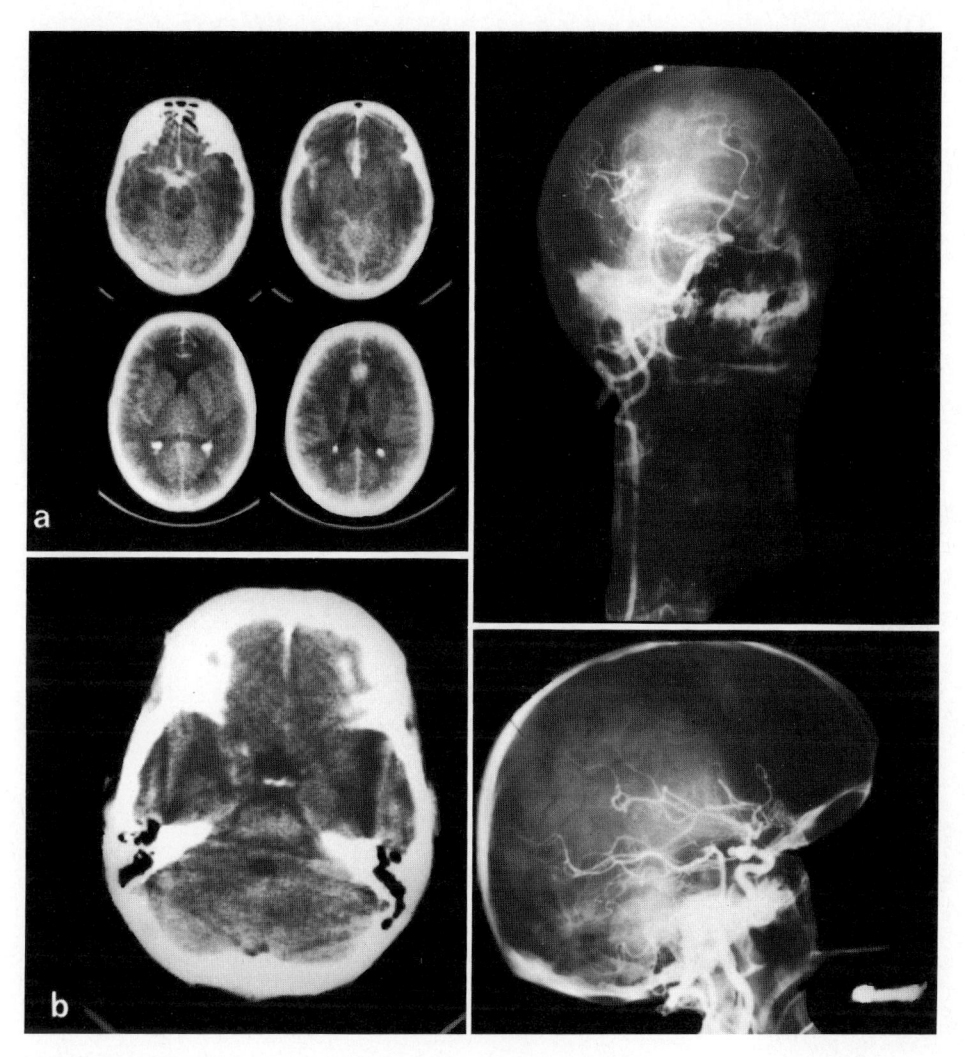

Fig. 1. a Aneurysm of the anterior communicating artery, computertomographic and angiographic findings. b Hemorrhage into the left parasellar cistern demonstrated by computerized tomography caused by an angiographically demonstrated aneurysm of the supraclinoid segment of the internal carotid artery

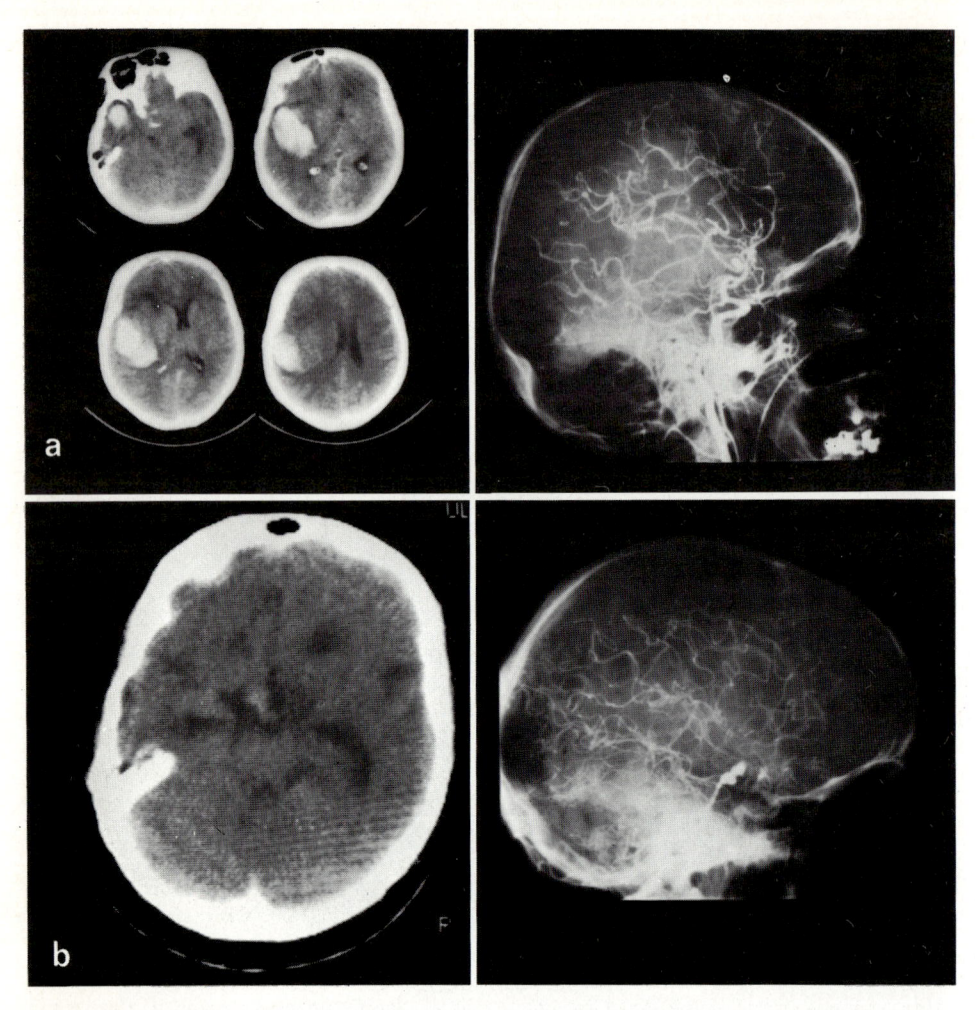

Fig. 2. a Hemorrhage in the Sylvian fissure and left temporal lobe caused due to an aneurysm of the left middle cerebral artery. b Aneurysm of the basilar artery with bleeding into the interpeduncular cistern.

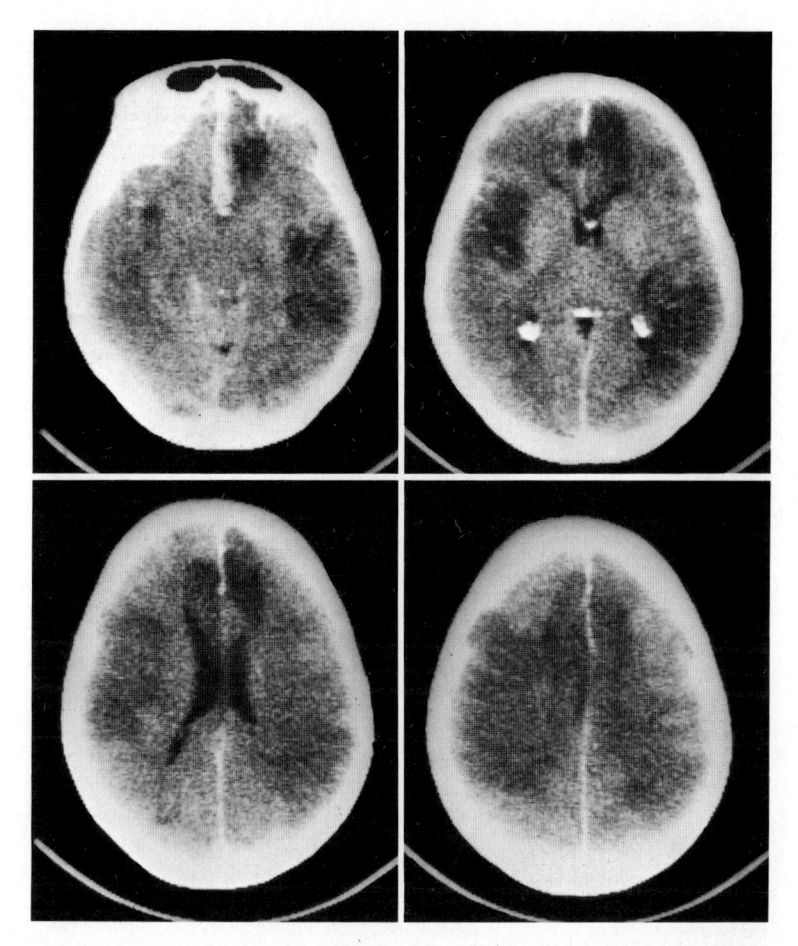

Fig. 3. Bilateral infarcts of the frontal and temporal region caused by spasms of the anterior and middle cerebral arteries after subarachnoid bleeding from an aneurysm of the anterior communicating artery

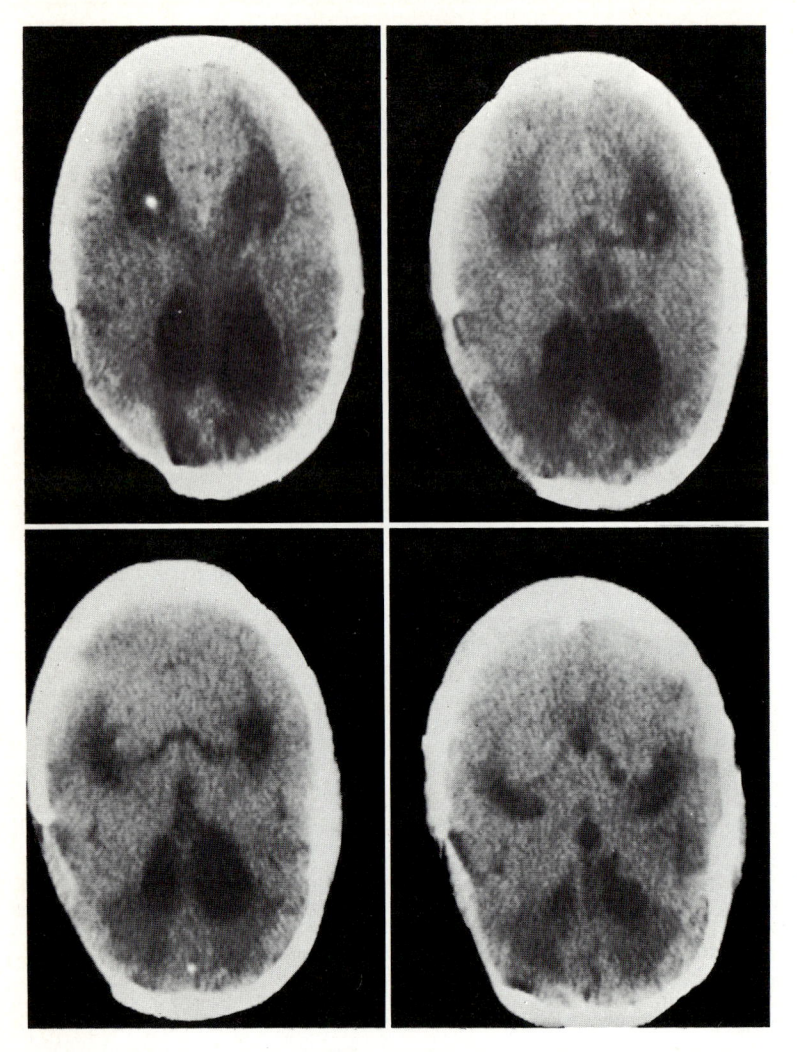

Fig. 4. Massive posthemorrhagic hydrocephalus with marked periventricular lucency and occlusion of cortical sulci

Computerized Tomography in the Operative Treatment of Cerebrovascular Disease

H. Wassmann, R. Bollbach, and E. Lins

Introduction

The indication and timing for carotid endarterectomy or extra-intracranial arterial bypass (EIAB) surgery in patients suffering from occlusive cerebrovascular disease has come mainly from clinical follow-ups and angiographic findings up to the present. Difficult questions were, on the one hand to decide on surgery in patients with partial recovery of completed stroke and, on the other hand, to assess the blood-brain-barrier (BBB) damage with regard to operative timing. Visualization of cerebral infarcts was rendered possible for the first time by computerized tomography (CT). The early visualization of infarcts depends on the amount of water in the tissue, in that a 3% increase in water content gives a fall in the absorption coefficient of 2 Houndsfield Units (4). A contrast medium enhancement in the infarcted area is detectable by CT in 40% of patients in the first stages, rising to 70% by the 3rd week and decreasing continuously until the 6th week. The existence of a hypodense lesion is found in 18% of the patients with a transient ischemic attack (TIA), in 76% of the patients with prolonged reversible ischemic neurological deficit (PRIND) and in 95% of the patients with completed stroke (CS) (3).

Method and Results

Since the introduction of CT in our clinic in 1978 all patients suffering from occlusive cerebrovascular disease have been examined preoperatively by this method in addition to neurological, EEG-, angiographic, Doppler sonographic and psychometric examinations.

With regard to indication and timing of the operation, our patients are classified into different stages according to the course of clinical symptoms and CT findings (Table 1).

Patients in *stage I* have suffered no ischemic symptoms. The diagnosis of the obstruction has been made accidentally. CT shows no ischemic lesion. In patients younger than 60 years, we consider a stenosis of the internal carotid artery (ICA) of more than 50% to be an indication for surgery. Patients are classified into *stage II*, if they suffered from TIAs with a maximum period of 24 hours. In some cases CT can show a small low-density area in a silent cerebral region. Surgery should be carried out as soon as possible, for one should always anticipate a complete stroke, which occurs in an average of 50% of the cases within one year (1).
Stage III is defined as a prolonged reversible ischemic neurological deficit. In stage III a the neurological deficits subside completely within 48 hours. In stage III b, mild neurological symptoms persist and CT findings show a small sub-/cortical infarction in most of

Table 1. Classification of cerebrovascular disease with regard to surgical indication and operative timing

Stage	Neurological symptoms	CT-findings	Indication for surgery	Timing for surgery
I	No	Normal	Patient younger than 60 years stenosis more than 50%	At any time
II TIA	Reversible within 24 h	Normal, small hypodense area in a silent cerebral region possible	Urgent, pre-apoplectic signs!	In a free interval
III PRIND a)	Reversible within 48 h			
b)	Reversible except mild remaining symptoms	Small infarction in a sub-/cortical region		If no signs of blood-brain-barrier damage are existing, about 6-8 weeks after stroke
IV a)	Severe, partial reversibility	Distinct and/or multiple infarctions	Eventually, if improvement under hyperbaric oxygenation	
b)	Severe, no reversibility	Distinct and/or infarctions within the internal capsule	No	No

these cases. Surgery is urgently indicated, provided that no signs of BBB damage are still present.

To illustrate this group of patients, the case of a 56-year-old patient is presented. Three months before surgery he had suffered an acute right-sided hemiparesis and dysphasia. When admitted to our clinic he only showed moderate dysphasia and latent hemiparesis. Angiography revealed an occlusion of the left ICA. In CT a small hypodense lesion was found in the area of the middle cerebral artery (MCA) (Fig. 1a). Signs of BBB damage were missing. EIAB surgery was successful (Fig. 1b).

Patients with a completed stroke and persistent distinct neurological deficits are grouped in *stage IV*. This can be subdivided into a stage IV a with a partial improvement of clinical symptoms and a stage IV b without any recovery. In almost all of these cases multiple lesions and contrast medium uptake can be detected by CT. That enhancement, as a sign of BBB damage, is a contraindication to surgery.

A characteristic case, illustrating stage IV a (Fig. 2) is a 58-year-old patient suffering from a stroke with a severe right-sided hemiparesis and total aphasia. An occlusion of the left MCA was found angiographically. Gradual recovery over more than a year resulted in a mild hemiparesis and slight dysphasia. CT scans revealed multiple hypodense lesions, e.g. in the left cortex but also in the left basal ganglia and the right hemisphere (Fig. 2a). After signs of further improvement by hyperbaric oxygen therapy (6) we decided to perform an EIAB - with satisfactory results (Fig. 2b).

CT scans in patients of stage IV b show either large and multiple infarcts or small hypodense lesions in the basal ganglia.

An example is a 51-year-old patient with a left-sided ICA occlusion who suffered a severe persistent right-sided hemiparesis. CT examinations showed small infarcts in the region of the caudate nucleus and the internal capsule (Fig. 3). Hyperbaric oxygenation turned out to be ineffective. Therefore no indication for surgery was seen.

All in all, since the introduction of CT in our clinic 70 patients have been treated by EIAB surgery and 30 patients by carotid endarterectomy, according to this classification. 26 patients were female, 74 were male, with an average age of 52.5 years. The post-operative course was complicated in one patient by subdural hematoma, in one by hemorrhagic infarction on the 14th postoperative day after an uneventful follow-up, and brain edema in another.

The other patients showed an uneventful clinical follow-up. In no case was a cerebral infarction or TIA observed. 60% of the patients grouped in stage III b or IV a showed a further improvement of their neurological deficits in post-operative controls (2).

Conclusions

It has to be assumed that preoperative CT diminishes the danger of too early vascular surgery that might provoke a hemorrhagic infarction or additional brain edema.

Moreover the knowledge of the extension of the infarcted area combined with the preoperative hyperbaric oxygenation allows, to a certain degree, a prediction about the reversibility of the neurological symptoms. So CT aids a correct decision concerning vascular surgery for cerebrovascular disease. These assumptions and the comparison with the pre-CT-era in the treatment of cerebrovascular disease must await a larger well-controlled study.

References

1. Fields, W.S., Bell, R.M., Campbell, J.M.: Computed tomography in the management of cerebrovascular disease. Stroke 6, 105-107 (1975)
2. Holbach, K.-H., Wassmann, H.: Extra-intracranial anastomosis operation associated with hyperbaric oxygenation in the treatment of completed stroke. In: Microsurgery for cerebral ischemia. Peerless, S.J., McCormick, C.W. (eds.), pp. 286-291. Berlin, Heidelberg, New York: Springer 1980
3. Ladurner, G., Sager, W.D., Iliff, L.D., Lechner, H.: A correlation of clinical findings and CT in ischemic cerebrovascular disease. Eur. Neurol. 18, 281-288 (1979)
4. Oettinger, W., Lanksch, W., Baethmann, A.: Korrelation zwischen Computer-Tomographie und Gewebsbefund beim Hirnödem. Vortrag a.d. Symposion: Craniale Computer-Tomographie, München 1976
5. Wassmann, H.: Quantitative Indikatoren des hirnelektrischen Wirkungsverlaufes bei hyperbarer Oxygenierung. Z. EEG-EMG 11, 97-101 (1980)

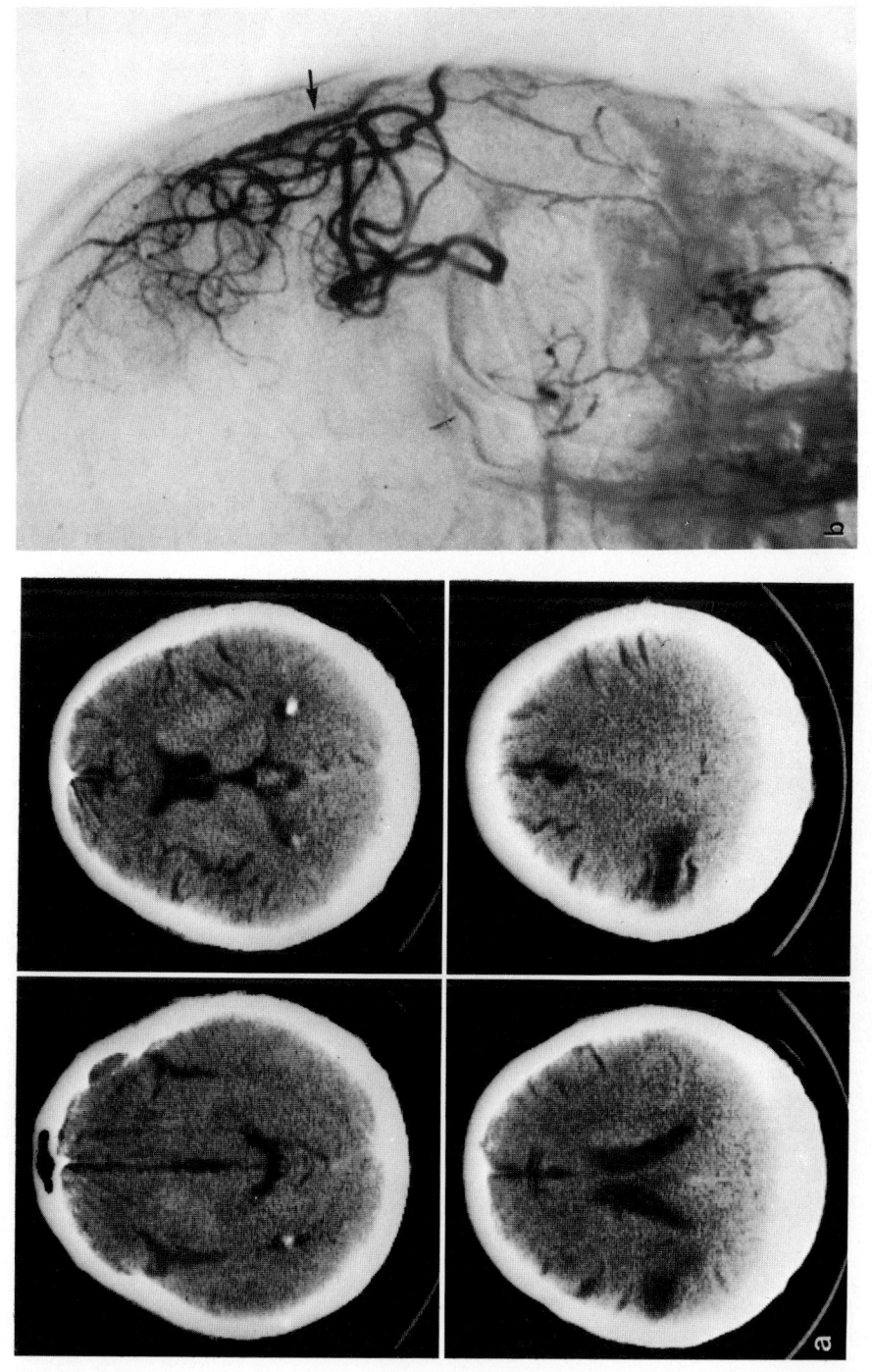

Fig. 1. a CT of a 56-year-old patient with occlusion of left internal carotid artery and a hypodense area in the territory of the left middle cerebral artery. b Left-sided angiography after extra-intracranial bypass surgery in this patient shows a filling of the left centro-parietal region through the bypass (*arrow*)

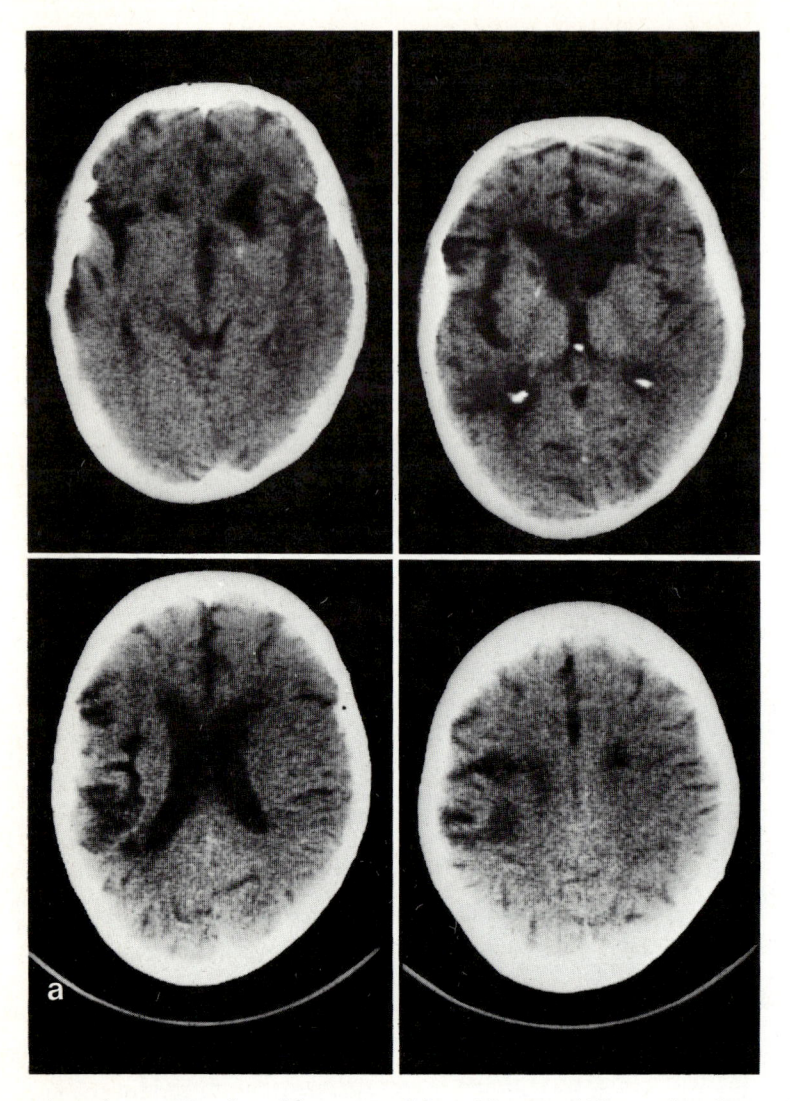

Fig. 2. a CT of a 58-year-old patient with occlusion of the left middle cerebral artery and multiple hypodense lesions

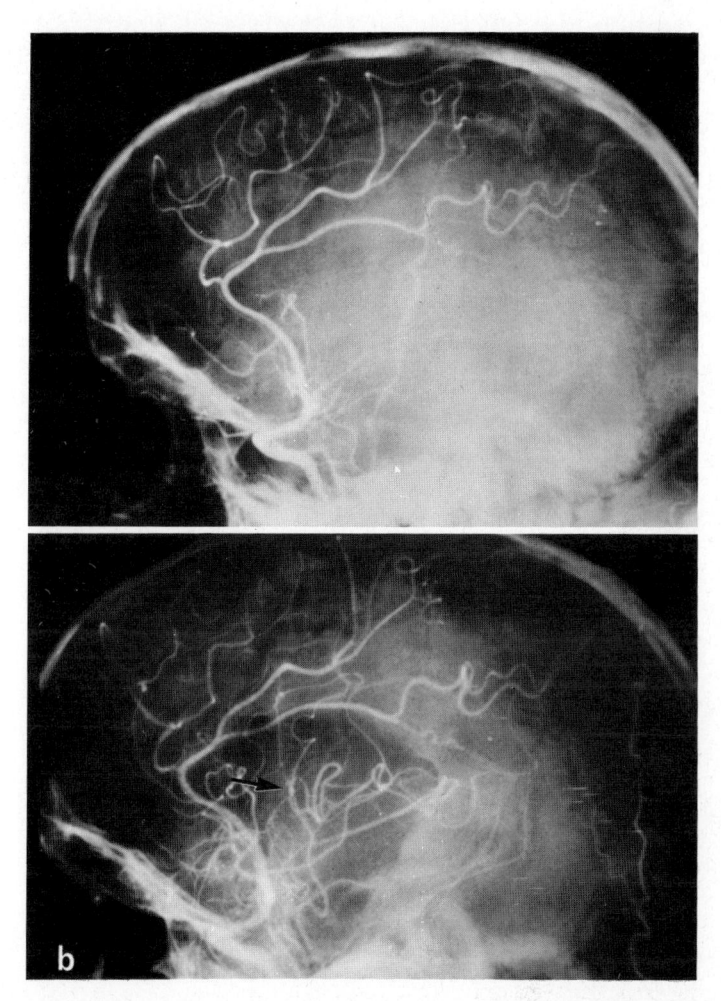

Fig. 2. b Angiography in this patient before (above) and after surgery shows filling of the perfusion area of the middle cerebral artery by anastomosis (→)

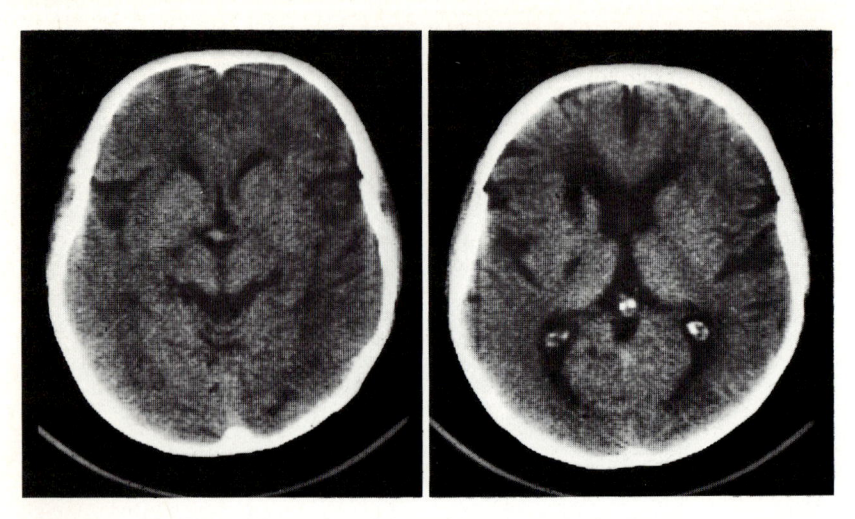

Fig. 3. CT of a 51-year-old patient with left internal carotid artery occlusion and small infarcts in the caudate nucleus and internal capsule

The Diagnostic Value of Computerized Tomography in Follow-Up Studies After CSF Drainage

TH. HERTER and H. ALTENBURG

Hydrocephalus has been treated operatively since the time of Hippokrates, but the drainage systems developed by NUSLEN and SPITZ (1952), SPITZ and HOLTER (1954) and PUDENZ and HEYER (1957) could not obviate all the difficulties; on the contrary, the CSF drainage operations still rank with those neurosurgical procedures most prone to complications (Fig. 1).

In judging the course after CSF drainage, computerized tomography (CT) offers the following possibilities:

Recognition of Postoperative Complications

Three main categories of complications detectable by CT can be distinguished.

Overdrainage Phenomena

Complications due to too low opening pressures constituted 1% of all complications according to LEEM and also KEUCHER, 2% and 5% according to STEINBOCK and GUIDETTI, respectively. STRAHL reported no case of overshunting using peritoneal catheters. The dependence of the valve function on the body height - siphon-effect - is also to be taken into account.

Symptoms of the overdraining phenomenon recognizable in the CT scan are: slit ventricles, subdural hygromas or hematomas, CSF tracts forming along the ventricular catheter, CSF cysts or general cerebral edema (15). Subdural hygromas or hematomas only very rarely are space-occupying. Mostly they are simply space-filling (6). According to the MONROE-KELLY doctrine the sum of the intracranial volumina is constant. It follows that subdural hygromas or hematomas, being merely space-filling, not causing increased intracranial pressure and therefore being without symptoms, are to be operated upon only in exceptional cases.

Concerning the therapeutic consequences, ventricle collapse and slit ventricles are more important, because occlusion of the catheter is favoured by opposed ventricular walls (Fig. 2).

Underdrainage Phenomena

Too high opening pressure were reported in 3%, 4% and 1% of all complications (18, 19, 26) respectively. Shift and occlusion of the ventricle catheter or/and the heart catheter amounts to 67%, 47%,

55%, 45%, 22%, 29% and 45% of all complications according to GUIDETTI, STEINBOCK, IGNELCI, KEUCHER, LEEM, JEFFREY and our own investigations, respectively. Further causes of underdraining to be considered are: shunt blockage, venous thrombosis, shift of the heart catheter e.g. due to growing of the patient, fracture, kinking and disconnection of the catheters, malfunction of the valve, and - with peritoneal drainage - peritoneal adhesions and malabsorptions, such as loss of peritoneal absorptive capacity and subcutaneous CSF accumulation. Compared with atrial catheters, disconnection was 4 times as frequent with peritoneal catheters, whereas atrial catheters became too short 8 times more frequently due to growth of the patient (27).

Computerized tomography merely demonstrates an increasing or non-improving hydrocephalus or a shift of the intracranial part of the catheter, e.g. a dislocation into the ependyma or the brain substance. The alterations mostly give only an indirect indication of the actual cause of the complication (Fig. 3).

Infections

Infections make up 12%, 17%, 13%, 12%, 29% and 21% of all complications according to GUIDETTI, STEINBOCK, IGNELCI, KEUCHER, JEFFREY and our own investigations, respectively. LEEM reported 9% with atrial and 20% with peritoneal drainage.

Apart from inadequate sterility, a shunt infection can be caused by a meningitis, pneumonia or sepsis. Further, an infection is favoured by repeated shunt revisions, an incorrect - mostly too low - position of an atrial catheter and skin erosions above the valve or the burr hole. Also - with peritoneal drainage - peritonitis can bring about shunt infection. Infection as one of the most common complications after CSF draining operations can be recognized in the CT scan only in special cases when an acute ependymitis in the hypervascular stage can be demonstrated by more intense staining with contrast medium. In later stages of an ependymitis the ependyma depicts itself altered in shape and is rigid. An infection often starts with occlusion of the catheters, thereby causing an underdrainage phenomenon seen in the CT scan (Figs. 4, 5).

Very rarely *intracerebral bleeding* occurs either directly caused by advancing the ventricular catheter or being the result of injury to the ependyma due to the development of ependymal adhesions to the catheter and their subsequent wrenching off (4). These haemorrhages are easily seen in the CT scan (Fig. 4).

Aeroceles or accumulations of air in the ventricle or intracranially are very rare. Usually, the air enters along the ventricle catheter in the course of overshunting or originates from an additional craniocerebral trauma. Because some valves are obstructed by air, a tension pneumencephalus can result. There are no problems in diagnosing the air in the CT scan (Fig. 5).

Computerized tomography enables an uncomplicated and low-risk re-evaluation of the diagnosis and surgical indication for the treatment of hydrocephalus. To be undertaken for example, a suspected but not yet confirmed tumor in the region of the aqueduct can be verified during the course of control examinations. If a moderate ventricular dilatation is noted in the postoperative course and a shunt obstruction is suspected, all that is involved could be a well tolerated compensated hydrocephalus. Unless there are severe manifestations of increased intracranial pressure, it is wise to await a control CT. Should a progressive ventricular dilatation be demonstrated at the time, a revision is mandatory; or the intracranial pressure should be checked.

Computerized tomography makes it possible to check therapeutic success. It enables an objective judgement of ventricular width to be formed and allows a critical comparison of clinical improvement and ventricle size. By a special computer program the volume of the brain and of the external and internal CSF spaces can be calculated and their relation be expressed as the so-called brain-CSF space index. In the course of control examinations the therapeutic success can be checked by alterations of this index (23).

Computerized tomography greatly facilitates diagnosis, surgical treatment and management of hydrocephalus, but often yields only indirect hints as to the cause of any disturbance. It supplements diagnosis in such a way that contrast ventriculography, measurement of CSF pressure, CSF dynamics, shunt depiction and other procedures still maintain their importance.

Summary

Computerized tomography is an important means of diagnosis, determining the indications for surgical treatment and checking the control of hydrocephalus. With regard to computerized tomography the complications are classified into five groups: over- and undershunting, infection, intracerebral haemorrhage and intracranial air accumulations. In some cases, computerized tomography only yields indirect evidence of the cause of complications. Apart from recognition of postoperative complications computerized tomography can detect pathological lesions developing during the course of monitoring the control of hydrocephalus and check the therapeutic success within certain limits.

References

1. Altenburg, H., Walter, W.: Vergleich ventrikulographischer und computertomographischer Befunde beim postmeningitischen Hydrocephalus internus. 16. JT d. Dtsch. Ges. f. Neurorad., München 1980
2. Altenburg, H., Brandt, M., Böhm, P.: Unusual development of chronic subdural hematomas after cerebrospinal fluid shunting. In: Advances in neurosurgery, Vol. 9. Schiefer, W., Klinger, M., Brock, M. (eds.). Berlin, Heidelberg, New York: Springer 1981
3. Bagston, R., Spitz, L.: Infective and cystic causes of malfunctions of ventriculoperitoneal shunts for hydrocephalus. Z. Kinderchir. Grenzgeb. 22/4, 419-424 (1977)
4. Becker, D., Nulsen, F.: Control of hydrocephalus by valve-regulated venous shunt: Avoidance of complications in prolonged shunt maintenance. J. Neurosurg. 28, 215-226 (1968)
5. von Beusekom, G.: Complications in hydrocephalus shunting procedures. In: Advances in neurosurgery, Vol. 6. Wüllenweber, R., Wenker, H., Brock, M., Klinger, M. (eds.), pp. 28-29. Berlin, Heidelberg, New York: Springer 1978

6. Faulhaber, K., Schmitz, P.: Overdrainage phenomena in shunt treated hydrocephalus. Acta Neurochirurgica 45, 89-101 (1978)
7. Forrest, D., Cooper, D.: Complications of ventriculo-atrial shunts. J. Neurosurg. 29, 506-512 (1968)
8. George, P., Leibrock, L., Epstein, M.: Long-term analysis of cerebrospinal fluid shunt infections. J. Neurosurg. 51, 804-811 (1979)
9. Grote, E., Zieski, J., Klinger, M., Grohmann, G., Markakis, E.: Complications following ventriculo-cisternal shunts. In: Advances in neurosurgery, Vol. 6. Wüllenweber,, R., Wenker, H., Brock, M., Klinger, M. (eds.), pp. 10-16. Berlin, Heidelberg, New York: Springer 1978
10. Guidetti, B., Occhipinti, E., Riccio, A.: Ventriculo-atrial shunt in 200 cases of non tumoural hydrocephalus in children: Remarks on the diagnostic criteria, postoperative complications and long-term results. Acta Neurochirurgica 21, 295-308
11. Hemmer, R.: Surgical treatment of hydrocephalus: complications, mortality, developmental prospects. Z. Kinderchir. 22, 443-452 (1977)
12. Hockley, A., Holmes, A.: Computerized axial tomography and shunt dependency. In: Advances in neurosurgery, Vol. 6. Wüllenweber, R., Wenker, H., Brock, M., Klinger, M. (eds.), pp. 48-51. Berlin, Heidelberg, New York: Springer 1978
13. Ignelzi, R., Kirsch, W.: Follow-up analysis of ventriculo peritoneal- and ventriculo-atrial shunts for hydrocephalus. J. Neurosurg. 42, 679-682 (1975)
14. Illingworth, R., Logue, V., Symon, L., Vemuru, K.: The ventriculo-caval shunt in the treatment of adult hydrocephalus. J. Neurosurg. 35, 681-685 (1971)
15. Janneck, C.: Lebensbedrohliche Hirndruckkrisen beim "überdrainierten" Hydrocephalus. Z. Kinderchir. 29, 4, 292-302 (1980)
16. Jeffrey, F., Chiv, M.: The complications of ventriculo-atrial shunting in hydrocephalus. In: Advances in neurosurgery, Vol. 6. Wüllenweber, R., Wenker, H., Brock, M., Klinger, M. (eds.), pp. 17-22. Berlin, Heidelberg, New York: Springer 1978
17. Jensen, F., Jensen, F.T.: Acquired hydrocephalus. Acta Neurochirurgica 46, 119-133, 243-257 (1978)
18. Keucher, T., Mealey, J.: Long-term results after ventriculo-atrial and ventriculo-peritoneal shunting for infantile hydrocephalus. J. Neurosurg. 50, 179-186 (1979)
19. Leem, W., Miltz, H.: Complications following ventriculo-atrial shungs in hydrocephalus. In: Advances in neurosurgery, Vol. 6. Wüllenweber, R., Wenker, H., Brock, M., Klinger, M. (eds.), pp. 1-4. Berlin, Heidelberg, New York: Springer 1981
20. MacGee, E.: Shunt position within the brain stem: A preventable complication. Neurosurgery 6, 1, 99-100 (1980)
21. Moussa, A., Sharma, S.: Subdural hematoma and the malfunctioning shunt. J. of Neurology, Neurosurgery and Psychiatry 41, 759-761 (1978)
22. Palmieri, A., Menichelli, F., Pasquini, U., Salvolini, U.: Role of computed tomography in the postoperative evoluation of infantile hydrocephalus. Neuroradiology 14, 257-262 (1978)

23. Sager, W.: Der Gehirn-Liquorraum-Index. Ein Parameter zur Diagnose des Hydrocephalus mit Hilfe der Computertomographie. Röntgen-Bl. 31, 567-574 (1978)
24. Salak, S., Sunder-Plassmann, M., Zaunbauer, F., Koos, W.: The use of the anti-siphon-value in prevention of functional complications of shunting system. In: Advances in neurosurgery, Vol. 6. Wüllenweber, R., Wenker, H., Brock, M., Klinger, M. (eds.), pp. 42-44. Berlin, Heidelberg, New York: Springer 1978
25. Savolaine, E., Gerber, A.: Need for complementary use of air ventriculography and computerized tomographic scanning in infected hydrocephalus. Neurosurgery 6, 1, 96-98 (1980)
26. Steinbock, P., Thompson, G.: Complications of ventriculo-vascular shunts: computer analysis of etiological factor. Surg. Neurol. 5, 31-35 (1976)
27. Strahl, E., Liesegang, I., Roosen, K.: Complications following ventriculo-peritoneal shunts. In: Advances in neurosurgery, Vol. 6. Wüllenweber, R., Wenker, H., Brock, M., Klinger, M. (eds.), pp. 6-9. Berlin, Heidelberg, New York: Springer 1978
28. Udvarhelyi, G.: Kritische Bewertung neurochirurgischer Behandlungsmethoden beim sogenannten Normaldruck-Hydrocephalus. Neurochirurgia 21, 1-8 (1978)
29. Venes, I.: Computerized axial tomography in the management of the child with shunted hydrocephalus. Z. Kinderchir. 25, 4, 330-335 (1978)
30. Villarejo, F.: Postoperative ventriculitis in hydrocephalus: treatment with external ventricular drainage. Acta Neurochirurgica 48, 41-45 (1979)

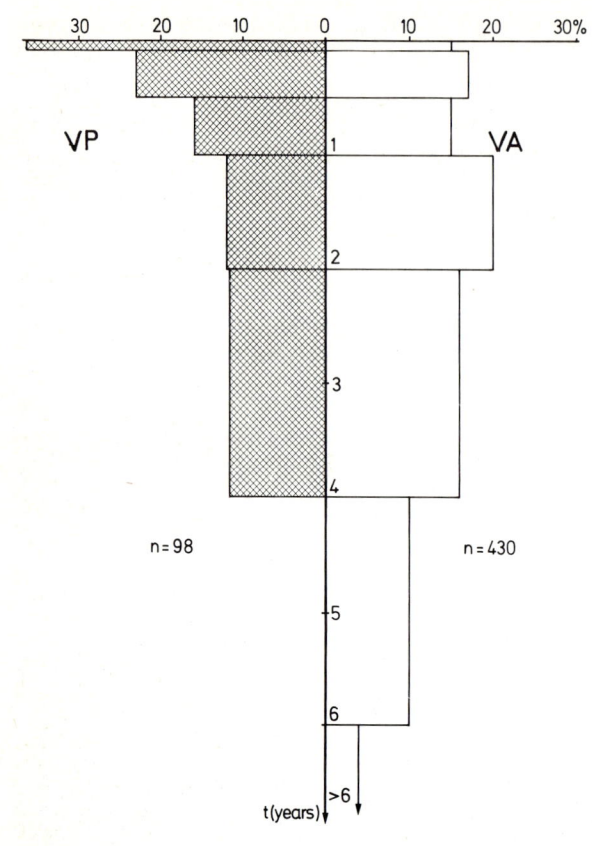

Fig. 1. Time interval between insertion and occurrence of complications in ventriculo-atrial (VA) and ventriculo-peritoneal (VP) shunt operations. With VP 77% of all complications occur within the first year, as compared to 48% with VA. After the fourth year complications were no longer observed with VP. (Mod. acc. to LEMAND STRAHL 1970-1976)

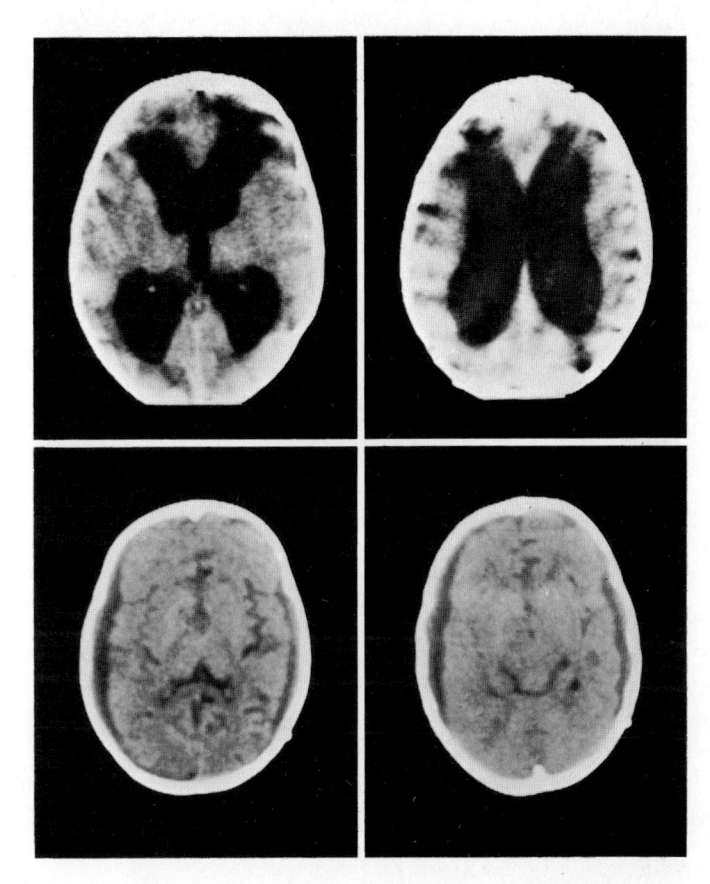

Fig. 2. 10-year-old girl with occlusive hydrocephalus. Immediate postoperative ventricular collapse, slit ventricles and bitemporal hygromas. Improvement after insertion of a Hakim-average-pressure valve

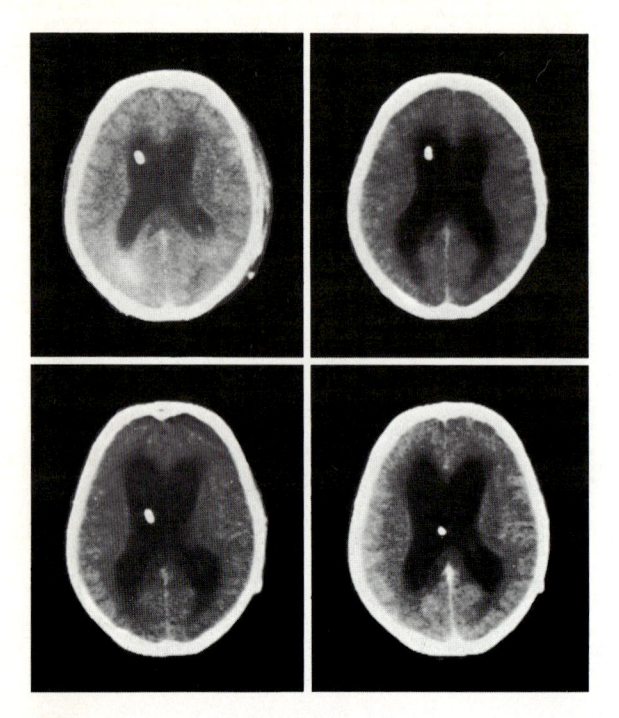

Fig. 3. 40-year-old man: CT scans made Dec. 30, Jan. 5, Jan. 14 and Feb. 26 do not demonstrate clear-cut decline of ventricular width. Patient was found to suffer from miliary tuberculosis with leptomeningeal involvement

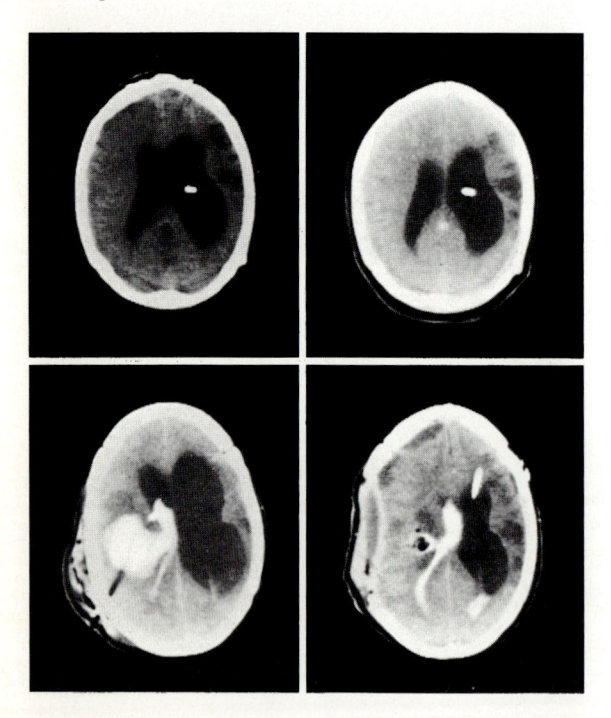

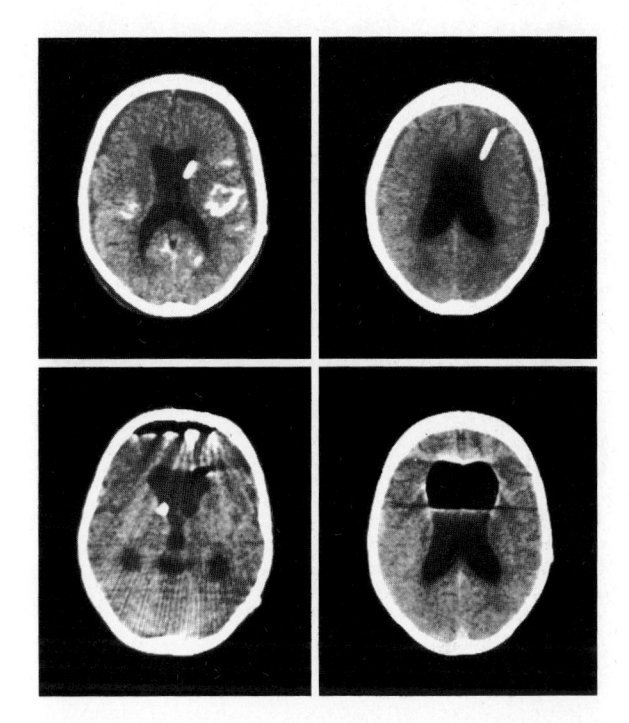

Fig. 5. 15-year-old girl with occlusive hydrocephalus. After insertion of a mini-low valve a relief-hygroma and ventriculitis supervened. After replacement of the valve air entered and a tension pneumencephalus developed

Fig. 4. 28-year-old woman: Hydrocephalus following operation for an aneurysm; insertion of a SPITZ-HOLTER drainage system which became inefficient in the course of a meningitis caused by staphylococcus aureus *(upper illustrations)*. After temporary external drainage it was attempted to re-insert a SPITZ-HOLTER drainage system, a resulting intracerebral hematoma *(left)* was emptied operatively *(lower right)*

Correlation of Postoperative Clinical Course and Ventricular Size Determined by Computed Tomography in Normal Pressure Hydrocephalus

C. Sprung and B. Schulz

Introduction

A generally accepted theory for the genesis of dilatation of ventricles of patients suffering from normal-pressure hydrocephalus (NPH) is the restriction of the capacity to absorb cerebro-spinal fluid (CSF). This restricted absorption of CSF is equalised by the implantation of a drainage system. Based on theoretical considerations it would be expected that the dilatation of the ventricles should decrease in parallel with the postoperative clinical improvement. However, our own experiences in the era of echo- and pneumoencephalography made us doubt this correlation, doubts which were confirmed by the evaluations of SHENKIN et al. (12). The methods offered by computed tomography (CT) which submit patients to less stress, enable us for the first time to carry out more exact examinations of the correlation between clinical improvement and postoperative decrease of the dilatation of the ventricles.

Methods

43 patients with typical clinical symptoms and signs of a normal-pressure hydrocephalus who, in addition, showed on lumbar or intraoperative ventricular measurement a CSF-pressure below 180 mm H_2O, could be submitted pre- and postoperatively to a computertomographic examination in the Klinikum Charlottenburg of the Free University, Berlin, since 1975. Contrary to SHENKIN (12), in our opinion the time interval between the date of operation and the final decision about the clinical outcome and grade of the decrease of the ventricular size is very important and should not be less than about 3 months. As a parameter for the determination of the width of ventricles preoperatively and the postoperative decrease of the ventricular dilatation the HUCKMAN-index proved superior to any other indices. Table 1 illustrates on the one hand the classification of our patients in groups depending on the clinical outcome and the 4 categories of reduction of ventricular size and on the other hand the schematic grading of the degree of correlation between these parameters.

Results

On Table 2 the postoperative clinical results of the whole series are summarized. 33 of our patients (77%) showed an excellent or good improvement after surgery, in 8 patients we did not find a significant improvement but no further deterioration while in two cases there was a further deterioration postoperatively. A further evaluation of our clinical results with respect to the etiology (Table 3) documents the

Table 1. Schematic illustration of our system of grading the correlation between clinical and computertomographic follow-up studies. + = complete correlation; (+) = discrepancy of one category or group; (-) = discrepancy of two classes between clinical and CT-findings postoperatively; - = no correlation at all between those parameters

Reduction of ventricular size Clinical response	Category 1 > 30%	Category 2 10% - 30%	Category 3 < 10%	Category 4 0%
Group I: excellent	+	(+)	(-)	-
Group II: good	(+)	+	(+)	(-)
Group III: poor	(-)	(+)	+	(+)
Group IV: no	-	(-)	(+)	+

Table 2. Grading of patients in four groups and overall postoperative clinical result. "Excellent" means that the patient resumed pre-illness activity and an improvement of all neurological symptoms and signs including dementia. "Good" means objective improvement of only single symptoms like gait disturbance or dementia. "Poor" means no change but also no worse clinical course postoperatively. "No" improvement means further deterioration of clinical symptoms postoperatively

Improvement	n
Group I: excellent	23
Group II: good	10
Group III: poor	8
Group IV: no	2

Table 3. Clinical improvement with respect to etiology. Noteworthy is the difference between the high rate of failures in the so-called "idiopathic" group of patients with NPH contrary to the patients with NPH following a subarachnoid hemorrhage or a traumatic lesion

Etiology of NPH improvement	Idiopathic	Posttraumatic	Subarachnoid hemorrhage	Meningitis	Total
Excellent	10	7	6	0	23
Good	3	5	1	1	10
Poor	6	2	0	0	8
No	1	0	1	0	2
Total	20	14	8	1	43

remarkably better results in patients with a definite etiological factor. We noted only in 13 of our 20 patients, suffering from idiopathic NPH, a sufficient clinical improvement, while 7 out of 8 cases with NPH following subarachnoid hemorrhage showed an excellent clinical response to shunting. Table 4 gives a survey on the decrease of the ventricular size in our 43 patients and the classification in four categories. A reduction of the HUCKMAN-index of 10 - 30% is the most frequent. 16, that is 37% of our patients in total, showed only a slight or no decrease at all of the ventricular dilatation in postoperative CT follow-up studies.

A clear correlation between the decrease of ventricular size and the preoperative dilatation of the ventricles or the preoperative duration of symptoms could not be identified. However, it was evident that out of 13 patients who showed at the same time a periventricular zone of low density, 11 had a really good improvement of clinical signs and symptoms postoperatively. 6 of our patients showed already in the preoperative CT-scans clear signs of an additional dilatation of the cortical sulci as well as of the basal cisterns. Out of this collection only 3 patients improved after insertion of a shunt, in only one case did we see a decrease of ventricular size of more than 10% postoperatively.

The outcome of our correlation between clinical results on the one hand and theoretically expected decrease of ventricular size on the other hand is documented in Table 5. Perfect correlation between both of the parameters could be stated in 18, i.e. 42%, of our patients. A relatively good correlation, that means that an individual patient was only little discrepant from a group or class, could be found in 15, i.e. 35%, of all cases. But 10 patients still showed a rather bad or no correlation at all. Seven of these patients had to be classified as those who showed an unimportant or no decrease of ventricular size in spite of an excellent clinical response postoperatively. Especially remarkable are those 3 cases which showed no improvement of neurological signs and symptoms in contrast to a considerable decrease of the size of the ventricles. Typical examples for the correlation between clinical and computertomographic follow-up studies are represented in Figs. 1 and 2.

Table 4. Grading of 43 patients in respect to the postoperative reduction of ventricular size. The different categories were established by measuring the reduction of the postoperative HUCKMAN-index in % of the preoperative value. In 16 cases there was only a very slight or no decrease of ventricular size

Reduction of ventricular size	n
Category 1: > 30%	11
Categroy 2: 10% - 30%	16
Category 3: < 10%	9
Category 3: 0%	7

Table 5. Correlation of clinical response and postoperative ventricular size

Correlation		n	%
Complete	+	18	42
Good	(+)	15	35
Poor	(-)	8	18,5
No	-	2	4,5
Total		43	100

Discussion

A great number of papers were published dealing with clinical improvement after shunting large series of patients suffering from NPH (1, 2, 11, 14, 16), but the authors did not stress the correlation of clinical outcome and postoperative ventricular size. Following the basic evaluation of KATZMAN and colleagues (4, 7) and the more sophisticated methods of LORENZO (9), the main reason for the development of ventricular dilatation in patients with NPH is a cerebrospinal fluid absorption deficit. According to that theory the improvement of the clinical state after correction of that defect by implanting a shunt should be paralleled by a corresponding decrease of ventricular size. This was only significant in small series (3, 15) but not valid in others (5, 6, 8, 12).

In comparison with other published results (1, 2, 3, 8, 10, 14, 16) our relatively good clinical response to shunting in a total of 33 patients or 77%, is mainly due to our strict criteria for the indication to perform shunt operations (13).

Comparable significant differences in the clinical outcome, depending on the duration of symptoms preoperatively, as described by other authors (2, 16), were not found. The higher percentage of clinical improvement among the group of NPH following trauma or subarachnoid hemorrhage is dependent more on the definite etiological factor than on the length of the clinical history before shunting, which was considerably shorter in this series. This result does not correspond with the findings of WOOD (16), but is in agreement with BLACK (1).

JACOBS and KINKEL (6) could find an objective clinical improvement in 6 out of 7 patients with additional signs of cortical atrophy. This excellent outcome does not correspond with our results of improvement of 3 cases out of 6 (50%). But our findings are in agreement with LAWS (8) and even better than those of BLACK (1). On the other hand, according to our results additional signs of cortical atrophy do not prevent an excellent or good clinical result as could be assumed by the evaluation of GUNASEKERA (3), who did not find any improvement in 6 patients out of that group.

In the series of JACOBS and KINKEL (6) 40% of the patients showed ventricles that remained enlarged in CT follow-up studies in spite of a significant clinical improvement. This corresponds with 10 of our cases. SHENKIN (12) also reported on 2 patients, who had postoperative clinical improvement although the ventricular size did not decrease after the shunt operation. Vice versa he was able to demonstrate a reduction of the ventricles in 10 patients without any clinical response to shunting. In the 3 patients of our series showing this phenomenon, the additional neurological symptoms (2 patients with polytrauma, 1 patients with parkinsonism) could have affected the disappointing clinical outcome. LAWS (8) found 5 patients who did not improve in spite of reduction of the width of the ventricles and 4 patients who improved without corresponding decrease of ventricular size, but he did not give an explanation for that phenomenon. Although we could find a better correlation compared to the authors mentioned above (5, 8, 12), we have to conclude that

1. The lack of a postoperative decrease of the ventricular size is suspicious of a blockade of the shunting system, but does not prove it and is often correlated with a continuous improvement of clinical state.
2. The reduction of ventricular size in patients with NPH is not necessarily followed by an improvement of clinical signs and symptoms.

In spite of thorough analysis of those cases with insufficient correlation, especially with reference to the genesis of normal-pressure hydrocephalus, to the preoperative neurologic state as well as to additional symptoms of cerebral atrophy, an incontestable interpretation of the missing correlation between clinical and computertomographic development could not be found. Consequently, in our opinion, the reduced absorption of CSF cannot be the origin of normal-pressure hydrocephalus.

Summary

Out of 43 patients suffering from NPH, 77% showed an excellent or good clinical response to shunting. The clinical result depended more on the etiology than on the duration of symptoms preoperatively. Signs of cortical atrophy on preoperative CT-scans worsened the prognosis of the clinical outcome, but do not exclude an improvement of the neurological state. In only 27 (63%) of our cases there was a distinct decrease of ventricular size. The failure to find an incontestable interpretation for the missing correlation (23%) between clinical and computertomographic postoperative findings proves, in our opinion, that reduced absorption of CSF cannot be the main or sole pathogenetic factor of NPH (Table 6).

Table 6. Comparison of our results and series with pre- and postoperative radiological evaluation of patients with norma-pressure-hydrocephalus. This table includes only those cases out of the series, which had systematic radiological examinations before and after the shunt operation

Authors	Year	n	Clinical improvement n	%	Reduction of ventricular size n	%	Correlation
SHENKIN et al.	1975	19	9	47	14	74	No
JACOBS and KINKEL	1976	20	16	80	12	60	No
WANNAMAKER et al.	1977	5	5	100	5	100	Complete
GUNASEKERA and RICHARDSON	1977	11	4	36	5	45	Good
LAWS and MOKRI	1977	30	17	57	18	60	Poor
SPRUNG and SCHULZ	1981	43	33	77	27	63	Poor

References

1. Black, P. McL.: Idiopathic normal-pressure hydrocephalus. Results of shunting in 62 patients. J. Neurosurg. 52, 371-377 (1980)
2. Greenberg, J.O., Shenkin, H.A., Adam, R.: Idiopathic normal-pressure hydrocephalus - a report of 73 patients. J. Neurosurg. Psychiatry 40, 336-341 (1977)
3. Gunasekera, L., Richardson, A.E.: Computerized axial tomography in idiopathic hydrocephalus. Brain 100, 749-754 (1977)
4. Hussey, F., Schanzer, B., Katzman, R.: A simple constant-infusion manometric test for measurement of CSF absorption. II. Clinical-studies. Neurology 20, 665-680 (1970)
5. Jacobs, L., Conti, D., Kinkel, W.R., Manning, E.: Normal-pressure hydrocephalus: Relationship of clinical and radiographic findings to improvement following shunt surgery. JAMA 235, 510-512 (1976)
6. Jacobs, L., Kinkel, W.: Computerized axial transverse tomography in normal pressure hydrocephalus. Neurology 26, 501-507 (1976)
7. Katzman, R., Hussey, F.: A simple constant-infusion manometric test for measurement of CSF absorption: I. Rational and method. Neurology (Minneap.) 20, 534-544 (1970)
8. Laws, E.R., Mokri, B.: Occult hydrocephalus: Results of shunting correlated with diagnostic tests. Clin. Neurosurg. 24, 316-333 (1977)
9. Lorenzo, A.V., Bresnan, M.J., Barlow, C.F.: Cerebrospinal fluid absorption deficit in normal-pressure hydrocephalus. Arch. Neurol. 30, 387-393 (1974)
10. Messert, B., Wannamaker, B.B.: Reappraisal of the adult occult hydrocephalus syndrome. Neurology 224-231 (1974)
11. Salmon, J.H.: Adult hydrocephalus: Evaluation of shunt therapy in 80 patients. J. Neurosurg. 37, 423-428 (1972)
12. Shenkin, H.A., Greenberg, J.O., Grossman, Ch.B.: Ventricular size after shunting for idiopathic normal pressure hydrocephalus. J. Neurol., Neurosurg. Psych. 38, 833-837 (1975)
13. Sprung, Ch., Grumme, Th.: Use of CT cisternography, RISA cisternography, and the infusion gest for predicting shunting results in normal pressure hydrocephalus (NPH). Advances in neurosurgery, Vol. 7. Marguth, F., Brock, M., Kazner, E., Klinger, M., Schmiedek, P. (eds.), pp. 350-360. Berlin, Heidelberg, New York: Springer 1979
14. Udvarhelyi, G.B.: Kritische Bewertung neuro-chirurgischer Behandlungsmethoden beim sogenannten Normaldruck-Hydrocephalus. Neurochirurgia 21, 1-8 (1978)
15. Wannamaker, B.B., Hungerford, G.D., Rawe, S.E.: Computed tomography in patients with successfully shunted normal pressure hydrocephalus. Computed axial tomography 1, 175-181 University Park Press USA (1977)
16. Wood, J.H., Bartlet, D., James, A.E., Udvarhelyi, B.: Normal-pressure hydrocephalus: diagnosis and patient selection for shunt surgery. Neurology 517-526 (1974)

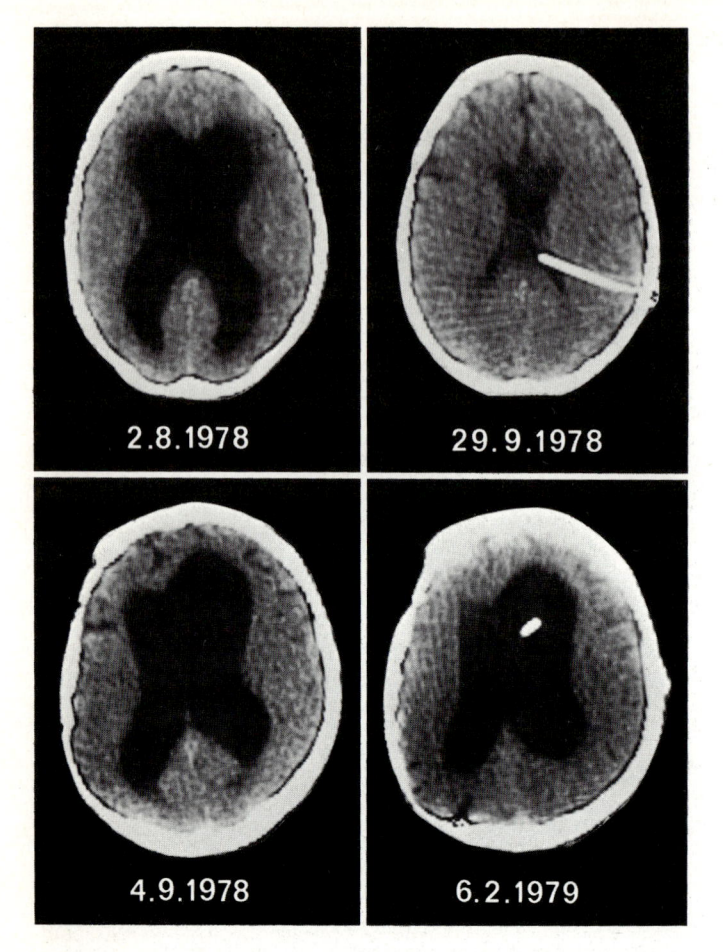

Fig. 1. Examples for complete and good correlation. *Above:* K.S., 70 years, idiopathic NPH. Note the periventricular rim of decreased attenuation values preoperatively. Six weeks (29.9.1978) after the implantation of a ventriculo-atrial shunt a decrease of more than 30% of ventricular size paralleled the excellent clinical improvement. *Below:* B.P., 33 years, posttraumatic NPH. Five months after the operation there was no reduction in ventricular size corresponding to no improvement of the clinical signs of dementia and gait disturbance in spite of a functioning Low-pressure-Holter-Shunt

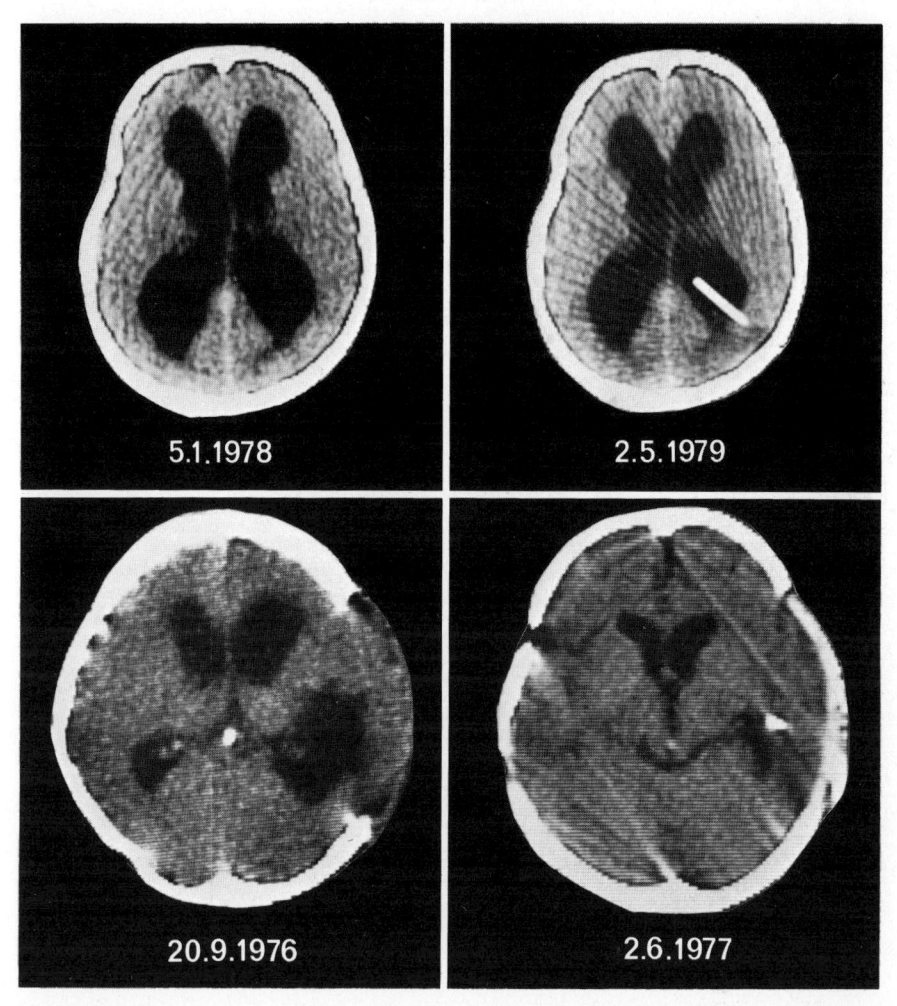

Fig. 2. Examples for poor and no correlation between clinical and CT follow-up studies. *Above:* S.B., 65 years, idiopathic NPH. More than 14 months postoperatively there is only a very slight reduction of ventricular size but he showed an excellent clinical response to shunting. *Below:* H.S., 44 years, posttraumatic NPH. In spite of the apparent decrease of the ventricular size 9 months after the Shunt-operation the patient showed no significant improvement of his neurological deficits

B-Waves and Periventricular Lucency (PVL) in Intermittently Normotensive Hydrocephalus

H.-J. SCHMITZ, M. BROCK, and G. B. BRADAC

Introduction

Since its description by ADAMS et al. in 1965 (1) Normal Pressure Hydrocephalus (NPH) has been considered the cause of a syndrome consisting of: dementia, gait disturbances, and urinary incontinence as a rule in the elderly. Its successful treatment by cerebrospinal fluid (CSF) drainage can often lead to curves. Various designations were proposed for this syndrome: *symptomatic hydrocephalus* (1), *surgically treatable dementia* (26), *intermittent pressure hydrocephalus* (7), *episodically raised pressure hydrocephalus* (26), and *intermittently normotensive hydrocephalus* (5). These difficulties in nomenclature arise from the poor understanding of the pathophysiology of this kind of ventricular enlargement (VE).

SYMON and HINZPETER (28), summarizing the literature, found 8 papers describing beneficial effects of CSF-shunting on NPH, while 18 papers, however, reported difficulties or disappointing results from CSF drainage. Therefore, proper selection of cases of ventricular enlargement which could be expected to improve following CSF-shunting still is of immediate practical importance. Due to these controversial results, a series of studies has been undertaken to design preoperative tests or criteria for the prediction of response to shunting in patients with NPH.

The clinical syndrome has been considered the most important criterium for surgical treatment (3, 4, 8, 12, 28). When gait disturbances are primary and predominate, shunting is believed to be successful. In response to CSF diversionary procedures (8) gait disturbances preceded impaired mentation in 12/16 cases, whereas in shunt failure mentation disorders had developed first in 9/11 patients.

Ventricular width, the callosal angle, dilation of sulci, and reaction to pneumencephalography (PEG) were also admitted to be of some help. The lumbar infection test is not always reliable for patient selection (24). Surgical treatment of NPH of known aetiology (i.e. following head injury, meningitis, subarachnoid hemorrhage) is accompanied by an 80% success rate (22, 23, 25). There is strong evidence that outcome is better and selection of patients more satisfactory if data from continuous preoperative intracranial pressure (ICP) measurement are taken into consideration for patient selection. Several authors (2, 5, 7, 27, 28) studied the variations of ICP associated with NPH. They reported "A"-waves and "B"-waves in patients responding to CSF-shunting.

Therefore, long term pressure studies appear mandatory especially in idiopathic NPH.

The results of a prospective study of STEIN and LANGFITT (25) cast doubt on the reliability of any other preoperative test or combination of tests for predicting shunt response. In NPH, the cisternogramm demonstrates the absence of isotope propagation into the ventricles possibly associated with deficient CSF reabsorption. In studies on experimental hydrocephalus (1, 11, 21), an alternate transventricular CSF-absorption pathway was suggested as a possible mechanism for compensation of impaired resorptive capacity. LUX et al. (14) reported an increase in periventricular water content in cats with chronic hydrocephalus and suggested that fluid from the ventricles penetrated the extracellular space of the brain to a depth of about 600 µm beyond the ependymal lining before it was removed by the blood. Partial destruction of the ependymal cells and loosening in the subependymal areas were thought to explain some of the morphological changes associated with transventricular absorption (10, 14, 19).

The equivalent of these changes on CT appears to be the periventricular lucency (PVL) (18). The aim of the present study is to investigate the importance of PVL in predicting the results of shunting procedures in intermittently normotensive hydrocephalus.

Material and Approach

Twenty-nine patients (19 men and 10 women, mean age 60.4 years), who had hydrocephalus on CT and were suspected to suffer from NPH were studied retrospectively. VFP was continuously recorded for a period of 27.5 to 358 hours in 28 cases. The recordings were analyzed for mean daily pressure, pulse amplitude and incidence as well as duration and nature of waves. PVL was judged present or absent on CT. Charts were revised for assessment of gait disturbances, mental disorders, and urinary incontinence. Supplementary sequelae such as ataxia, headache, vertigo, dysphasia, or clouding of consciousness were noted. The etiology of VE was considered. The minimum criteria for shunting included 1. VE on CT, 2. presence of either B- and/or ram-(R-)waves (5) and/or 3. PVL together with 4. the typical clinical syndrome. In most cases the ICP measurement was continued postoperatively, usually for 24 hours, to verify shunt function.

Results

Twenty of the 29 patients included in the study were suffering from idiopathic NPH; two had hydrocephalus following subarachnoid hemorrhage and 4 after head injury. Two had developed VE after posterior fossa surgery and one was caused by prior radiation therapy.

Patients showing the classical triad were assigned to group I. In six patients these symptoms were associated with additional sequelae (group II). Patients with head injury were gathered in a third group (Fig. 1).

Preoperative CT scans revealed PVL in more than half of the cases (Fig. 1). VE ceased completely after shunting in only 7 cases. Despite evident clinical improvement, 15 patients showed either only moderate decrease in ventricular size or none at all. PVL, however, disappeared after CSF shunting in all cases (Fig. 3).

Intermittent B-waves occurred in 27 patients (Figs. 1, 4). Analysis of the continuous pressure recordings revealed no significant difference in daily mean pressure values between groups I, II, and III. During periods of wave activity the pulse pressure amplitude tended to increase in all three groups. The pulse pressure ratio (pressure amplitude of B- or R-waves/pressure amplitude in the absence of waves (2) was about 2 in all groups. B- and/or R-waves amounted to 58.7% of the total recording time in group I, 10.6% in group II and to 39.1% in group III. A-waves were observed in only 2 cases. In a patient with head injury we recorded one A-wave in a 3-day monitoring period. Three A-waves in 3 days of ICP recording were observed in the case of NPH following radiation therapy. Twenty-four patients were shunted. Two died prior to shunting, one of pulmonary embolism and the other of lung cancer. Twenty-two ventriculoatrial (VA) and two ventriculoperitoneal (VP) shunts were implanted. Three patients were excluded from shunting, two because of absence of PVL and periodic waves only during less than 5% of recording time, and one because calculating of the pressure-volume-index (PVI) and outflow resistance (15, 16) yielded normal values.

Of the 24 patients shunted, 21 showed substantial improvement and 3 remained unchanged, as did the patients not operated on (Fig. 2). Continuous monitoring of ICP by CSF pressure measurement involved only minor complications. One patient developed an acute meningitis, while 1/3 of the group had elevated cell-counts without clinical signs of infection, in agreement with the figures of PÖLL et al. (20). In three cases, shunt operations were followed by chronic subdural collections, which could be treated successfully.

Discussion

A close correlation was found between PVL and B-waves. SHIGENO and coworkers (22, 23) demonstrated the presence of PVL in 7 cases of NPH following subarachnoid hemorrhage, whereas PVL was observed only once when no NPH developed. The occurrence of PVL in more than half of the patients with B- or R-waves thus renders it an important diagnostic phenomenon in NPH. An improvement rate of 21 out of 24 compares well with percentages reported in literature (28). The ratio of wave/non-wave periods of 58.7% is also in agreement with figures reported by SYMON (26, 28). In 1976 BELLONI and coworkers (2) stated that the pulse pressure ratio (pressure amplitude during waves/amplitude in absence of waves) is the most reliable parameter to indicate surgery. He found that in all cases where the pulse pressure ratio was greater than 2, successful shunting was achieved. We could not confirm this finding, since patients with ratios of 1.0 and 1.25 were shunted successfully in our series.

Conclusions

We feel that PVL reinforces the diagnosis and indication for surgical treatment of intermittently normotensive hydrocephalus in cases with clinical symptoms or known etiology of ventricular enlargement, particularly in the presence of B-waves and/or R-waves. One must, however, consider that PVL may possibly occur in cases where surgery would not be indicated, e.g. meningitis, multiple sclerosis, and leucodystrophies.

References

1. Adams, R.D., Fisher, C.M., Hakim, S. et al.: Symptomatic occult hydrocephalus with "normal" cerebrospinal fluid pressure. A treatable syndrome. N. Engl. J. Med. 273, 117-126 (1965)
2. Belloni, G., di Rocco, C., Focacci, C., Galli, G., Maira, G., Rossi, G.F.: Surgical indications in normotensive hydrocephalus. A retrospective analysis of the relations of some diagnostic findings to the results of surgical treatment. Acta Neurochir. 33, 1-21 (1976)
3. Black, P.M., Sweet, W.H.: Normal pressure hydrocephalus - idiopathic type selection of patients for shunt procedures. In: Advances in neurosurgery, Vol. 4. Wüllenweber, R., Brock, M., Hamer, J., Klinger, M., Spoerri, O. (eds.), pp. 106-114. Berlin, Heidelberg, New York: Springer 1977
4. Black, P.M.: Idiopathic normal-pressure hydrocephalus. J. Neurosurg. 52, 371-377 (1980)
5. Brock, M.: Klinik und Therapie des intermittierend normotensiven Hydrocephalus. Radiologe 17, 460-465 (1977)
6. Brock, M., Tamburus, W.M., Telles Ribeiro, C.R., Dietz, H.: Circadian occurrence of pathologic cerebropsinal fluid pressure waves in patients with brain tumor. In: Advances in neurosurgery, Vol. 6. Frowein, R.A., Wilcke, O., Karimi-Nejad, A., Brock, M., Klinger, M. (eds.), pp. 188-193. Berlin, Heidelberg, New York: Springer 1978.
7. Chawla, J.C., Hulme, A., Cooper, R.: Intracranial pressure in patients with dementia and communicating hydrocephalus. J. Neurosurg. 40, 376-380 (1974)
8. Fisher, C.M.: The clinical picture in occult hydrocephalus. Clin. Neurosurg. 24, 270-284 (1977)
9. Hemmer, R.: Dynamics of cerebrospinal fluid and pathophysiology of the hydrocephalus in the adult. In: Advances in neurosurgery. Vol. 4. Wüllenweber, R., Brock, M., Hamer, J., Klinger, M., Spoerri, O. (eds.), pp. 99-102. Berlin, Heidelberg, New York: Springer 1977
10. Hochwald, G.M., Sahar, A., Sadik, A.R., Ransohoff, J.: Cerebrospinal fluid production and histological observations in animals with experimental obstructive hydrocephalus. Exp. Neurol. 25, 190-199 (1969)
11. Kumar, A.J., Hochwald, G.M., Kricheff, I., Chase, N.: Positive contrast ventriculography in cats with experimental obstructive hydrocephalus. Investigative Radiology 11, 605-611 (1976)
12. Laws, E.R., Mokri, B.: Occult hydrocephalus: Results of shunting correlated with diagnostic tests. Clin. Neurosurg. 24, 316-333 (1977)
13. Lundberg, N.: Continuous recording and control of ventricular fluid pressure in neurosurgical practice. Acta Psychiatr. Neurol. Scand. 149, 1-193 (1960)
14. Lux, W.E. Jr., Hochwald, G.M., Sahar, A., Ransohoff, J.: Periventricular water content: effect of pressure in experimental chronic hydrocephalus. Arch. Neurol. 23, 475-479 (1970)
15. Marmarou, A., Shulman, K., LaMorgese, J.: Compartmental analysis of compliance and outflow resistance of the cerebrospinal fluid system. J. Neurosurg. 43, 523-534 (1975)

16. Marmarou, A., Shulman,K., Rosende, R.M.: A nonlinear analysis of the cerebrospinal fluid system and intracranial pressure dynamics. J. Neurosurg. 48, 332-344 (1978)
17. McCullough, D.C., Fox, J.L.: Negative intracranial pressure hydrocephalus with shunts and its relationship to the production of subdural hematoma. J. Neurosurg. 40, 372-375 (1974)
18. Mori, K., Murata, T., Nakano, Y., Hanada, H.: Periventricular lucency in hydrocephalus on computerized tomography. Surg. Neurol. 8, 337-340 (1977)
19. Ogata, J., Hochwald, G.M., Cravioto, H., Ransohoff, J.: Distribution of intraventricular horseradish peroxidase in normal and hydrocephalic cat brains. J. Neuropathol. Exp. Neurol. 31, 454-463 (1972)
20. Pöll, W., v. Waldthausen, W., Brock, M.: Infection rate of continuous monitoring of ventricular fluid pressure with and without open cerebrospinal fluid drainage. In: Advances in neurosurgery, Vol. 9. Schiefer, W., Brock, M., Klinger, M. (eds.). Berlin, Heidelberg, New York: Springer 1981
21. Sahar, A., Hochwald, G.M., Ransohoff, J.: Alternate pathway for cerebrospinal fluid absorption in animals with experimental obstructive hydrocephalus. Exp. Neurol. 25, 200-206 (1969)
22. Shigeno, T., Saito, I., Aritake, K., Kaneko, M., Mima, T., Sasaki, M., Nagashima, T., Sano, K.: Hydrocephalus following early operation on ruptured cerebral aneurysms. Neurologia Medico. chirurgica 19, 529-535 (1979)
23. Shigeno, T., Aritake, K., Saito, I., Sano, K.: Hydrocephalus following early operation on ruptured cerebral aneurysms: Significance of long-term monitoring of intracranial pressure. In: Intracranial pressure IV. Shulman, K., Marmarou, A., Miller, J.D., Becker, D.P., Hochwald, G.M., Brock, M. (eds.), pp. 235-240. Berlin, Heidelberg, New York: Springer 1980
24. Sprung, Ch., Collmann, H., Fuchs, E.C., Suwito, S., Duisberg, R.: Pre- and postoperative evaluation of hydrocephalus using the infusion test. In: Advances in neurosurgery, Vol. 4. Wüllenweber, R., Brock, M., Hamer, J., Klinger, M., Spoerri, O. (eds.), pp. 161-167. Berlin, Heidelberg, New York: Springer 1977
25. Stein, S.C., Langfitt, T.W.: Normal pressure hydrocephalus. Predicting the results of cerebrospinal fluid shunting. J. Neurosurg. 41, 463-470 (1974)
26. Symon, L., Dorsch, N.W.C., Stephens, R.J.: Pressure waves in so-called low-pressure hydrocephalus. The Lancet II, 1291-1292 (1972)
27. Symon, L., Dorsch, N.W.C.: Use of long-term intracranial pressure measurement to assess hydrocephalic patients prior to shunt surgery. J. Neurosurg. 42, 258-273 (1975)
28. Symon, L., Hinzpeter, T.: The enigma of normal pressure hydrocephalus: Tests to select patients for surgery and to predict shunt function. Clin. Neurosurg. 24, 285-315 (1977)

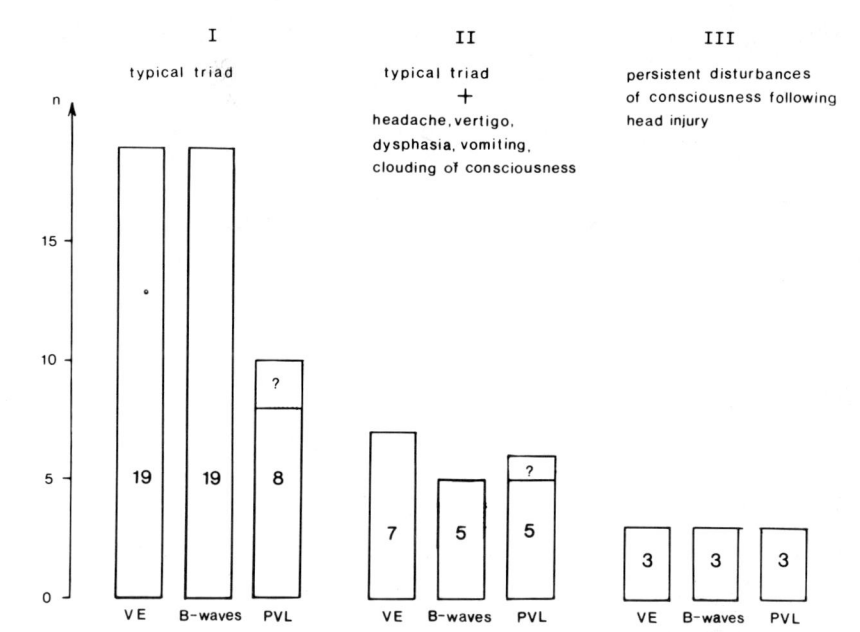

Fig. 1. Patients were subdivided into three groups according to clinical symptoms. Group I showed the typical clinical triad: disturbances of gait, disturbances of mentation, and urinary incontinence. In group II the typical triad was accompanied by additional symptoms. Group III consisted of patients with persistent disturbances of consciousness following head injury. The incidence of ventricular enlargement (VE), B-waves, and periventricular lucency (PVL) is symbolized by columns

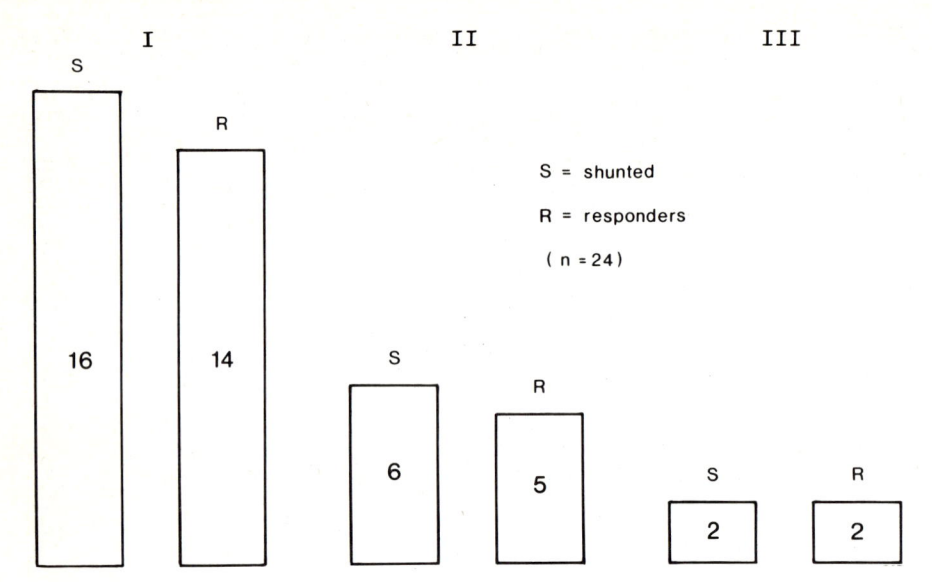

Fig. 2. Outcome of CSF shunting procedures. This figure shows the number of patients shunted (S) in the various groups as well as the number of patients who improved (R) after CSF shunting

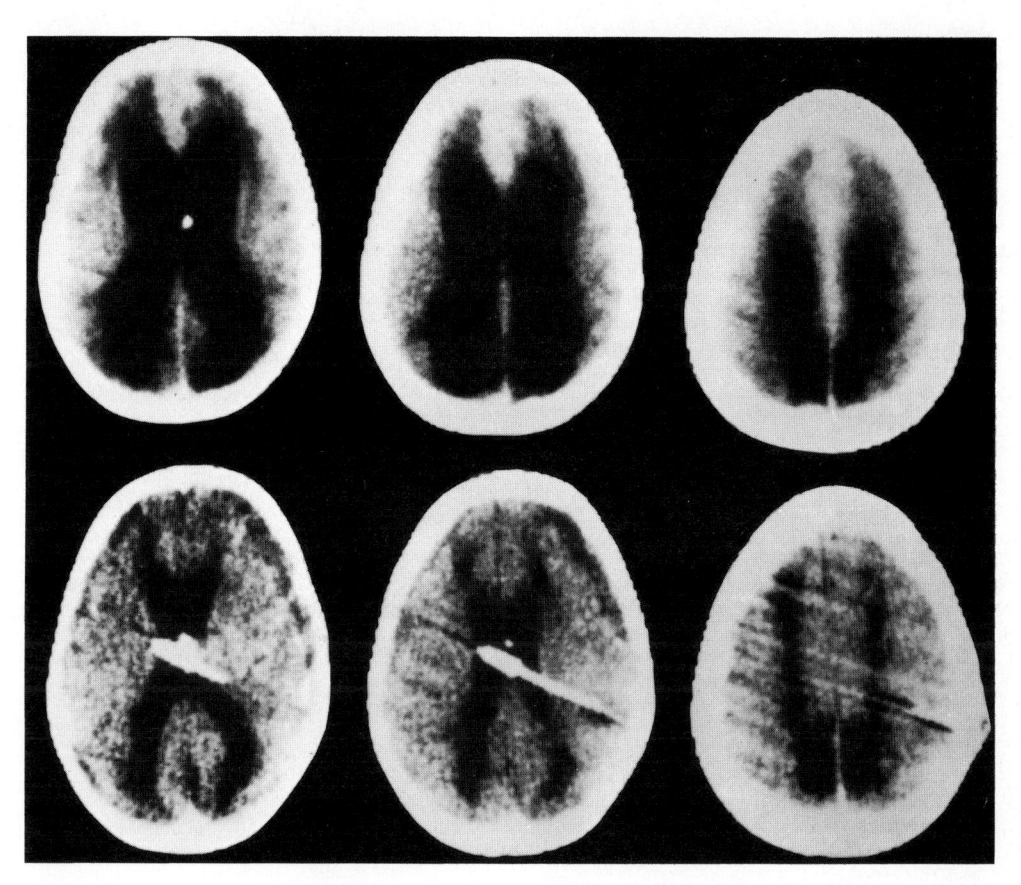

Fig. 3. Preoperative PVL (upper CT images). Ventricular enlargement (VE) and PVL ceased after shunting (lower CT images)

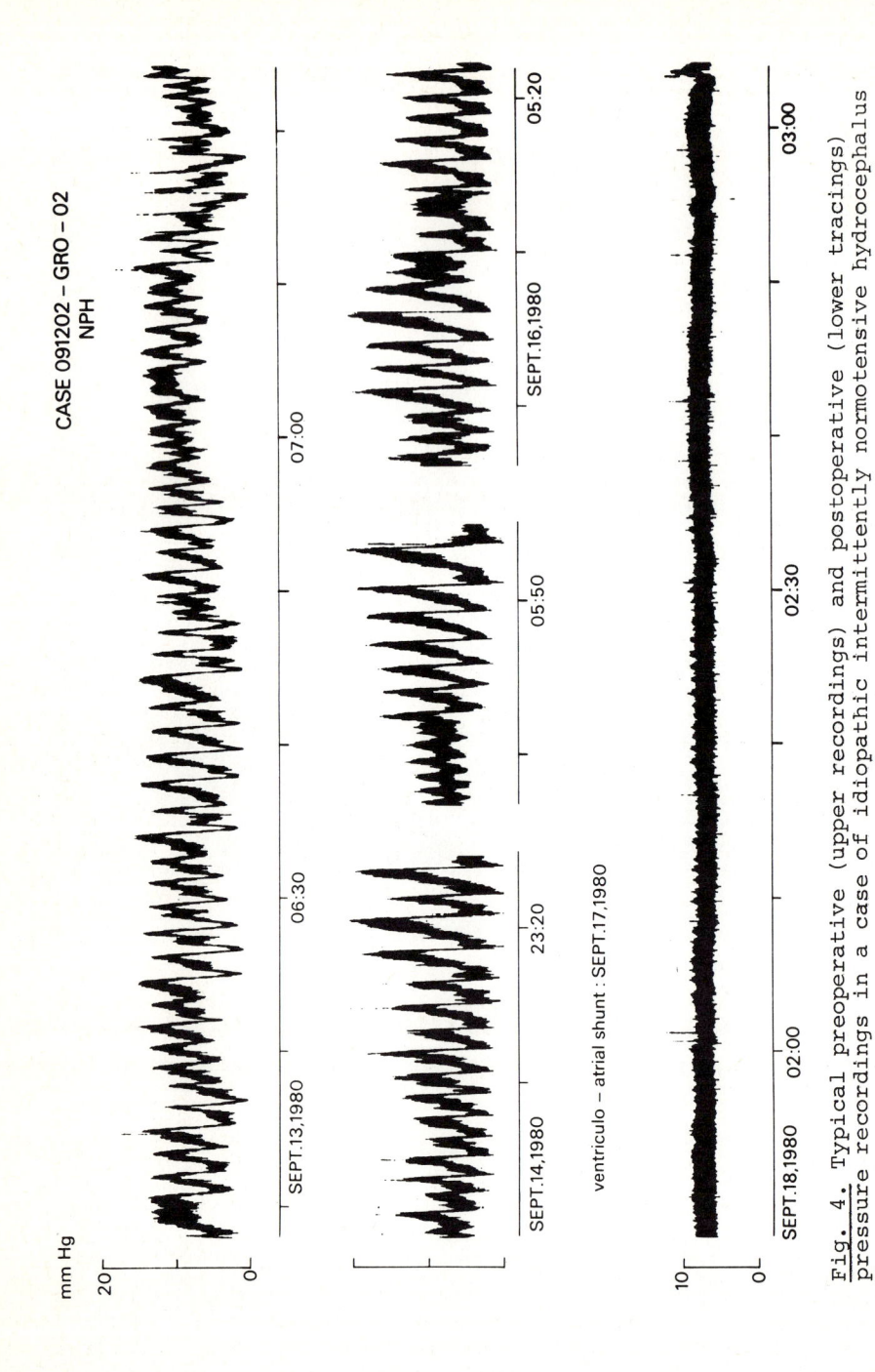

Fig. 4. Typical preoperative (upper recordings) and postoperative (lower tracings) pressure recordings in a case of idiopathic intermittently normotensive hydrocephalus

Slit Ventricle Syndrome – Computerized Tomography Aid in the Evuluation and Management

S. Tiyaworabun, H. H. Kramer, R. Kiekens, and H. K. Seibert

Prior to the introduction of check valve for regulation of mechanical redirection of cerebro-spinal fluid (CSF) from ventricle in hydrocephalus, over-drainage of the ventricular fluid with its subsequent complications, were the challenging problems left unresolved (1, 2, 7). After the invention of valves (HAKIM, HOLTER, PUDENZ, PORTNOY valve) with various opening pressures there is no doubt that many children are not only saved but their psychomotor development can be improved or even a normal level achieved, depending on the etiology of their hydrocephalus. However, they still provide considerable early and late complications, which remain the problems for further investigations. Among these many complications, overdraining phenomena have been found in a small but significant group of patients. With the aid of computerized tomography (CT), this phenomena leading to ventricular collapse can be promptly and accurately recognized, as small or slit-like ventricle (SLV) associated with slight dilatation of subarachnoid space. Moreover its course of treatment can be adequately evaluated and followed up.

The purpose of this communication is to review and analyse the clinical course, physical and neuro-radiological examinations, therapeutic approach and follow-up results of this subgroup of shunt-dependent hydrocephalus patients.

Material and Approach

From July 1979 until now, 560 hydrocephalus shunt-treated patients have been followed up in the hydrocephalus and spina bifida out-patient division of the neuro-pediatric and neurosurgical department of the university hospital at Düsseldorf. Among these, 38 patients were detected to have small or SLV in our CT/EMI 1010 Scanner, according to the measurement evaluated by PEDERSEN in 1979 (14). There are 26 male patients and 12 female. Their age ranged from 8 months to 18 years. 15 patients suffered from hydrocephalus associated with myelomeningocele (MMC), 18 from communicating and 5 from obstructive hydrocephalus of various causes. They received their first shunt at the mean age of 2, 9, 31 months respectively (Table 1). 29 and 9 patients received their first shunts and 9 and 29 cases their last shunts as ventriculo-atrial (V-A) and ventriculo-peritoneal (V-P) shunts respectively. The tip of the ventricular catheters resided in the anterior horn of right ventricle or third ventricle in 15 cases and in the posterior horn in 23 patients. Medium opening pressure valves were used in all cases except in 2 patients who received low (opening) pressure valves. Shunt revisions were carried out in 30 patients while 8 cases did not need them. Seven children received valvulography with Amipaque^R for suspicion of shunt obstruction.

Table 1. Type of hydrocephalus and age at first shunt of 38 patients

Type of hydrocephalus	No.	Age Range	Mean
Hydrocephalus myelomeningocele	15	3 days – 6 months	2 months
Communicating hydrocephalus:	18		
idiopathic	10	3 months – 5 years 3 months	1 year 6 months
post-meningitis	6	1 month – 1 year 4 months	5 months
neonatal intracranial hemorrhage	2	1 month – 7 months	4 months
Obstructive hydrocephalus:	5		
aqueduct stenosis	3	3 months – 8 years 2 months	2 years 10 months
idiopathic	2	2 weeks – 4 years 8 months	2 years 4 months

Pediatric, neurological and ophthalmological examinations were carried out regularly at 3 to 6 months intervals. The filling of time of reservoir prior to CT examinations during the periods with and without clinical symptoms were recorded.

We divided our patients in two groups. Patients in the symptomatic group are those who have a past history of one or more intermittent episodes of complaints, suggesting overdrainage. Those who never had any symptoms despite CT demonstration of SLV, belong to the asymptomatic group.

Results

In our series, 25 cases (66%) are symptomatic while others 13 patients (34%) are still asymptomatic. The most common symptoms were headache, nausea, vomiting, loss of appetite, malaise or irritability. There was only one case with disturbance of consciousness. The episodes usually lasted from a few hours to many days. Their frequency ranged from 4 episodes per week to once yearly. The intervals between the first clinical symptoms and signs after the last shunt in the two groups are shown in Tabe 2.

Only 2 patients (5.2%) developed their first clinical complaints within the first 6 months after shunting.

The correlation of the filling time of reservoir to the two groups of patients is shown in Table 3.

Table 2. Correlation of the duration of symptom-free interval since last shunt to two groups of patients with V-A and V-P shunts

Type of preceding shunt	(n)	Duration of symptom-free interval since last hunt (months)	
		Range	Mean
Asymptomatic group	(13)		
Ventriculo-atrial	(6)	13 - 154	95
Ventriculo-peritoneal	(7)	24 - 106	59
Symptomatic group	(25)		
Ventriculo-atrial	(15)	1 - 98	50.5
Ventriculo-peritoneal	(10)	5 - 71	31.4

Table 3. The relation of the filling time of reservoir at the time of CT SLV to the two groups of patients

CT - SLV	(n)	Filling time of reservoir		
		0" - 20"	20" - 3'	> 3'
Asymptomatic group	(13)	16	6	5
Symptomatic group	(25)			
Asymptomatic period		14	4	6
Symptomatic period		12	20	8

Ventricular catheters have been revised once or more times in 18 out of 38 patients prior to CT confirmation of SLV; 6/13 out of asymptomatic group and 12/25 out of symptomatic group. 3 shunt revisions were due to infection of the system.

Neuroradiological findings: 36 symmetrical and 2 asymmetrical SLV; 1 enlargement of 4th ventricle (Fig. 1); 1 subdural fluid collection (Fig. 2); 15 fronto-occipital diameter over 95.5 percentile (9) some scaphocephalic deformation of head, and 2 microcephaly. Valvulography was performed in 7 patients; 3 proved to have obstructive shunts, while the others 4 showed intact function of the systems.

All patients were treated conservatively with satisfactory results. Until now, no surgical correction was needed. Eight patients with previously known SLV developed shunt obstructions. Six of them showed hydrocephalic change in CT (Fig. 3), while 2 patients showed *normal* ventricular size (Fig. 4). Acute irreversible obstruction of the ventricular catheters was detected in 4 cases, who required surgical correction. Overrapid decompression was observed in 3 infants.

Discussion (Fig. 5)

Since the advent of CT, the ventricular configuration and their anatomical relationships to the surrounding brain could be promptly and accurately determined. Many investigations have been done to measure the normal ventricular system and the associated subarachnoid space. Among these, the results reported by PEDERSEN (14) are accepted by us for establishing our CT diagnosis of small or SLV. Some patients with CT-SLV may remain asymptomatic for a long period of time. However, some of them suffer intermittent symptoms and signs of shunt malfunction without substantial ventricular enlargement. This is known as *SLIT-VENTRICLE-SYNDROME* (SVS).

Some theories concerning the pathogenesis of SVS have been reported. EPSTEIN (4) explains that, with the passage of time, this potential collapse of the ventricular cavity may cause intermittent shunt obstruction leading to increased intraventricular pressure and thus dilate the ventricle, which again frees the trapped catheter. When the shunt again resumes its previous function, this vicious cycle is likely to be reactivated. Moreover, FAULHABER (7) proposed that the evacuation of the spatial buffer, which is mainly represented by the CSF, and the decrease of brain compliance, may be additional factors causing loss of the adapting properties of the brain to the minimal change of intracranial pressure (ICP). COLLMANN (3), however, states that it is probably the specific change within the parenchyma, which leads to rigidity of the ventricular walls, causing intermittent rises of ICP when shunt malfunction occurs. Our observations provide conflicting opinions to those of EPSTEIN:
1) About one third of our patients do not have any clinical complaints suggesting increased or decreased of ICP.
2) Only 4 patients have obstructed ventricular catheter after episodic SVS.
3) Fundoscopic examinations at the period of SVS does not provide signs of increased ICP and at the same time CT revealed unchanged ventricular size.
2 patients, who had catheter obstruction and manifested acute clinical symptoms and signs of increased ICP, have *normal* ventricular size, similar to those cases observed by COLLMANN (Fig. 4). However, another 6 patients have the CT picture of hydrocephalus, 2 with periventricular lucency; these contradict the theory of COLLMANN (Fig. 3). Thus,

based on the above observations, it can be said that, in cases of SLV with irreversible catheter obstruction manifested acute symptomatology of increased ICP, the morphological changes of the ventricular volume may be variable. This may be due to the reserve-volume of CSF and brain, the degree of stenosis or obstruction of the catheter, rate of CSF production and absorption, state of compensation and shunt-dependency of the hydrocephalus as well as the time interval and pressure contribute towards the build up of excessive positive pressure (ICP).

Intermittent headache, which is not associated with other symptoms, may sometimes be difficult to evaluated and thus need caution in approach and analysis. This problem has also been pointed out by EPSTEIN (5).

Usually, manual testing of the reservoir may give information about the patency of the shunt. However, as noted in Table 3, the filling time of the reservoir may give false positive as well as false negative results in cases of SLV.

Hence, in our experience, it lacks the clinical parameters to predict the existence of SLV and is often difficult or almost impossible to foretell the nature of ICP during the period of SVS.

Contrast medium study of the valves provide a great help and reliability, especially in cases with severe clinical complaints.

Some possible factors, which provoke the occurrence of SVS have been observed as follows:

1. dehydration after infectious fever, vomiting and diarrhea;
2. excessive negative pressure in right atrium in cases with respiratory distress and sport;
3. iatrogenic after overmanipulation of the reservoir.

However, they lack the objective confirmation.

Although we have not undertaken ICP monitoring in these children, it seems to us that the results in Table 2 may be influenced by the siphon effect (13, 15).

Much to our surprise, the majority of the patients have a long-term of symptom-free intervals since last shunt. Why this is so, remains unanswered.

The incidence of revisions of ventricular catheters prior to SLV in both groups of patients are almost the same. Thus, this factor seems not to have any significant influence on the development of SVS.

Overrapid decompression of CSF was observed in 3 cases in our series; they may be due to uncontrolled loss of CSF during operation in 1 case and the applying of low opening pressure valve in 2 cases. All children were treated promptly with lowering the head in supine position and i.v. fluid supply. They recovered within a few hours to days.

Prolonged hyperdrainage in infants may cause changes in the cranial volume and shape; mostly with scaphocephaly. Some of them were due to secondary synostosis of the sutures (7, 11). In our series, children with scaphocephaly were not the result of secondary craniosynostosis. Microcephaly (head circumference below 3 percentile) are observed in 2 cases, who show the typical skull changes as mentioned by KAUFMAN (11).

Secondary aqueduct stenosis or obstruction as was observed by FOLTZ (6), has not been detected in our collection. But its possibility does exist and requires further long-term observation.

Enlargement of the fourth ventricle in cases with shunting-hydrocephalus due to obstruction of the outlet of the 4th ventricle has been reported (8). Our case as shown in Fig. 1 shows no obstruction of the outlet of 4th ventricle at the initial pneumoencephalogram prior to shunting. This change was observed after CT defined SLV and evaded aqueduct after shunting.

Chronic subdural fluid collection was a rather common complication found by many authors (6, 10, 12). However, only one case was detected in our patients. It was found accidentally years after shunting and is not space-occupying but rather space-filling.

In comparison to the other series, our complication rate was rather low. This is probably due to the fact that low opening pressure valves were used more frequently than in other series. On the contrary, we prefer medium opening pressure valves.

All of our patients, except for the 8 cases with shunt obstructions, required no further surgical correction and were treated conservatively with satisfactory results. They are usually free from symptoms after lowering of the head in supine position, fluid supply and avoidance of reservoir manipulation. In cases which fail to recover after this trial, a further evaluation and management as shown in Fig. 4 should be considered.

In summary, there is no doubt that CT provides the only non-invasive investigation in detection of SLV. 38 children with shunt-treated hydrocephalus have been found with SLV. 13 patients are still asymptomatic while 25 children suffered from one or more episodes of intermittent symptoms probably due to over-drainage. This is called SVS. Until now, all children recovered from the complaints after the trial of conservative treatment. The fact that relatively few complications occurred in our series may be due to the insertion of medium opening pressure valves in these children. In cases with irreversible catheter-obstruction in SLV, CT may not reflect proportionally the manifested acute symptomatology.

Reference

1. Becker, D.P., Nuslen, F.E.: Control of hydrocephalus by valve-regulated venous shunt: Avoidance of complications in prolonged shunt maintenance. J. Neurosurg. 28, 215-225 (1968)
2. Carteri, A., Longatti, P.L., Geroga, M. et al.: Complications due to incongruous drainage of shunt operations. Adv. neurosurg. 8, 199-203 (1980)
3. Collmann, H., Mauersberger, W., Mohr, G.: Clinical observations and CSF absorption studies in the slit ventricle syndrome. Adv. Neurosurg. 8, 183-186 (1980)
4. Epstein, F.J., Fleischer, A.S., Hochwald, G.M. et al.: Subtemporal craniectomy for recurrent shunt obstruction secondary to small ventricles. J. Neurosurg. 41, 29-31 (1974)

5. Epstein, F.J., Marlin, A.E., Wald, A.: Chronic headache in the shunt-dependent adolescent with nearly normal ventricular volume: Diagnosis and treatment. Neurosurg. 3, 351-355 (1978)

6. Foltz, E.L., Shurtleff, D.B.: Conversion of communicating hydrocephalus to stenosis or occlusion of the aqueduct during ventricular shunt. J. Neurosurg. 24, 520-529 (1966)

7. Faulhauer, K., Schmitz, P.: Overdrainage phenomena in shunt treated hydrocephalus. Acta Neurochir. 45, 89-101 (1978)

8. Hawkins, J.C. III, Hoffman, H.J., Humphreys, R.P.: Isolated fourth ventricle as a complication of ventricular shunting. Report of three cases. J. Neurosurg. 49, 910-913 (1978)

9. Haas, L.L.: Roentgenological skull measurements and their diagnostic applications. Am. J. Roentgenol. 67, 197-202 (1952)

10. Illingworth, R.D.: Subdural haematoma after the treatment of chronic hydrocephalus by ventriculocaval shunts. J. Neurol. Neurosurg. Psychiat. 33, 95-99 (1970)

11. Kaufman, B., Weiss, M.H., Young, H.F. et al.: Effects of prolonged cerebrospinal fluid shunting on the skull and brain. J. Neurosurg. 38, 288-297 (1973)

12. Mc Collough, D.C., Fox, J.L.: Negative intracranial pressure hydrocephalus in adults with shunts and its relationship to the production of subdural hematoma. J. Neurosurg. 40, 372-375 (1974)

13. Portnoy, H.D., Tripp, L.: Antisiphon and reversible occlusion valves for shunting in hydrocephalus and preventing post-shunt subdural haematomas. J. Neurosurg. 38, 729-738 (1973)

14. Pedersen, H., Gyldensted, M., Gyldensted, C.: Measurement of the normal ventricular system and supratentorial subarachnoid space in children with computerized tomography. Neuroradiolog. 17, 231-237 (1979)

15. Yamyda, H., Tajima, M., Nagaya, M.: Effect of respiratory movement on cerebrospinal fluid dynamics in hydrocephalic infants with shungs. J. Neurosurg. 42, 194-200 (1975)

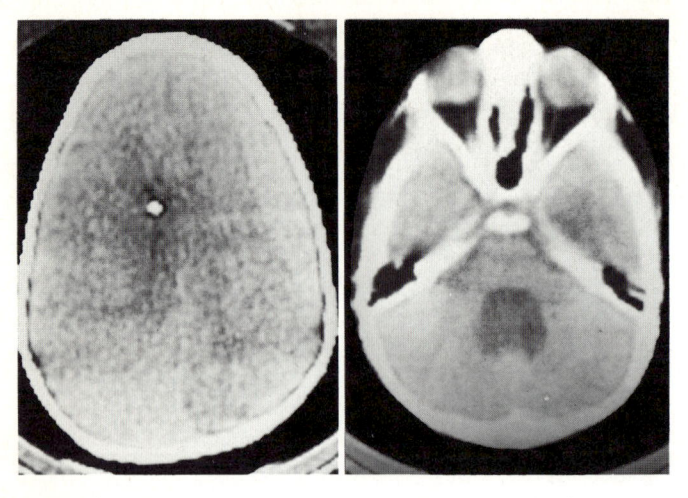

Fig. 1. Post-meningitis communicating hydrocephalus: Overdrainage leads to SLV *(left)* and secondary enlargement of the 4th ventricle *(right)*, possible due to secondary functional aqueduct stenosis

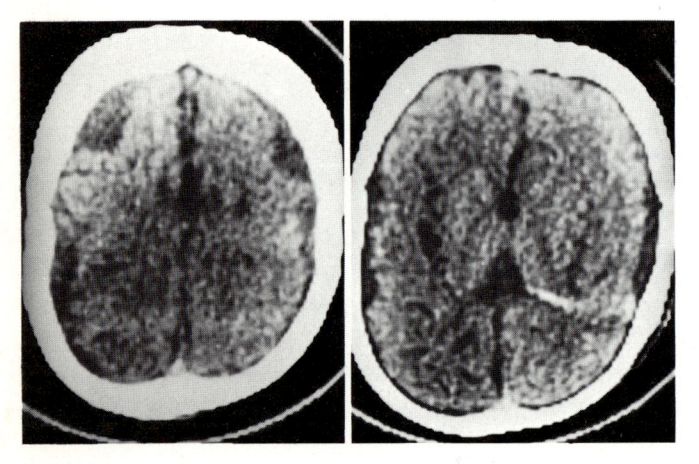

Fig. 2. Communicating hydrocephalus. Subdural fluid collection *(left and right)* after overdrainage with SLV *(right)*

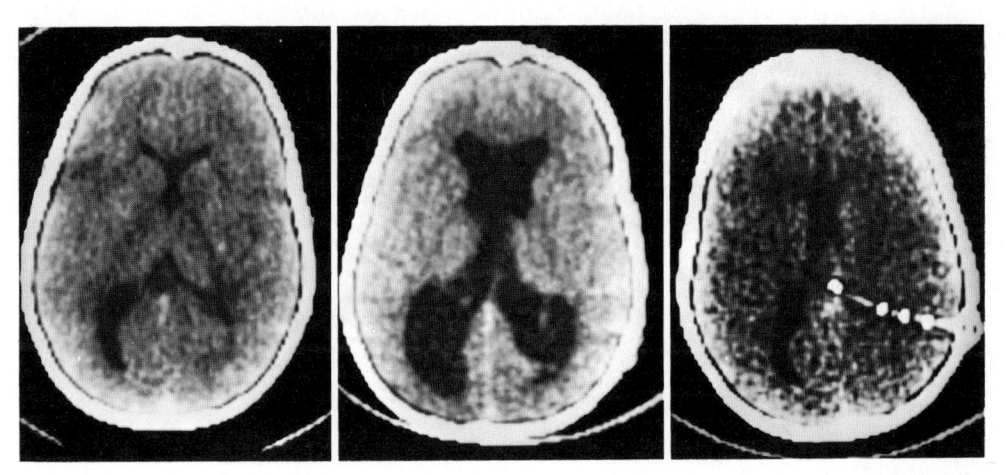

Fig. 3. Post-meningitis hydrocephalus. *Right:* SLV after shunting; *middle:* hydrocephalus with increased ICP due to ventricular catheter obstruction. After revision, slight dilatation *(right)* of ventricular system as compared to those of the left CT

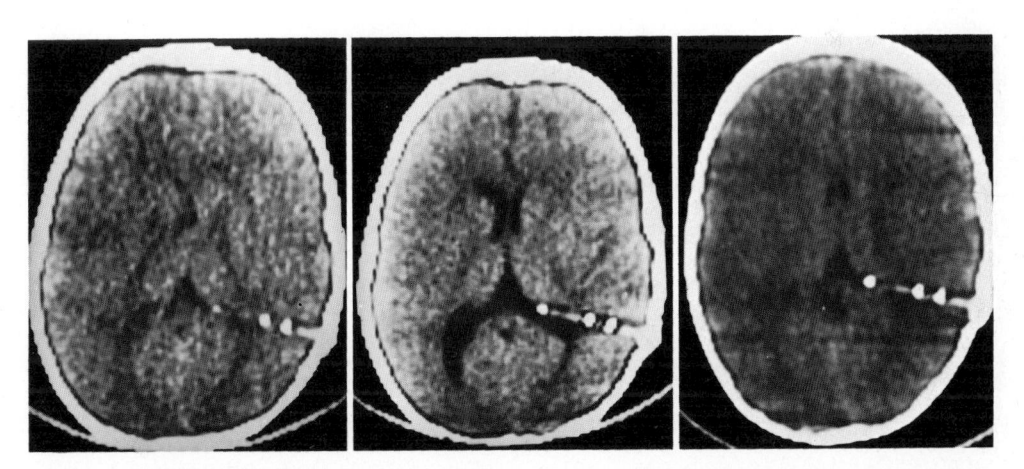

Fig. 4. Communicating hydrocephalus. *Left:* SLV after shunting; *middle:* normal ventricles with increased ICP due to ventricular catheter obstruction; *right:* after revision

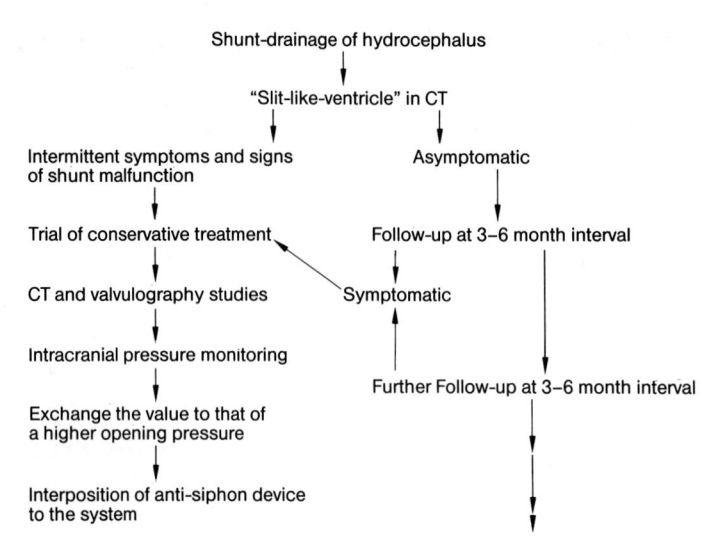

```
                    Shunt-drainage of hydrocephalus
                                  ↓
                      "Slit-like-ventricle" in CT
                       ↓                  ↓
Intermittent symptoms and signs     Asymptomatic
of shunt malfunction                      ↓
            ↓
Trial of conservative treatment    Follow-up at 3-6 month interval
            ↓                ↘            ↓
CT and valvulography studies    Symptomatic
            ↓                      ↑
Intracranial pressure monitoring   ↓
            ↓                  Further Follow-up at 3-6 month interval
Exchange the value to that of
a higher opening pressure                 ↓
            ↓
Interposition of anti-siphon device       ↓
to the system
```

Fig. 5. Therapeutic procedures of slit ventricle syndrome after shunting of hydrocephalus

Radiological Diagnosis Before and After Introduction of Computerized Tomography

H. K. SEIBERT, D. P. LIM, W. J. BOCK, and C. LUMENTA

Introduction

The introduction of computerized tomography has induced a decisive change in neuroradiological diagnosis. The number of examinations made at our hospital demonstrates the kind of changes that have occurred, and they reveal which conventional methods have retained their value.

In 1977, a computerized tomograph was put into operation at our hospital. We have compared the nature and the number of the diagnostic investigations made during the four years before the introduction of the computerized tomography, and in the course of the four years thereafter. We did not take into consideration the increase of the number of patients treated, after January 1, 1979.

Approximately 3,800 computerized tomographs are performed every year. This number has remained almost unchanged in the course of four years, with slight variations in either direction.

Figure 1 shows a graphic representation of the numbers of angiograms, encephalograms after insufflation of air, and ventriculograms made at our clinic (Fig. 1).

The number of the angiograms of cerebral vessels has declined but slightly, but its indications have changed considerably. Angiography has retained its value in elucidating subarachnoid and intracerebral haemorrhages, i.e. in the search of vascular anomalies. Moreover, angiography together with sonography is of value invariably in the diagnosis of disorders of cerebral blood flow. In the presence of tumorous lesions that displace the neighbouring tissues, an angiogram is often made use of to determine the vascularisation of neoplasms that narrow the intracranial space and that have already been demonstrated by computerized tomography. Encephalography after insufflation of air has practically been abandoned.

The number of the ventriculograms performed at our clinic has remained unchanged. This is especially true of pathological changes in the median line that narrow the intracranial space, of intraventricular tumors and of lesions narrowing the space in the brain stem and of the posterior cranial fossa. If an external drain has been placed to relieve increased intracranial pressure, the indication for ventriculography is self-evident. Thereafter, contrast ventriculography can be performed via the external drain. We suppose that ventriculography will keep its value in this field, for the number of ventriculograms performed at our hospital before and after the introduction of computerized tomography, has remained almost unchanged.

Figure 2 shows enlargement of the third ventricle in the dorsal direction revealed by contrast computerized tomography, although the tomogram does not allow recognition as to whether the tumor is located intra- or extraventricularly (Fig. 2).

Ventriculography shows a tumor with a cystic component in the dorsal part of the third ventricle (Fig. 3).

The computerized tomogram made after the ventriculography visualized the cysts that had not been opacified.

In the future, it will become possible to make use of scanners having good resolution, in order to obtain results by sagittal and coronal reconstruction.

In selected cases, ventriculography will be, now as ever, the superior method for the demonstration of lesions that displace neighbouring tissues, especially in the region of the median line, and in the ventricles.

Summary

Neuroradiological diagnosis has undergone a fundamental change after the introduction of computerized tomography. The number of air encephalograms, has almost come down to zero; angiography has retained its former value more or less, while ventriculography remains indicated in some selected cases, for the demonstration of intraventricular tumors and tumors located in the median line. The indications for ventriculography are simplified in those cases in which a ventricular drainage has been established for therapeutic reasons to relieve increased intracranial pressure.

References

1. Anderson, F.M., Segall, H.D., Caton, W.L.: Use of computerized tomography scanning in supratentorial arachnoid cysts. J. Neurosurg. 50, 333 (1979)
2. Black. H.: Intracranial epidermoids occurring simultaneously below and above the tentorium. Arch. Neurol. Psychiatry 49, 214 (1943)
3. Kishore, P.R.S., Krishna Rao, C.V.G., Williams, J.P., Vines, F.S.: The limitation of computerized tomographic diagnosis of intracranial midline cysts
4. Strand, R.D., Baker, R.A., Idahosa, J.O., Arkins, T.J.: Metrizamide ventriculography and computed tomography in lesions about the third ventricle. Radiology 128, 405 (1978)

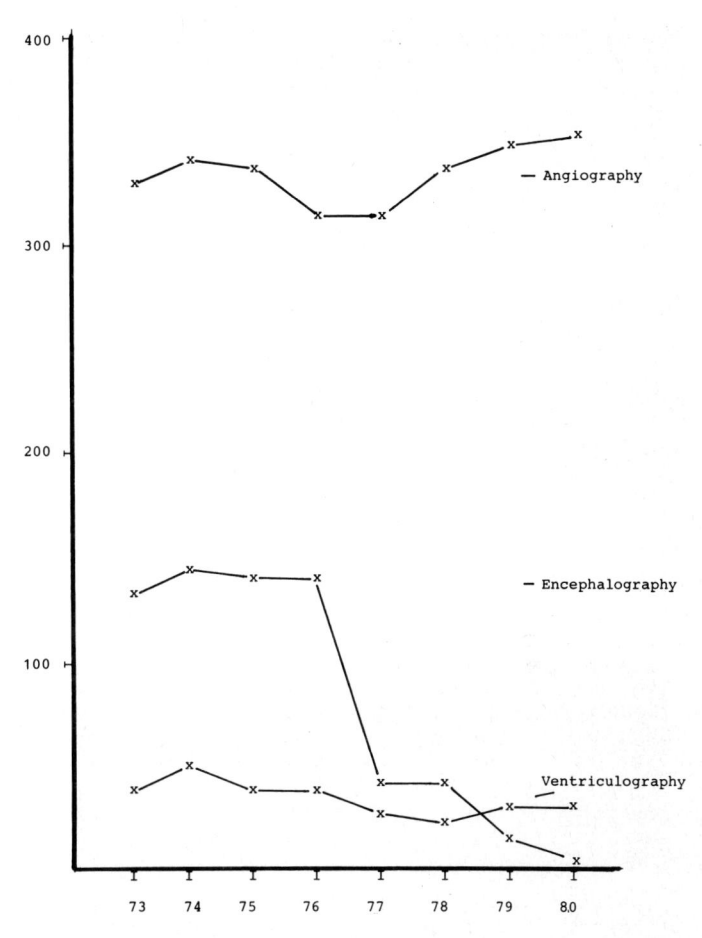

Fig. 1. Numbers of examinations in 1973 - 1980

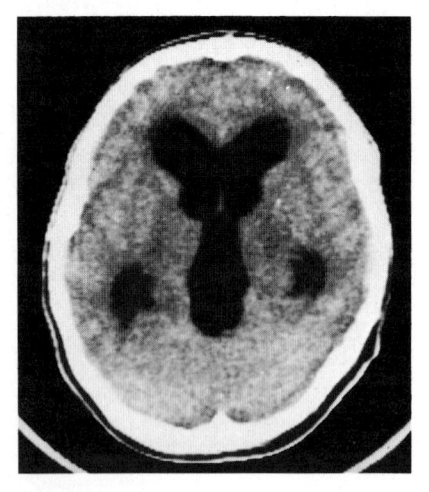

Fig. 2. Computer tomography. Enlargement of the third ventricle. The CT does not allow one to recognize whether the tumor is located intra- or extraventricularly

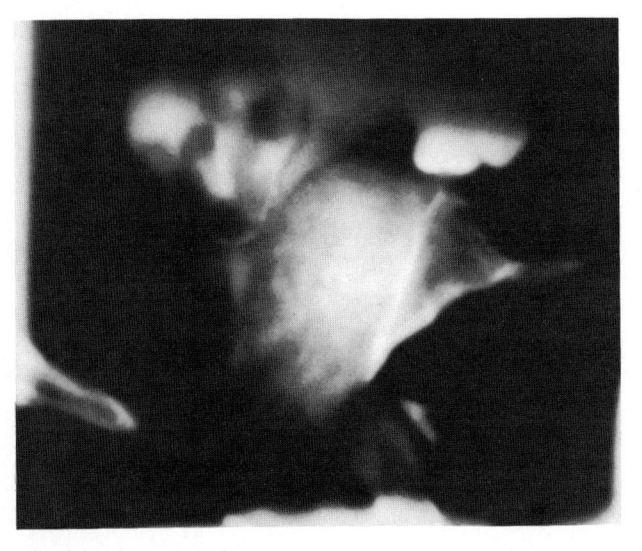

Fig. 3. Ventriculography displays a tumor with a cystic component, in the dorsal part of the third ventricle

Brain Metabolism

Normal and Abnormal Oxidative Brain Metabolism

S. HOYER

The mature and healthy human brain normally weighs around 1400 g. This is about 2 to 3% of the normal body weight. The brain is perfused by about 1000 l of blood daily and it uses about 70 l of oxygen and about 100 g of glucose in the same period. This corresponds to about 20% of the cardiac output and to about 20% of the needs for oxygen and to about 25% for glucose, respectively, of the whole organism.

It is well documented that these great requirements of the brain are ensured mainly by two important biological parameters which control blood flow and metabolism of the brain:
1. the cerebral perfusion pressure and
2. the partial pressure of carbon dioxide in arterial blood ($paCO_2$).

The partial pressure of oxygen in arterial blood has also been found to influence cerebral blood flow and metabolism but does not control them.

Under physiological conditions, the brain oxidizes only glucose to obtain energy and thus to meet functional and structural tasks (31, 32, 48). Glucose is transported from arterial blood across the blood brain barrier into the brain cells by means of a carrier-facilitated mechanism. Only 5% of the total amount of glucose used in the brain passes the blood brain barrier by diffusion (6-10, 21, 70, 77-79).

In the cytoplasm of the brain cells, glucose is metabolized glycolytically to pyruvate (90). Glycolysis is mainly regulated by the allosteric enzyme phosphofructokinase which works in concert with hexokinase and pyruvate kinase (71, 96). About 7% of the amount of glucose taken up by the brain is converted into lactate and released into the venous blood (18, 25, 32, 48, 96). In the mitochondria, pyruvate is metabolized by means of the citric acid cycle which is extended by a gamma-aminobutyric acid (GABA) shunt which is connected with an amino acid pool (87-89). The breakdown of one mole glucose by complete aerobic oxidation, i.e. oxidative decarboxylation and oxidative phosphorylation thus yields 36 mole ATP (60).

In neurosurgery, both disturbances in brain tissue itself, i.e. brain edema, changes in blood brain barrier function or increased intracranial pressure and variations in the transportation system, i.e. disturbances in arterial blood pressure or in the composition of the arterial blood may be responsible for abnormal reactions in odixative brain metabolism and may thus be of importance in a similar manner.

Reduction of cerebral perfusion pressure by means of increased intracranial pressure or by decreased mean arterial blood pressure does not seem to change cerebral blood flow over a wide range of cerebral

perfusion pressure from about 50 to about 150 mm Hg (17, 23, 38, 41
43, 45, 49, 52, 53, 56, 59, 68, 69, 102-104, 109, 111, 112). If autoregulation of cerebral blood flow is preserved no abnormal changes
in oxidative and energy metabolism of the brain were observed within
the range of cerebral perfusion pressure mentioned (49, 54, 99, 101,
110).

When cerebral perfusion pressure has been reduced below 40 mm Hg,
decreases in creatine phosphate and ATP and increased concentrations
in ADP, AMP, lactate and pyruvate in brain tissue were observed (54,
85, 86, 100, 101) along with reductions in both oxygen and glucose
consumption of the brain (16, 43, 49). From the view of cerebral
blood flow, it has been suggested that a reduction of brain blood
flow by about 50% is tolerated. Reductions below this threshold were
found to cause a decrease in cerebral energy state (24, 64). In
moderate arterial hypotension when autoregulation of cerebral blood
flow and the cerebral metabolic rates of both oxygen and glucose
were unchanged, both lactate output from the brain and lactate concentration in the cerebral cortex were found to be increased, but
the concentrations of adenine nucleotides had not changed (106).

It is well established that cerebral blood flow changes almost linearly with $paCO_2$ from about 20 to about 80 mm Hg: it decreases in hypocapnia and increases in hypercapnia (1-3, 5, 39, 46, 55, 66, 80, 83,
94, 107, 108).

The cerebral metabolic rates of both oxygen and glucose as well as
the energy metabolism of the brain remain unchanged in both moderate
hypo- and hypercapnia (4, 19, 20, 26, 33-37). However, the more hypercapnia increases, the more the concentration of glucose increases
and the more the concentrations of citric acid cycle intermediates
and creatine phosphate decrease in cortical brain tissue. On the
other hand, the energy charge of the adenyl(te) system remains unchanged even in extreme hypercapnia (26, 27, 97). It could be demonstrated that the glycolit flux is inhibited at the phosphofructokinase step, leading to a decrease in glucose consumption, but not
in oxygen consumption and thus resulting in a reduced formation of
pyruvate. Therefore, the CO_2 fixation rate is decreased at the pyruvate carboxylase step leading to a depletion of citric acid cycle
intermediates. Furthermore, it was observed that endogenous substrates such as carbohydrates and amino acids were oxidized instead
of glucose when $paCO_2$ values were further raised (14, 28, 29, 67).

In arterial hypocapnia, an increased glycolytic flux due to an activation of the phosphofructokinase step was observed along with a
gradually increasing pool size of citric acid cycle intermediates
with duration of hypocapnia due to a rise in pyruvate concentration
and to enhanced CO_2 fixation at the pyruvate carboxylase step (73).
Excessively low arterial partial pressures of CO_2 below 15 mm Hg
give rise to additional hypoxic lesions in brain tissue as demonstrated by a small rise in ADP and a small fall in creatine phosphate concentrations (63).

In arterial hypoxemia, cerebral blood flow initially increases slowly but progressively, with decreasing arterial partial pressure of
oxygen (paO_2). When paO_2 drops below 50 mm Hg, cerebral blood flow
increases abruptly, indicating a threshold phenomenon. However, oxygen consumption was found to remain unchanged until paO_2 had decreased
below 25 mm Hg, but both the cerebral uptake of glucose and cerebral
release of lactate were enhanced (18, 42, 44, 51, 58, 61, 72, 95).

In arterial hypoxemia, the glycolytic flux is obviously increased to maintain energy homeostasis at the onset of tissue hypoxia. Some ATP may be formed from glycolysis. Lactacidosis may shift the pH dependent creatine kinase reaction to maintain ATP stores at the expense of creatine phosphate. At the onset of arterial hypoxemia, an activation of the phosphofructokinase step was found to be responsible for increased flux (74, 75). After 30 minutes duration of arterial hypoxemia, the increased glycolytic flux seems to be maintained by activation of the other flux-controlling steps hexokinase and pyruvate kinase (44). As mentioned above, no changes could be observed in the concentrations of adenine nucleotides by decreasing paO_2 to about 25 mm Hg, but there was a decrease in creatine phosphate concentration (11, 62, 76, 98). It may be postulated that the well-established increase in cerebral blood flow may represent an important homeostatic mechanism (13).

When moderate arterial hypoxemia is associated with moderate arterial hypotension - a not uncommon situation under clinical conditions - autoregulation of cerebral blood flow has been found to be abolished and the oxygen consumption of the brain was reduced (39, 106). The pool of adenine nucleotides remained unchanged (106). In severe arterial hypoxemia with paO_2 below 30 mm Hg and ischemia due to carotid clamping (graded oligemia), a decrease in the cortical concentrations of creatine phosphate, ATP, and energy charge potential, and an increase in ADP, AMP and lactate could be observed (91).

In neurosurgery, vasogenic brain edema is of much greater importance than cytotoxic brain edema. Available data on oxidative metabolism in vasogenic brain edema are difficult to interpret: 1) in brain edema secondary effects due to increased intracranial pressure are often present and not easy to separate and 2) white matter, the cerebral region most affected by vasogenic brain edema (84) has surprisingly been investigated less than cerebral cortex.

Recent studies on metabolic changes in vasogenic brain edema showed no alterations of creatine phosphate and ATP in edematous white matter if dilution due to edematous water content was taken into account. However, lactate concentrations had increased (105). These findings were consistent with investigations in brain cortex (30, 65, 92).

The blood brain barrier has to fulfill two important functions. First, it protects the brain from deleterious substances which may be present in arterial blood, and second, it manages the exchange of substrates between blood and brain and vice versa by means of carrier-mediated transport mechanisms or pinocytosis (77, 78). Under pathological conditions, the barrier can be opened and permeability can be increased by shrinkage of the endothelial cells due to hypertonic solutions (81, 82). This process is mostly reversible. On the other hand, extreme dilatation of the capillaries may open tight junctions and thus alter junctional permeability.

This may occur in arterial hypertension beyond the autoregulative threshold (40, 47, 50) and also in absence of autoregulation of cerebral blood flow along with cerebral hyperemia due to other impairments in the brain such as head injuries (57, 93) or tumors (15), or convulsions (12, 22). Since it may be assumed that it is cerebral hyperemia and not seizure activity which causes the increased permeability across the blood brain barrier, it may be suggested that cerebral hyperemia due to hypoxemia or hypercapnie may also produce changes in blood brain barrier function.

References

1. Alberti, E., Hoyer, S., Hamer, J., Stoeckel, H., Packschiess, P., Weinhardt, F.: The effect of carbon dioxide on cerebral blood flow and cerebral metabolism in dogs. Br. J. Anaesth. 47, 941-947 (1975)

2. Alexander, S.C., Cohen, P.J., Wollman, H., Smith, T.C., Reivich, M., van der Molen, R.A.: Cerebral carbohydrate metabolism during hypocarbia in man. Studies during nitrous oxide anesthesia. Anesthesiology 26, 624-632 (1965)

3. Alexander, S.C., Marshall, B.E., Agnoli, A.: Cerebral blood flow in the goat with sustained hypocapnia. Scand. J. Clin. Lab. Invest. 22, Suppl. 102, VIII C (1968)

4. Alexander, S.C., Smith, T.C., Strobel, G., Stephen, G.W., Wollman, H.: Cerebral carbohydrate metabolism of man during respiratory and metabolic alkalosis. J. Appl. Physiol. 24, 66-72 (1968)

5. Alexander, S.C., Wollman, H., Cohen, P.J., Behar, M.: Cerebrovascular response to $paCO_2$ during halothane anesthesia in man. J. Appl. Physiol. 19, 561-565 (1964)

6. Bachelard, H.S.: Specificity and kinetic properties of monosaccharide uptake into guinea pig cerebral cortex in vitro. J. Neurochem. 13, 213-222 (1971)

7. Bachelard, H.S.: Glucose transport and phosphorylation in the control of carbohydrate metabolism in the brain. In: Brain hypoxia. Brierly, J.B., Meldrum, B.S. (eds.), pp. 251-260. London: Heinemann 1971

8. Bachelard, H.S.: How does glucose enter brain cells? In: Brain work. The coupling of function, metabolism and blood flow in the brain. Ingvar, D.H., Lassen, N.A. (eds.), pp. 126-141. Copenhagen: Munksgaard 1975

9. Bachelard, H.S., Daniel, P.M., Love, E.R., Pratt, O.E.: The in vivo influx of glucose into the brain of the rat compared with the net cerebral uptake. J. Physiol. (London) 222, 149-150 P (1972)

10. Bachelard, H.S., Daniel, P.M., Love, E.R., Pratt, O.E.: The transport of glucose into the brain of the rat in vivo. Proc. Roy. Soc. B. 183, 71-82 (1973)

11. Bachelard, H.S., Lewis, L.D., Ponten, U., Siesjö, B.K.: Mechanisms activating glycolysis in the brain in arterial hypoxia. J. Neurochem. 22, 395-405 (1974)

12. Bolwig, T.G., Westergaard, E.: Permeability of blood-brain barrier during electrically induced epileptic seizures. In: Cerebral vascular disease. Meyer, J.S., Lechner, H., Reivich, M. (eds.), pp. 256-259. Amsterdam, Oxford: Excerpta Medica 1977

13. Borgström, L., Johannson, H., Siesjö, B.K.: The relationship between arterial pO_2 and cerebral blood flow in hypoxic hypoxia. Acta Physiol. Scand. 93, 423-432 (1975)

14. Borgström, L., Norberg, K., Siesjö, B.K.: Glucose consumption in rat cerebral cortex in normoxia, hypoxia and hypercapnia. Acta Physiol. Scand. 96, 569-574 (1976)

15. Brock, M., Hadjidimos, A.A., Schürmann, K., Ellger, M., Fischer, F.: Regional cerebral blood flow in cases of brain tumor. In: Cerebral blood flow. Brock, M., Fieschi, C., Ingvar, D.H., Lassen, N.A., Schürmann, K. (eds.), pp. 169-171. Berlin, Heidelberg, New York: Springer 1969

16. Bruce, D.A., Schutz, H., Vapalahti, M., Langfitt, T.W., Gunby, N.: An intrinsic metabolic mechanism to protect the brain during progressive cerebral ischemia. In: Cerebral circulation and metabolism. Langfitt, T.W., McHenry Jr., L.C., Reivich, M., Wollman, H. (eds.), pp. 203-206. New York, Heidelberg, Berlin: Springer 1975

17. Carlyle, A., Grayson, J.: Blood pressure and the regulation of brain blood flow. J. Physiol. (London) 127, 15-16 P (1955)

18. Cohen, P.J., Alexander, S.C., Smith, T.C., Reivich, M., Wollman, H.: Effects of hypoxia and normocarbia on cerebral blood flow and metabolism in conscious man. J. Appl. Physiol. 23, 183-189 (1967)

19. Cohen, P.J., Alexander, S.C., Wollman, H.: Effects of hypocarbia and of hypoxia with normocarbia on cerebral blood flow and metabolism in man. Scand. J. Clin. Lab. Invest. 22, Suppl. 102, IV A (1968)

20. Cohen, P.J., Wollman, H., Alexander, S.C., Chase, P.E., Behar, M.G.: Cerebral carbohydrate metabolism in man during halothane anesthesia. Effects of $paCO_2$ on some aspects of carbohydrate utilization. Anesthesiology 25, 185-191 (1964)

21. Crone, C., Thompson, A.M.: Permeability of brain capillaries. In: Capillary permeability. Crone, C., Lassen, N.A. (eds.), pp. 446-455. Copenhagen: Munksgaard 1970

22. Cutler, R.W.P., Lorenzo, A.V., Barlow, C.F.: Changes in blood brain barrier permeability during pharmacologically induced convulsions. Progr. Brain Res. 29, 367-384 (1968)

23. Dinsdale, H.B., Robertson, D.M., Haas, R.A.: Cerebral blood flow in acute hypertension. Arch. Neurol. 31, 80-87 (1974)

24. Eklöf, B., Siesjö, B.K.: The effect of bilateral carotid artery ligation upon the blood flow and the energy state of the rat brain. Acta Physiol. Scand. 86, 155-165 (1972)

25. Erbslöh, F., Klärner, P., Bernsmeier, A.: Die Milchsäureabgabe des menschlichen Gehirns. Pflüger's Arch. ges. Physiol. 268, 120-133 (1958)

26. Folbergrova, J., MacMillan, V., Siesjö, B.K.: The effect of moderate and marked hypercapnia upon the energy state and upon the cytoplasmatic $NADH/NAD^+$-ratio of the rat brain. J. Neurochem. 19, 2497-2505 (1972)

27. Folbergrova, J., MacMillan, V., Siesjö, B.K.: The effect of hypercapnic acidosis upon some glycolytic and Krebs cycle-associated intermediates in the rat brain. J. Neurochem. 19, 2507-2517 (1972)

28. Folbergrova, J., Norberg, K., Quistorff, B., Siesjö, B.K.: Carbohydrate and amino acid metabolism in rat and cerebral cortex in moderate and extreme hypercapnia. J. Neurochem. 25, 457-462 (1975)

29. Folbergrova, J., Ponten, U., Siesjö, B.K.: Patterns of changes in brain carbohydrate metabolites, amino acids and organic phosphates at increased carbon dioxide tensions. J. Neurochem. 22, 1115-1125 (1974)

30. Frei, H.J., Wallenfang, Th., Pöll, W., Reulen, H.J., Schubert, R., Brock, M.: Regional cerebral blood flow and regional metabolism in cold induced oedema. Acta Neurochir. (Wien) 29, 15-28 (1973)

31. Gibbs, E.L., Lennox, W.G., Nims, L.F., Gibbs, F.A.: Arterial and cerebral venous blood. Arterial-venous differences in man. J. Biol. Chem. 144, 325-332 (1942)

32. Gottstein, U., Bernsmeier, A., Sedlmeyer, I.: Der Kohlenhydratstoffwechsel des menschlichen Gehirns. I. Untersuchungen mit substratspezifischen enzymatischen Methoden bei normaler Hirndurchblutung. Klin. Wschr. 41, 943-948 (1963)

33. Gottstein, U., Gabriel, F.H., Held, K., Textor, Th.: Continuous monitoring of arterial and cerebral venous glucose concentrations in man. Advantage, procedure and results. In: Blood glucose monitoring. Methodology and clinical application of continuous in vivo glucose analysis, pp. 127-135. Sttuttgart: Thieme 1977

34. Gottstein, U., Zahn, U., Held, K., Gabriel, F.H., Textor, Th., Berghoff, W.: Einfluß der Hyperventilation auf Hirndurchlbutung und cerebralen Stoffwechsel des Menschen. Untersuchungen bei fortlaufender Registrierung der arterio-hirnvenösen Glucosedifferenz. Klin. Wschr. 54, 373-381 (1976)

35. Granholm, L., Lukjanova, L., Siesjö, B.K.: The effect of marked hyperventilation upon tissue levels of NADH, lactate, pyruvate, phosphocreatine and adenosine phosphates of rat brain. Acta Physiol. Scand. 77, 179-199 (1969)

36. Granholm, L., Siesjö, B.K.: The effects of hypercapnia and hypocapnia upon the cerebrospinal fluid lactate and pyruvate concentrations and upon the lactate, pyruvate, ATP, ADP, phosphocretine and creatine concentrations of cat brain tissue. Acta Physiol. Scand. 75, 257-266 (1969)

37. Granholm, L., Siesjö, B.K.: The effect of combined respiratory and non-respiratory alkalosis on energy metabolites and acid-base parameters in rat brain. Acta Physiol. Scand. 81, 307-314 (1971)

38. Häggendal, E.: Blood flow autoregulation of the cerebral grey matter with comments on its mechanism. Acta Neurol. Scand. 41, Suppl. 14, 104-110 (1965)

39. Häggendal, E., Johannson, B.: Effects of arterial carbon dioxide tension and oxygen saturation on cerebral blood flow autoregulation in dogs. Acty Physiol. Scand. 66, Suppl. 258, 27-53 (1965)

40. Häggendal, E., Johannson, B.: On the pathophysiology of the increased cerebrovascular permeability in acute arterial hypertension in cats. Acta Neurol. Scand. 48, 265-270 (1972)

41. Häggendal, E., Löfgren, J., Nilsson, N.J., Zwetnow, N.N.: Effects of varied cerebrospinal fluid pressure on cerebral blood flow in dogs. Acta Physiol. Scand. 79, 262-271 (1970)

42. Hamer, J., Hoyer, S., Alberti, E., Weinhardt, F.: Cerebral blood flow and oxidative brain metabolism during and after moderate and profound arterial hypoxaemia. Acta Neurochir. 33, 141-150 (1976)

43. Hamer, J., Hoyer, S., Stoeckel, H., Alberti, W., Weinhardt, F.: Cerebral blood flow and cerebral metabolism in acute increase of intracranial pressure. Acta Neurochir. 28, 95-110 (1973)

44. Hamer, J., Wiedemann, K., Berlet, H., Weinhardt, F., Hoyer, S.: Cerebral glucose and energy metabolism, cerebral oxygen consumption and blood flow in arterial hypoxaemia. Acta Neurochir. 44, 151-160 (1978)

45. Harper, A.M.: Autoregulation of cerebral blood flow: Influence of the arterial blood pressure on the blood flow through the cerebral cortex. J. Neurol. Neurosurg. Psychiat. 29, 398-403 (1966)

46. Harper, A.M., Glass, H.J.: Effect of alteration in the arterial carbon dioxide tension on the blood flow through the cerebral cortex at normal and low arterial blood pressure. J. Neurol. Neurosurg. Psychiat. 28, 449-452 (1965)

47. Hossmann, K.-A., Hossmann, V., Takagi, S.: Blood flow and blood brain barrier in acute hypertension. In: Cerebral vascular disease. Meyer, J.S., Lechner, H., Reivich, M. (eds.), pp. 260-265. Amsterdam, Oxford: Excerpta Medica 1977

48. Hoyer, S.: Der Aminosäurenstoffwechsel des normalen menschlichen Gehirns. Klin. Wschr. 48, 1239-1243 (1970)

49. Hoyer, S., Hamer, J., Alberti, E., Stoeckel, H., Weinhardt, F.: The effect of stepwise arterial hypotension on blood flow and oxidative metabolism of the brain. Pflüger's Arch. ges. Physiol. 351, 161-172 (1974)

50. Johannson, B., Olsson, Y., Klatzo, I.: The effect of acute arterial hypertension on the BBB to protein tracers. Acta Neuropath. (Berlin) 16, 117-124 (1970)

51. Johansson, H., Siesjö, B.K.: Cerebral blood flow and oxygen consumption in the rat in hypoxic hypoxia. Acta Physiol. Scand. 93, 269-276 (1975)

52. Johnston, I.H., Rowan, J.O., Harper, A.M., Jennett, W.B.: Raised intracranial pressure and cerebral blood flow. Cisterna magna infusion in primates. J. Neurol. Neurosurg. Psychiat. 35, 285-296 (1972)

53. Jones, J.V., Strandgaard, S., MacKenzie, E.T., Fitch, W., Lawrie, T.D.V., Harper, A.M.: Autoregulation of cerebral blood flow in chronic hypertension. In: Blood flow and metabolism in the brain. pp. 5.10-5.13. Harper, A.M., Jennett, W.B., Miller, J.D., Rowan, J.O. (eds.). Edinburgh, London, New York: Churchill Livingstone 1975

54. Kaasik, A.E., Nilsson, L., Siesjö, B.K.: The effect of arterial hypotension upon the lactate, pyruvate and bicarbonate concentrations of the brain tissue and cisternal CSF and upon the tissue concentrations of phosphocreatine and adenine nucleotides in anesthetized rats. Acta Physiol. Scand. 78, 448-458 (1970)

55. Kety, S.S., Schmidt, C.F.: The effects of altered arterial tensions of carbon dioxide and oxygen on cerebral blood flow and cerebral oxygen consumption of normal young men. J. Clin. Invest. 27, 484-492 (1948)

56. Kjällquist, A., Siesjö, B.K., Zwetnow, N.: Effects of increased intracranial pressure on cerebral blood flow and on cerebral venous pO_2, pCO_2, pH, lactate and pyruvate in dogs. Acta Physiol. Scand. 75, 267-275 (1969)

57. Klatzo, I., Wisniewski, H., Smith, D.E.: Observations on penetration of serum proteins into the central nervous system. Progr. Brain Res. 15, 73-88 (1965)

58. Kogure, K., Scheinberg, P., Reinmuth, O.M., Fujishima, M., Busto, R.: Mechanisms of cerebral vasodilation in hypoxia. J. Appl. Physiol. 29, 223-229 (1970)

59. Lassen, N.A.: Control of cerebral circulation in health and disease. Circulation Res. 34, 749-760 (1974)
60. Lehninger, A.L.: Bioenergetik. Molekulare Grundlagen der biologischen Energieumwandlungen, S. 79-105. Stuttgart: Thieme 1974
61. MacDowall, D.G.: Interrelationship between blood oxygen tension and cerebral blood flow. In: Oxygen measurements in blood and tissues, pp. 205-214. Payne, J.D., Hill, D.W. (eds.). London: Churchill Livingstone 1966
62. MacMillan, V., Siesjö, B.K.: Brain energy metabolism in hypoxemia. Scand. J. Clin. Lab. Invest. 30, 126-136 (1972)
63. MacMillan, V., Siesjö, B.K.: The influence of hypocapnia upon intracellular pH and upon some carbohydrate substrates, amino acids and organic phosphates in the brain. J. Neurochem. 21, 1283-1299 (1973)
64. Marshall, L.F., Welsh, F., Durity, F., Lounsbury, R., Graham, D.J., Langfitt, T.W.: Experimental cerebral oligemia and ischemia produced by intracranial hypertension. Part 3: Brain energy metabolism. J. Neurosurg. 43, 323-328 (1975)
65. Matsumoto, A., Kogure, K., Utsunomiya, Y., Busto, R., Scheinberg, P., Reinmuth, O.M.: Energy metabolism and CBF in cold-induced brain edema: Comparison of the effect of dexamethasone under nitrous oxide and under pentobarbital anesthesia. In: Blood flow and metabolism in the brain, pp. 6.29-6.30. Harper, A.M., Jennett, W.B., Miller, J.D. Rowan, J.O. (eds.). Edinburgh, London, New York: Churchill Livingstone 1975
66. Meyer, J.S., Gotoh, F., Tazaki, Y., Hamaguchi, K., Ishikawa, S., Novailhat, F., Symon, L.: Regional cerebral blood flow and metabolism in vivo. Effects of anoxia, hyperglycemia, ischemia, acidosis, alkalosis and alterations of blood pCO_2. Arch. Neurol. 7, 560-581 (1962)
67. Miller, A.L., Hawkins, R.A., Veech, R.L.: Decreased rate of glucose utilization by rat brain in vivo after exposure to atmospheres containing high concentrations of CO_2. J. Neurochem. 25, 553-558 (1975)
68. Miller, J.D., Stanek, A.E., Langfitt, T.W.: A comparison of autoregulation to changes in intracranial and arterial pressure in the same preparation. Europ. Neurol. 6, 34-38 (1971/72)
69. Miller, J.D., Stanek, A., Langfitt, T.W.: Concepts of cerebral perfusion pressure and vascular compression during intracranial hypertension. Progr. Brain Res. 35, 411-432 (1972)
70. Nemoto, E.M., Stezoski, S.W., MacMurdo, D.: Glucose transport across the rat blood-brain barrier during anesthesia. Anesthesiology 49, 170-176 (1978)
71. Newsholme, E.A., Start, C.: Regulation in metabolism. Chichester, New York, Brisbane, Toronto: Wiley 1973
72. Noell, W., Schneider, M.: Über die Durchblutung und die Sauerstoffversorgung des Gehirns im akuten Sauerstoffmangel. Pflüger's Arch. ges. Physiol. 246, 181-249 (1942)
73. Norberg, K.: Changes in the cerebral metabolism induced by hyperventilation at different blood glucose levels. J. Neurochem. 26, 353-359 (1976)

74. Norberg, K., Quistorff, B., Siesjö, B.K.: Effects of hypoxia of 10-45 seconds duration on energy metabolism in the cerebral cortex of unanaesthetized and anaesthetized rats. Acta Physiol. Scand. 95, 301-310 (1975)

75. Norberg, K., Siesjö. B.K.: Cerebral metabolism in hypoxic hypoxia. I. Pattern of activation of glycolysis, a re-evaluation. Brain Res. 86, 31-44 (1975)

76. Norberg, K., Siesjö, B.K.: Cerebral metabolism in hypoxic hypoxia. II. Citric acid cycle intermediates and associated amino acids. Brain Res. 86, 45-54 (1975)

77. Oldendorf, W.H.: Brain uptake of radiolabeled amino acids, amines and hexoses after arterial injection. Am. J. Physiol. 221, 1629-1639 (1971)

78. Oldendorf, W.H.: Blood-brain barrier. In: Brain metabolism and cerebral disorders, pp. 163-180. Himwich, H.E. (ed.). New York: Spectrum 1976

79. Pardridge, W.M., Oldendorf, W.H.: Transport of metabolic substrates through the blood-brain barrier. J. Neurochem. 28, 5-12 (1977)

80. Raichle, M.E., Posner, J.B., Plum, F.: CBF during and after hyperventilation. Arch. Neurol. 23, 394-403 (1970)

81. Rapoport, S.J.: Effect of concentrated solutions on the blood-brain barrier. Am. J. Physiol. 219, 270-274 (1970)

82. Rapoport, S.J., Hori, M., Klatzo, I.: Testing of a hypothesis for osmotic opening of the blood-brain barrier. Am. J. Physiol. 223, 323-331 (1972)

83. Reivich, M.: Arterial pCO_2 and cerebral hemodynamics. Am. J. Physiol. 206, 25-32 (1964)

84. Reulen, J.J.: Vasogenic brain oedema. Br. J. Anaesth. 48, 741-752 (1976)

85. Reulen, H.J., Steude, U., Brendel, W., Medzihradsky, F.: Elektrolyt- und Metabolitkonzentrationen im Gehirn nach normovolämischer Drucksenkung. Z. Ges. Exp. Med. 146, 241-260 (1968)

86. Roth, E., Schüler, W., Suleder, O., Sobol, B.: Metabolitkonzentrationen in Herz, Gehirn, Niere und Leber des Hundes bei kontrollierter Hypotension. Z. Ges. Exp. Med. 144, 258-272 (1967)

87. Sacks, W.: Cerebral metabolism of isotopic glucose in normal human subjects. J. Appl. Physiol. 10, 37-44 (1957)

88. Sacks, W.: Cerebral metabolism of doubly labeled glocuse in humans in vivo. J. Appl. Physiol. 20, 117-130 (1965)

89. Sacks, W.: Cerebral metabolism in vivo. In: Handbook of Neurochemistry, Vol. 1, pp. 301-324. Lajtha, A. (ed.). New York: Plenum 1969

90. Sacks, W.: Human brain metabolism in vivo. In: Brain metabolism and cerebral disorders, pp. 89-127. Himwich, H.E. (ed.). New York: Spectrum 1976

91. Salford, L.G., Plum, F., Siesjö, B.K.: Graded hypoxia-oligemia in rat brain. I. Biochemical alterations and their implications. Arch. Neurol. 29, 227-233 (1973)

92. Schmiedek, P., Baethmann, A., Sippel, G., Oettinger, W., Enzenbach, R., Marguth, F., Brendel, W.: Energy state and glycolysis in human cerebral edema. J. Neurosurg. 40, 351-364 (1974)

93. Schutta, H.S., Kassell, N.F., Langfitt, T.W.: Brain swelling produced by injury and aggravated by arterial hypertension. A light and electromicroscopic study. Brain 91, 281-294 (1968)

94. Severinghaus, J.W., Lassen, N.A.: Step hypocapnia to separate arterial from tissue pCO_2 in the regulation of cerebral blood flow. Circulation Res. 20, 272-278 (1967)

95. Shimojyo, S., Scheinberg, P., Kogure, K., Reinmuth, O.M.: The effects of graded hypoxia upon transient cerebral blood flow and oxygen consumption. Neurology (Minneap.) 18, 127-133 (1968)

96. Siesjö, B.K.: Brain energy metabolism. Chichester, New York, Brisbane, Toronto: Wiley 1978

97. Siesjö, B.K., Folbergrova, J., MacMillan, V.: The effect of hypercapnia upon intracellular pH in the brain, evaluated by the bicarbonate-carbonic acid method and from the creatine phosphokinase equilibrium. J. Neurochem. 19, 2483-2495 (1972)

98. Siesjö, B.K., Nilsson, L.: The influence of arterial hypoxemia upon labile phosphates and upon extracellular and intracellular lactate and pyruvate concentrations in the rat brain. Scand. J. Clin. Lab. Invest. 27, 83-96 (1971)

99. Siesjö. B.K., Nilsson, L., Rokeach, M., Zwetnow, N.N.: Energy metabolism of the brain at reduced cerebral perfusion pressures and in arterial hypoxaemia. In: Brain hypoxia, pp. 79-93. Brierley, J.B., Meldrum, B.S. (eds.). London: Heinemann 1971

100. Siesjö, B.K., Zwetnow, N.N.: Effects of increased cerebrospinal fluid pressure upon adenine nucleotides and upon lactate and pyruvate in the rat brain. Acta Neurol. Scand. 46, 187-202 (1970)

101. Siesjö, B.K., Zwetnow, N.N.: The effect of hypovolemic hypotension on extra- and intracellular acid-base parameters and energy metabolism in the rat brain. Acty Physiol. Scand. 79, 114-124 (1970)

102. Strandgaard, S., Mackenzie, E.T., Sengupta, D., Rowan, J.O., Lassen, N.A., Harper, A.M.: Upper limit of autoregulation of cerebral blood flow in the baboon. Circulation Res. 34, 435-440 (1974)

103. Strandgaard, S., Olesen, J., Skinhøj, E., Lassen, N.A.: Autoregulation of brain circulation in severe arterial hypertension. Br. Med. J. 1, 507-510 (1973)

104. Strandgaard, S., Sengupta, D., Mackenzie, E.T., Rowan, J.O., Olesen, J., Skinhøj, E., Lassen, N.A., Harper, A.M.: The lower and upper limits for autoregulation of cerebral blood flow. In: Cerebral circulation and metabolism, pp. 3-6. Langfitt, T.W., McHenry Jr., L.C., Reivich, M., Wollman, H. (eds.). Berlin, Heidelberg, New York: Springer 1975

105. Sutton, L.N., Bruce, D.A., Welsh, F.A., Jaggi, J.L.: Metabolic and electrophysiologic consequences of vasogenic edema. In: Advances in Neurology, Vol. 28, pp. 241-254. Cervôs-Navarro, J., Ferszt, R. (eds.). New York: Raven 1980

106. Wiedemann, K., Weinhardt, F., Hamer, J., Wund, G., Berlet, H., Hoyer, S.: Einfluß von gleichzeitiger mäßiger arterieller Hypoxamie und mäßiger hypovolämischer Hypotension auf Gehirndurchblutung, oxidativen und Energiestoffwechsel des Gehirns beim Hund. Anaesthesist 28, 290-298 (1979)

107. Wollman, H., Alexander, S.C., Cohen, P.J., Smith, T.C., Chase, P.E., van der Molen, R.A.: Cerebral circulation during anesthesia and hyperventilation in man. Thiopental induction to nitrous oxide and d-tubocurarine. Anesthesiology 26, 329-334 (1965)

108. Wollman, H., Smith, T.C., Stephen, G.W., Colton, E.T., Gleaton, H.E., Alexander, S.C.: Effects of extremes of respiratory and metabolic alkalosis on cerebral blood flow in man. J. Appl. Physiol. 24, 60-65 (1968)

109. Wüllenweber, R., Gött, U., Szántó, J.: Beobachtungen zur Regulation der Hirndurchblutung. Acta Neurochir. 16, 137-163 (1967)

110. Zwetnow, N.N.: The influence of an icreased intracranial pressure on the lactate, pyruvate, bicarbonate, phosphocreatine, ATP, ADP and AMP concentrations of the cerebral cortex of dogs. Acta Physiol. Scand. 79, 158-166 (1970)

111. Zwetnow, N.N.: Effects of increased cerebrospinal fluid pressure on the blood flow and on the energy metabolism of the brain. Acta Physiol. Scand. Suppl. 339, 1-31 (1970)

Neuroendocrinological Aspects in Cases of Brain Death After Severe Brain Injury

G. KLINGELHÖFFER and E. HALVES

Introduction

In evaluating the clinical state of patients with a severe brain injury, the actual brain function can be determined by an examination of the central and the peripheral reflexes (5, 11). Additional information is obtained from the course of the laboratory and clinical findings, the electroencephalogram (EEG) and the cerebral angiogram. In practice, not all of these investigations will always be available or necessary (7). In case of the brain death e.g. of a kidney-donor however, the absent blood supply to the brain must be demonstrated by cerebral angiography. If the contrast-medium stops before reaching the base of the skull, one can conclude that there is also a failure of the blood supply to the Hypothalamic-Pituitary-System, and as a result of this, the whole neuroendocrine system is not perfused. The purpose of the present investigation was to find out whether patients after a severe brain injury with signs of brain death can be stimulated neuroendocrinologically, and if so, whether there are certain patterns of behaviour.

Material

Twenty patients were investigated, 6 female and 14 male aged between 15 and 63 years (average age 31,3 years). Seven patients were surgically treated, whilst in the other 13 patients surgical treatment was either not necessary or not possible. Because of technical reasons, or rather because of cessation of the circulation of the blood, brain death could not be documented by angiography or EEG in all of the patients. None of the patients however showed any central reflexes when they were examined. In two patients, angiography showed contrast medium in the area of the "PICA" (posterior inferior cerebellar artery), three showed a retarded internal carotid artery picture. The stimulation test was performed with 200 µg TRH (thyrotrophin-releasing hormone), 100 µg LH-RH (luteinizing hormone releasing hormone) and 500 ml of a 6 percent Arginin-Hydrochloride solution infused over a period of 30 minutes. After the determination of the basal level, blood was taken at intervals of 15, 30, 60, 90 and 120 minutes. The determination of the hormones was accomplished by Radioimmunoassay (RIA). The human growth hormone (HGH), prolactin (hPRL), luteinizing hormone (LH) and thyrotropin (TSH) were ascertained. In evaluating the TSH, a co-existent hyperthyroid metabolic state was excluded by a simultaneous analysis of triiodothyronine (T_3) and thyroxine (T_4). In addition, the spontaneous fluctuations of cortisol were measured.

Results

From the neuroendocrinological point of view the patients with brain death behave differently. Even the individual specific functions may differ within the same patient. There are, however, nearly always elevated basal levels in patients who have only a short survival time; whilst patients who are treated over a longer period show lower basal levels. This fact is also demonstrated by the fall in the average values when examinations are repeated within the same patient. In contrast to the HGH where one can see a weak or delayed response in only two of 20 patients, the levels of hPRL, TSH and LH occasionally show a distinct response. Patients with high hPRL levels resulting from the absence of prolactin-inhibiting-factor (PIF) can be partly stimulated by the TRH in the anterior pituitary lobe. The intact function of adenohypophysis for hPRL is recorded also in this particular case by a simultaneous increase in TSH. In case of a low hPRL, two groups of patients can be identified. One group shows a general pituitary insufficiency whilst the other one shows only a partial pituitary insufficiency. This phenomenon can be explained by a dependence on the dosage of the administered TRH. After the administration of LH-RH there is a definite tendency for the level of LH to rise. For example an eighteen years old female patient showed a distinct increase of LH in response to LH-RH, at a time when brain death had already been confirmed for over 24 hours. Even in one patient who had been treated for over 8 days a release of LH can be achieved. This effect is specific for LH, since all the other hormones mentioned above showed no response. A definite response from TSH was achieved only twice, 80 percent of the patients examined showed spontaneous fluctuations at or below basal levels. Apart from the above-mentioned dependence on the dosage of the releasing hormone for TSH response, pharmacological effects of current medication (e.g. phenytoin, steroids [1, 9]) have to be taken into consideration. Finally the measured cortisol levels show only random fluctuations around a variety of individual values. This leads to the assumption that the corticotrophin (ACTH)-cortisol-axis has been disrupted. If there are excessively high measured cortisol levels, these will not be observed to fall following therapeutic dexamethasone.

Discussion

It has to be noted that with so-called brain death, documented by angiography and EEG, a loss of function of the Hypothalamic-Pituitary-system need not be present in every case ([6]). Even if one excludes a documented intracerebral blood supply, the releasing hormones which have been given intravenously seem to be able to reach the hypothalamic-system by vascular or non-vascular means. The traumatic events at the adenohypophysis and at the hypothalamus itself which can cause a dissociated partial function, are especially important ([2 - 4, 8, 10]). The weak or delayed response of the levels of hormones and the random fluctuation cannot always be rigidly separated. Furthermore it has to be said that it cannot be the topic of this investigation to modify or discuss the clinically defined concept of brain death but to find out whether homogenous neuroendocrinological patterns of behaviour can be recognized whenever brain death occurs. This does not seem to be the case.

Conclusion

Twenty patients who had suffered from severe brain injury were examined in the phase of brain death. The stimulation of the hypothalamic-pituitary system was attempted by means of releasing hormones. The levels of HGH, hPRL, TSH and LH show not only various insufficiencies, but also a dissociation between specific functions within the same patient. Patients with a short survival time show higher hormone levels than those with a long survival time.

References

1. Brandt, M., Wagner, H., Walter, W.: Wachstumshormon, LH und FSH unter funktionsdynamischen Bedingungen im Serum sowie basale Kortisol- und Testosteron-Serumspiegel bei Schädel-Hirnverletzten unter Dexamethasonbehandlung. Act. Neuroch. 20, 79-83 (1977)
2. Ceballos, R.: Pituitary changes in head trauma (Analysis of 102 consecutive cases of head injury). Ala. J. Med. Sci. 3, 185-189 (1966)
3. Crompton, R.M.: Hypothalamic lesions following closed head injury. Brain 94, 165-172 (1971)
4. Daniel, P.M., Prichard, M.M.L., Treip, C.S.: Traumatic infarction of the anterior lobe of the pituitary gland. Lancet 927-930 (Nov. 1959)
5. Gerstenbrand, F.: Die klinische Symptomatik des irreversiblen Ausfalls der Hirnfunktionen (Das Vorstadium und die spinalen Reflexe). In: Die Bestimmung des Todeszeitpunktes. Kröse, W., Kröse, E. (eds.), pp. 33-38. Wien: Scherzer 1973
6. Grote, E.: Neuroendocrinological differential diagnosis of cerebral death. Summary No. 664, 253, Weltkongreß Sao Paulo (1977)
7. Ingvar, D.H.: Bestimmung des Sistierens der Gehirnzirkulation bei Hirntod. In: Die Bestimmung des Todeszeitpunktes. Kröse, W., Kröse, E. (eds.), pp. 195-198. Wien: Scherzer 1973
8. Kornblum, R.N., Fisher, R.S.: Pituitary lesions in craniocerebral injuries. Arch. Path. 88, 242-248 (1969)
9. Labhart, A.: Klinik der inneren Sekretion, 3. Aufl., S. 80. Berlin, Heidelberg, New York: Springer 1978
10. Oppenheimer, D.R.: Microscopic lesions in the brain following head injury. J. Neurol. Neurosurg., Psych. 31, 299-306 (1968)
11. Penin, H., Käufer, C.: Kriterien des cerebralen Todes aus neurologischer Sicht. In: Die Bestimmung des Todeszeitpunktes. Kröse, W., Kröse, E. (eds.), pp. 19-24. Wien: Scherzer 1973

Criteria for the Choice of Drugs Suitable for Controlled Hypotension in Neuroanaesthesia

D. HEUSER, P. J. MORRIS, and D. G. MCDOWALL

Introduction

Controlled hypotension for the improvement of intraoperative conditions is able to minimize operative blood loss, operative time and mortality as well as contributing to a shorter course of disease in patients undergoing neurosurgical procedures. Besides volatile anaesthetic agents (e.g. halothane), two groups of chemical substances are commonly used, which achieve low pressure conditions, either via a direct relaxing effect on vascular smooth muscle cells or by blocking ganglia belonging to the autonomic nervous system. In order to meet the essential requirements of the anaesthetist confronted with critical intraoperative conditions, the drug producing hypotension should ideally have the following basic properties:

1. easy to control,
2. no increase of intracerebral blood volume,
3. short half-life,
4. no change in cerebral blood flow (CSF) autoregulation,
5. no toxicity.

Some of the drugs presently available which claim to meet these criteria are:

1. pentolinium tartrate,
2. glyceryl trinitrate,
3. trimetaphan camsylate,
4. sodium nitroprusside.

However, as a result of many experimental studies, it has become obvious that none of these drugs possess all of the above mentioned ideal properties.

From studies of MAEKAWA et al. (6) we have learned that CBF and oxygen supply to the cerebral cortical tissue vary considerably under systemic hypotension at comparable levels of systemic blood pressure induced by the two drugs commonly used for induction of hypotension: trimetaphan (TMP) and sodium nitroprusside (SNP). The aim of the present investigation was to find out whether these rather large differences would be reflected in changes in cerebral extracellular ion homeostasis which can be regarded as a sensitive indicator of cellular hypoxia (1).

Material and Approach

Experiments were performed on 12 cats which were anaesthetized with halothane (0.6 - 1.0 Vol%) relaxed (pancuronium bromide 0.05 mg/kg·hr) and artificially ventilated (N_2O/O_2 2:1). Measurements of regional cerebral blood flow (rCBF) were performed by means of the Kr^{85}-clearance method. Administration of the isotope (dissolved in physiological saline) was performed via a polyethylene tube advanced within the lingual artery to its initial point of origin. Continuous measurements of extracellular K^+- and H^+-activities were performed by means of ion selective microelectrodes (3) which had been implanted about 800 µm into the cortical tissue in the area of the suprasylvian or marginal gyrus. Information about cerebral electrical activity was obtained from the Cerebral Function Monitor (CFM) which amplified and integrated signals from four electrodes placed in a fronto-occipital position on the skull. Mean arterial blood pressure (MABP) was measured in the abdominal aorta with a Statham transducer and end-expiratory CO_2 content was registered with an URAS. In addition, intermittent blood gas analysis was performed. Directly before the induction of hypotension, we administered Practolol (0.2 mg/kg), a beta-blocking agent, after control measurements of CBF had been performed and steady state conditions had been established. Then we induced systemic hypotension, either by continuous infusion of TMP (maximal dose 10 mg/kg·hr) or SNP (1 mg/kg), until we reached blood pressure levels of 30 mm Hg. This low pressure condition was maintained for 15 minutes while CBF measurements were performed. Subsequently, we again lowered the MABP to values between 26 and 28 mmHg which was usually possible by a withdrawl of limited amounts of blood. After this condition had been maintained for 15 minutes, we stopped the hypotensive drug infusion, retransfused the blood and attempted to recover the animals by suitable therapeutic treatment.

Results

There is no doubt that cerebral perfusion during systemic hypotension is maintained much better with SNP than with TMP. A statistically significant posthypotensive hyperemia could only be observed in the SNP group (Fig. 1). Measurements of cortical extracellular pH demonstrated the development of progressive tissue acidosis (Fig. 2) which seems to be less in the SNP group. However, the difference between both groups was not statistically significant. In contrast, measurements of extracellular K^+-activity demonstrated highly significant differences between both groups (Fig. 3). Cellular K^+ release occurred only during TMP-induced hypotension, probably because of anoxic cell depolarization, whereas in the SNP group no deviation from the initial value was ever detected. The critical flow level for the occurrence of the K^+-release varied from animal to animal under these experimental conditions. The breakdown in cerebral extracellular ionic homeostasis was usually reversible during the recovery period.

Discussion

Our experiments give evidence that the pathophysiological problem of cerebral ischemia is closely linked to those conditions which we observe during induced hypotension, especially when extremely low perfusion pressures are desirable. Under those circumstances the application of SNP for induction of controlled hypotension seems to be preferable to TMP administration. In this case not only CBF and pO_2 are maintained at a more favorable level, as has been shown in earlier studies (6), but also the extracellular ionic homeostasis as measured by pH and K^+ is more stable. Only during application of TMP can a break-down of cellular energy sources occur, followed by anoxic depolarisation indicating critical flow levels below 10 ml/100 g·min (4). Undesired side effects of SNP administration, e.g. the posthypotensive hyperperfusion (2), possibly due to an increase in plasma-Renin-activity, can be adequately treated. The acidosis we observed in both groups of animals can be sufficiently explained only in the TMP-group as a consequence of cerebral ischemic hypoxidosis. During SNP administration however an acidosis due to cyanide intoxication should be discussed, though we remained below the critical dose of 1 mg/kg under our experimental conditions. However this will be the subject of further investigations.

Conclusion

The local continuous registration of extracellular ion activities offers, at least in the experimental animal model, excellent possibilities for gathering "on line" information about cerebral metabolic states during critical perfusion conditions achieved during controlled systemic hypotension. This information is relevant in determining risks involved in the use of a specific drug during neuroanaesthetic management.

References

1. Astrup, J., Heuser, D., Lassen, N.A., Nilsson, B., Norberg, K., Siesjö, B.K.: Evidence against H^+ and K^+ as main factors for the control of cerebral blood flow: a microelectrode study. In: Cerebral vascular smooth muscle and its control; Ciba Foundation Symposion 56 (new series), pp. 313-337. Amsterdam: Elsevier Excerpta Medica 1978

2. Cottrell, J.E., Casthely, P., Brodie, J.D.: Prevention of nitroprusside-induced cyanide toxicity with hydroxocobalamin. N. Engl. J. Med. 298, 809-814 (1978)

3. Heuser, D.: Local ionic control of cerebral microvessels. In: The application of ion-selective microelectrodes. Zeuthen, T. (ed.), pp. 85-102. Amsterdam: Elsevier Biomedical Press 1971

4. Heuser, D., Morris, P.J., McDowall, D.G.: Ionic changes in the brain with ischemia. In: Anaesthesiology; International Congress Series No. 538. Zindler, M., Rügheimer, E. (eds.), pp. 821-826. Amsterdam: Excerpta Medica 1981

5. Khambatta, N.J., Stone, J.A., Khan, L.U.: Hypertension following sodium nitroprusside. Physiologist 21, 64-69 (1978)

6. Maekawa, T., McDowall, D.G., Okuda, Y.: Brain surface oxygen tension and cerebral cortical blood flow during hemorrhagic and drug-induced hypotension in the cat. Anaesthesiology 51, 313-320 (1979)

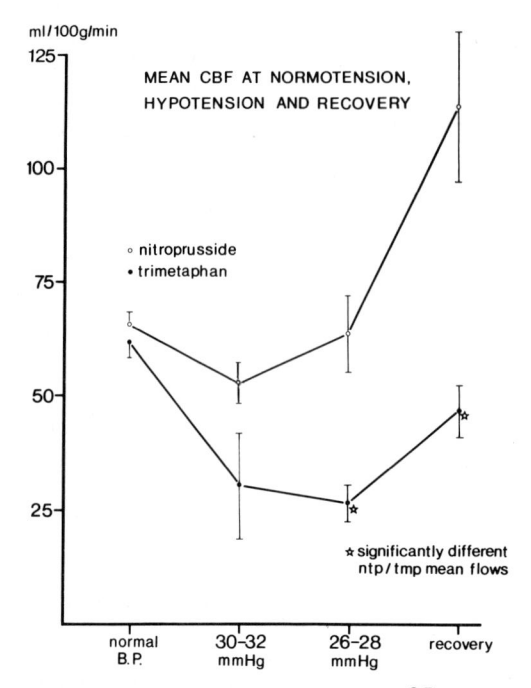

Fig. 1. Mean CBF values (Kr^{85}-clearance) in 12 cats before, during and after induction of controlled hypotension with SNP and TMP. (With kind permission: Verlag G. Witzstrock, Baden-Baden - Köln - New York)

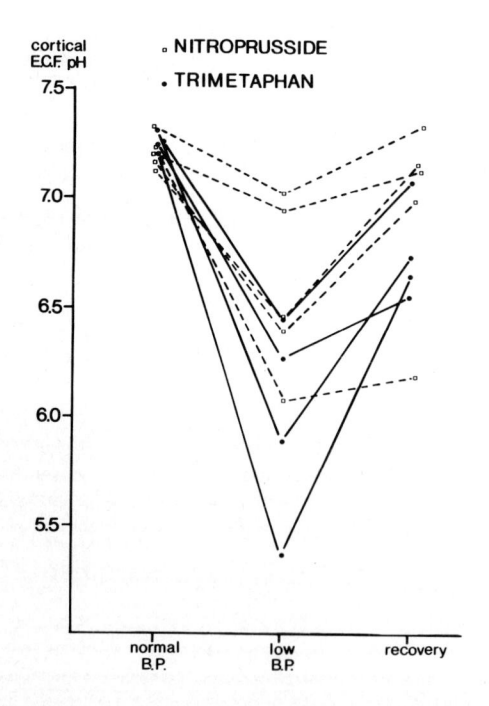

Fig. 2. Cerebral cortical extracellular pH values in cats during systemic hypotension induced by TMP *(straight, solid lines)* or SNP *(dotted lines)*

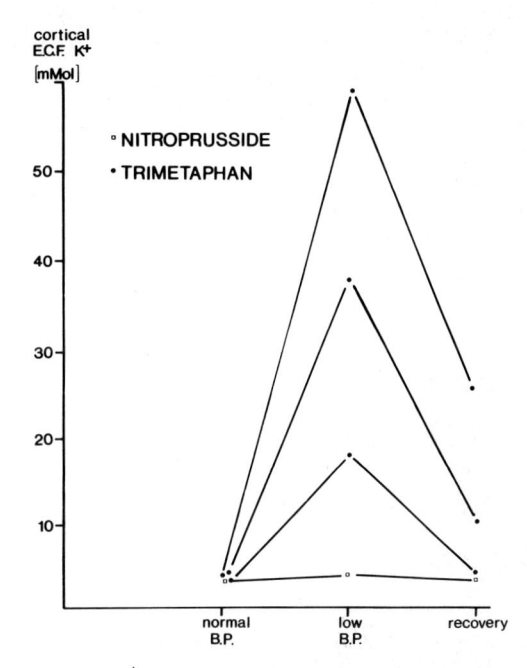

Fig. 3. Cerebral cortical extracellular K⁺-activity in cats during systemic hypotension induced by TMP *(filled circles)* or SNP *(open squares)*. The SNP line represents mean values of 6 animals

Sphingolipids in the Progress of Head Injury – A Preliminary Report
R. Preger and G. Schwarzmann

Introduction

Sphingolipids are complex lipids with one long chain sphingoid base containing one amino group. Glycosphingolipids such as cerebroside (ce) as well as sulfatide (su) and sphingomyelin (spm), a phosphosphingolipid, are the main constituents of the white matter of the brain. The main glycolipids of the white matter of the brain are galactolipids whereas almost all systemic organs e.g. serum contain glucolipids i.e. they are not synthesized in the brain but in different organs (4).

Analytical findings in brain reveal similar changes in destruction of myelin or in demyelination whether primary or secondary (7, 9). These changes due to an increase in water, a decrease in myelin constituents, esp. proteolipids, glycosphingolipids (gsl) and cholesterol and the occurrence of cholesterol esters. Because of the breakdown of the blood-brain-barrier one expects these constituents to be determined in serum and other biological samples. Numerous studies (5, 10) have demonstrated elevations of certain serum gsl in cases of specific storage diseases. In other disorders of the central nervours system the reports on the content in serum of gsl are contradictary.

The report on the serum levels of myelin-basic-protein in patients with head injury (15) encouraged us to investigate the serum levels of sphingolipids, esp. su which is closely related to the upper proteolipid and is normally absent in serum.

This study was done to elaborate a method for measuring small amounts of sphingolipids, esp. su in individual serum samples and to correlate these to the progress of myelin destruction.

Patients and Methods

Patients

To be sure that myelin breakdown products will be detected we examined serum samples from patients with severe myelin destruction after head injury (15 cases), brain tumor operation (5 cases), one case of an bleeding aneurysm, one case of a strangulation "coning", one case of cerebral concussion and as controls nine serum samples from healthy persons. Six patients with head injury suffered from intracerebral and subdural hemorrhages, four of them died. Nine patients suffered from severe cerebral contusions.

In the tumor bearing group of patients bleeding complications and severe brain edema were fatal in three cases, one patient developed a hydrocephalus malresorptivus.

Methods

From the patients mentioned above samples of serum were taken whenever possible. In this way 28 samples could be obtained during the first three days and 17 samples thereafter within four weeks following injury.

The lipid extraction from 1 ml serum samples was done by a method of ZÖLLNER/EBERHAGEN (18). For quantitative isolation of total gsl we used chromatography on Florisil columns following to described procedure (11). The separation of ce and su was achieved by DEAE-Sephadex chromatography (17). For quantification of sphingolipids their sphingoid bases are released by acid hydrolysis (1) followed by a new method of selective N-(1-^{14}C)-acetylation elaborated by SCHWARZMANN et al. (12). This procedure allows measurements of sphingolipids in the subnormal range. According to these procedures the sphingolipids of each serum sample have been measured as follows:

1. determination of total sphingolipids,
2. determination of total glycosphingolipids,
3. determination of cerebroside,
4. determination of sulfatide.

By calculation it was then possible to determine the amount of sphingomyelin.

For analytical studies and semiquantitative measurements of sphingolipids thin layer chromatography (14) on commercial silica gel plates was used.

Results

The content of total lipids in the samples of normal serum as gravimetrically measured is 6.96 mg/ml. In the average a decrease of total lipids down to 4.89 mg/ml (70.3%) could be demonstrated in patients with head injury, with a minimum of 31.3% of normal content of total lipids being observed.

In normal serum the small amount of spm with 90 nmol/ml, i.e. 7.2 µg/ml or 1.03% of total lipids was surprising. A slight increase of this lipid to 1.33% was found in patients with head injury.

The content of ce in normal serum was found to be 3.97 nmol/ml applying the isotope technique whereas a value of 5.59 nmol/ml has been obtained using densitometry subsequent to thin layer chromatography. Unexpectedly in the progress of myelin destruction in the acute phase of the disease the content of ce decreased as demonstrated in Fig. 1. However, in one case shortly after injury the serum content of ce was clearly above normal, but declining below normal levels during the following days. In some cases the content of ce went down to zero. The ce levels in the serum of the patient who died four days after "coning" varied from less than 0.29 nmol/ml on the day of injury to 2.73 nmol/ml on the 1st and to 1.58 nmol/ml on the 2nd day after injury.

Special regard was given to su determination. We were able to detect su in all pathological cases, including the case of cerebral concussion (Fig. 2). In three cases, however, su could only be found in serum samples taken on days 2, 7 and 28, respectively.

Two patients of those who died after head injury had su levels higher than 5 nmol/ml. In one case with a high value of 46 nmol/ml in the course of a posttraumatic meningitis 18 days after injury. The two patients with apallic syndrome 4 weeks after injury showed a su serum level of 5.29 nmol/ml and 1.73 nmol/ml, respectively. In contradistinction two patients with subdural hemorrhages died without showing great increase in su during the first 2 weeks. In the later progress of head injury up to the 4th week su could be detected only in case of severe injury.

In all patients after brain tumor operation su could be registered in amounts between less than 0.29 nmol/ml and 3.88 nmol/ml, the last value belonging to the patient who developed hydrocephalus. The two patients who died after operation had only small serum levels of su up to 0.58 nmol/ml.

In case of the patient with bleeding aneurysm in contradistinction to the serum ce level clearly increased levels of su up to 2.30 nmol/ml were observed.

The patient after strangulation also showed a continuous increase of su from 0.43 nmol/ml to 2.73 nmol/ml.

Discussion

The decrease of total lipids following different forms of head injury and brain diseases is well known (2) and can be explained by alimentary and metabolic factors.

PILZ (8) and KUNZ (6) reported on normal spm-levels of 7.9% of total lipids and compared these to values of 4.4% to 8.4%, i.e. 273 - 623 nmol/ml reported by other authors. In normal serum samples we found a spm content of 90 nmol/ml equivalent to 1.03% of total serum lipids which is significantly below the values mentioned above. If this discrepancy in the contents of spm observed is due to the different methods of determination has to be clarified.

In the literature different levels of ce in normal serum ranging from 53.17 nmol/ml to zero have been reported (5, 10, 13). In our study we found a ce content of 5.59 nmol/ml or 3.97 nmol/ml using densitometry or isotope technique, respectively.

In normal serum 87.8% of ce are made up by glucosyl-ceramide as reported by RATHKE and JONES (10). According to these authors these figures should not even change in cases of various neurological diseases. In view of our results these findings are quite surprising since we found a decrease in the serum levels of ce in all cases of myelin destruction studied. Therefore we have to assume that in the course of the demyelination glucosyl-ceramide vanishes from the blood, a phenomenon which cannot be explained as yet.

To the best of our knowledge there is no report on the occurrence of su in normal human serum. Numerous published studies demonstrate interactions of myelin-basic-protein and su (3, 16) and the occurrence of antibodies against ce and su in patients with multiple sclerosis (16).

Su and the antibodies can produce complement-dependent damage of membranes. Perhaps long time increases of su to myelin destruction as shown in a patient with apallic syndrome can lead to antibody production and progressive destruction of brain tissue.

Conclusion

A new method for the sphingoid base estimation based on selective N-(1-^{14}C)-acetylation of the sphingoid bases is very suitable to quantify sphingolipids in small serum samples of 1 ml, esp. for the small amounts of gsl. This report presents data on the increase of sulfatide in serum possibly due to breakdown of myelin following brain injury. This increase in su in serum seems to correlate to the degree of brain damage. Further investigations will be performed to support this view.

References

1. Gaver, R.C., Sweeley, C.C.: Methods for methanolysis of sphingolipids and direct determination of long-chain bases by gas chromatography. J. Am. Oil Chemists' Soc. 42, 294-298 (1965)
2. Heller, W., Stolz, Ch.: Veränderungen des Fettstoffwechsels bei hypoxischer Hypoxie. In: Deutsche Gesellschaft für Anästhesie und Wiederbelebung. Lawin, P., Morr-Strathmann, U. (eds.), pp. 212-216. Berlin, Heidelberg, New York: Springer 1974
3. Jones, A.J.S., Rumsby, M.G.: Localization of sites for ionic interaction with lipid in the C-terminal third of the bovine myelin basic protein. Biochem. J. 167, 583-591 (1977)
4. Kościelak, J., Krauze, R., Maśliński, W., Zdebska, E., Zieleński, J., Brudzyński, T., Miller-Podraza, H.: Neutral glycosphingolipids of serum and plasma. Arch. Immunol. Ther. Exp. 26, 119 (1979)
5. Kremer, G.J.: Nachweis der Sphingolipoide im Blutserum. Ärztl. Lab. 15, 209-215 (1969)
6. Kunz, F., Rumpl, E.: Phospholipids in Human Cerebrospinal Fluid. Z. Neurol. 203, 259-264 (1972)
7. Morell, P.: Diseases of myelin. In: Basic Neurochemistry. Albers, R.W., Siegel, G.J., Katzma-n, R., Agranoff, B.W. (eds.), pp. 497-516. Boston: Little, Brown and Company 1972
8. Pilz, H.: Die Lipide des normalen und pathologischen Liquor cerebrospinalis. Berlin, Heidelberg, New York: Springer 1970
9. Preger, R.: Changes in lipid metabolism in experimentally produced head injury: Qualitative and quantitative studies of lipids. In: Advances in neurosurgery, Vol. 5. Frowein, R.A., Wilcke, O., Karimi-Nejad, A., Brock, M., Klinger, M. (eds.), pp. 138-143. Berlin, Heidelberg, New York: Springer 1978
10. Rathke, E., Jones, M.: Serum cerebrosides in multiple sclerosis. J. Neurochem. 22, 311-313 (1974)
11. Saito, T., Hakomori, S.-I.: Quantitative isolation of total glykosphingolipids from animal cells. J. Lipid Res. 12, 257-259 (1971)

12. Schwarzmann, G., Schlemmer, U., Wiegandt, H.: A sensitive assay for gangliosides in the subnanomole range. In: Advances in experimental medicine and biology, Vol. 125. Svennerholm, L., Mandel, P., Dreyfus, H., Urban, P.-F. (eds.), pp. 199-205. New York: Plenum Press 1980

13. Seidel, D., Buck, R., Heipertz, R., Pilz, H.: Cerebrospinal fluid lipids in demyelinating disease. J. Neurol. 222, 171-176 (1980)

14. Stahl, E.: Dünnschichtchromatographie. Berlin, Göttingen, Heidelberg: Springer 1962

15. Thomas, D.G.T., Palfreyman, J.W., Ratcliffe, J.G.: Serum-myelin-basic-protein assay in diagnosis and prognosis of patients with head injury. Lancet 1, 113-115 (1978)

16. Uemura, K., Yuzawa-Watanabe, M., Kitazawa, N., Taketomi, T.: Immunochemical studies of lipids VI. J. Biochem. 87, 1221-1227 (1980)

17. Yu, R.K., Ledeen, R.W.: Gangliosides of human, bovine, and rabbit plasma. J. Lipid Res. 13, 680-686 (1972)

18. Zöllner, N., Eberhagen, D.: Untersuchung und Bestimmung der Lipoide im Blut. Berlin, Heidelberg, New York: Springer 1965

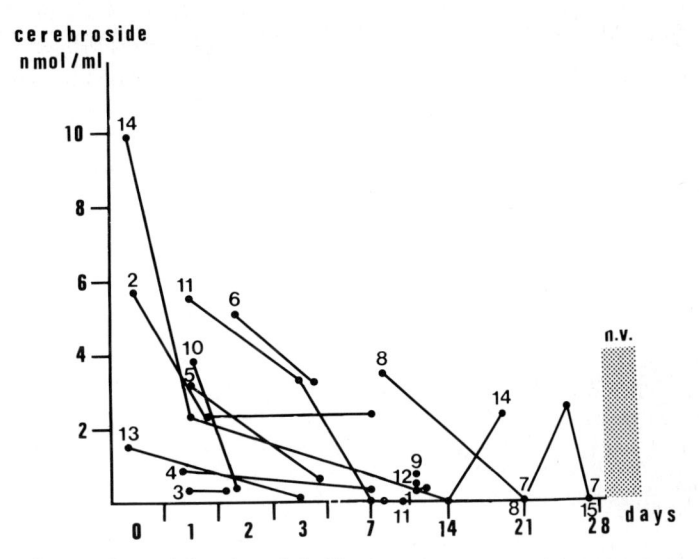

Fig. 1. Serum levels of cerebroside (nmol/ml) in the progress (days after injury) of 15 cases with severe head injury. n.v. = normal value. Diagnosis of case no.: 1 - 8 cerebral contusion, 9 - 13 intracranial hemorrhage, 14 open craniocerebral injury, meningitis, 15 apallic syndrome. Case no. 10, 11, 13, 14 died

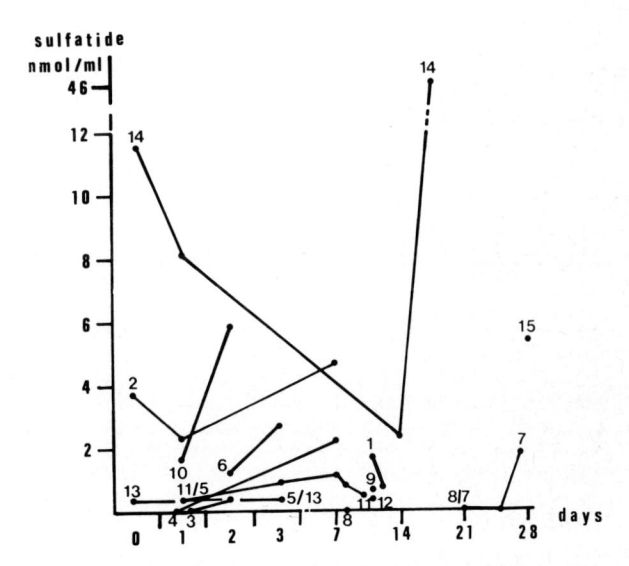

Fig. 2. Serum levels of sulfatide (nmol/ml) in the progress (days after injury) of 15 cases with severe head injury. Diagnosis of case no. see Fig. 1

The Relationship Between Brain Edema, Energy Metabolism, Glucose Content and rCBF Investigated by Artificial Brain Abscess in Cats

H. W. Bothe, Th. Wallenfang, A. Khalifa, and K. Schürmann*

Introduction

We developed the model of artificial brain abscess in cats to investigate quantitatively different forms of conservative management of acute brain abscess. First we compared antibiotic therapy alone with a combined therapy of antibiotics and glucocorticoids.

The application of this animal model is not limited to pharmacological problems. Additionally the model is advantageous to explore the relationship between brain edema, cerebral energy metabolism and rCBF:

The brain edema developing after inoculation of Staphylococcus aureus into cat's brain differs principally from other experimentally produced brain edema, e.g. cold lesion and water intoxication: After the development of brain abscess the form of brain edema is a slowly increasing one. The adaption of cerebral energy metabolism and rCBF corresponds to natural compensation more than in other experimentally produced brain edema (see discussion).

Material and Approach

Material. 42 adult, male cats weighing $\bar{x}$ = 3,7 kg (s_x = 0,5 kg) are grouped into 7 categories with 6 animals.

Approach. After inoculation of a bouillon-staphylococcus aureus A8 mixture all cats developed a brain abscess in the right white matter (4).

On the 7th day after inoculation the brain edema caused by the developing brain abscess reached its maximum. Therefore therapy was instituted on the 7th day. Cats were treated with a combination of 0,5 mg/kg/die dexamethasone and 50 mg/kg/die cefacedone or with 50 mg/kg/die cefacedone alone. Therapy was carried on over a period of either 3 or 13 days, so that animals could be killed on the 10th or 20th day after inoculation. Furthermore 3 groups of cats received no treatment. These animals were killed on the 7th day, 10th day or 20th day after inoculation.

After freezing the brain by the application of liquid nitrogen we measured in the white matter adjacent, remote and contralateral to the abscess the water content (10), the content of glucose (9), the ratio of reduced adenine dinucleotide to oxidized adenine dinucleotide, NADH/NAD (9, 11) and the energy charge potential, ECP (9, 1).

*The authors are indebted to JUTTA LUDWIG for her skillful technical assistance

In order to calculate NADH/NAD we measured the tissue content of lactate, pyruvate, arterial and CSF pCO_2 ($pCO_2 \rightarrow TCO_2$, see (11)).
The consideration of the results based on non-parametric rang-sum-tests for independent and dependent random sampling (8).

Results

Water Content (see Fig. 1). The region adjacent to the abscess shows the effect of the different kinds of therapy first (3). While the values of the untreated group measured adjacent to abscess remain pathologic until the 20th day after inoculation, the water content is normalized by the combined therapy within 3 days. The antibiotic therapy shows delayed effect until the 20th day after inoculation. The time cause of water content remote to the abscess is about the same in all groups of our experiment: From the 7th day to the 10th day after inoculation the water content decreases from high pathologic values to normal values, independent from a special treatment. From the 10th to the 20th day after inoculation the water content remote to the abscess shows no further changes.

NADH/NAD and ECP (see Fig. 2). The state of regional energy metabolism is critized by the changes of NADH/NAD and ECP (13). On the 7th, 10th and 20th day the untreated group established a decompensating O_2-deficit with increased NADH/NAD ratio and decreased ECP. With the application of combined therapy over a period of 3 days the value of ECP is normalized. High values of NADH/NAD show and anaerobe, compensating glycolysis. On the 20th day after combined therapy we find a normalisation of regional energy metabolism. An improvement of NADH/NAD and ECP values is not realised after 3 days of antibiotherapy alone, but after 13 days of antibiotic treatment an absolute normalisation of energy metabolism is achieved. Neither on the 10th nor on the 20th day hypoxic disturbances are measured in the region remote and contralateral to the abscess.

Content of Glucose (see Fig. 3). We can establish a positive correlation between glucose content and water content with a correlation coefficient $r = 0,65$ ($P(X = t_{r=0}) < 0,001$). Tissue concentrations of glucose (referenced to dry weight of brain to avoid dilution effects caused by the edema fluid) corresponds to the changes of the water content under the definite conditions of our experiment. Otherwise both quantities differ significantly at the application of statistical test. The differences of water content have a high probability of being more than that of glucose content.

Discussion

Water Content, NADH/NAD and ECP. Disturbances of energy metabolism are located only adjacent to the abscess. The danger of cell necrosis is not obvious (ECP slightly below normal level!). The deterioration of ECP is far less distinct than that of other experiments with the same content of water (7). In the situation of compensation, anaerobe glycolysis values of NADH/NAD ratio and the latter dates indicate the adaptation of brain metabolism following the developing of edema. The functional metabolism is inhibited in favour of energy metabolism.

Water Content and Content of Glucose. The maximum glucose content is measured on the 7th day after inoculation. It rates 7 mmol/kg wet weight. The difference between normal and pathological values is the concentration of blood glucose, 5 mmol/100 ml. To explain the correlation between water- and glucose content we can state the following:

1. The increase of glucose content in brain tissue is caused by isoosmotic glucose flow with the edema fluid across the disturbed BBB. Afterwards the extracellular concentration of glucose amounts to 5 mmol/100 ml H_2O. Because the volume of extracellular space amounts to 20% of the entire brain volume (2) an increase of glucose to 7 mmol/kg wet weight is not possible.

2. (see Fig. 4) Glucose escapes isoosmotic with the edema fluid and is taken up by the cells of neuroglia in a way the measured glucose content is attained by intracellular glucose accumulation. The rate constant of glucose uptake is determined by $k \cong 0,1$ min^{-1} (12). This value could be increased eight times (6). The high utilisation of glucose in anaerobe glycolysis is related to the measured glucose values.

Glucose Content and rCBF (see Fig. 4). Brain edema causes decreased rCBF (5). This relationship is not valid in all cases. Brain edema produced by infusion of isotonic NaCl solution is accompanied by increased rCBF as recently demonstrated by MARMAROU. An increased rCBF is logically required by the consideration of all of the following measured dates:

High glucose content, high NADH/NAD ratio and low ECP are possible only if rCBF is enhanced, - high glucose content and high NADH/NAD ratio include increased rCBF.

Conclusion

Brain edema is not necessarily a malignant event:

1. It changes over the aerobic glycolysis into anaerobic glycolysis. Metabolites of anaerobic glycolysis cause an inhibition of functional metabolism.
2. rCBF is increased by brain edema.

So brain edema provides a reparation of disturbed neuropile due to the stopping of functional metabolism in favour of energy metabolism and due to the increase of rCBF.

References

1. Atkinson, D.E.: The energy charge of the adenylate pool as a regulatory parameter. Biochemistry 7, 4030-4034 (1968)
2. Biesold, D.: Neurobiologie, pp. 500-504. Jena: Gustav Fischer 1977
3. Bohl, J., Wallenfang, Th., Bothe, H.W., Schürmann, K.: The effect of glucocorticoids in the combined treatment of experimental brain abscess in cats. In: Advances in neurosurgery, Vol. 9. Schiefer, W., Klinger, M., Brock, M. (eds.). Berlin, Heidelberg, New York: Springer 1981.
4. Bothe, H.W.: Der artifizielle Hirnabszeß bei der Katze und seine Therapie mit Antibiotika und Glukokortikoiden. Inaug. Diss. Med. Mainz (in press)

5. Bruce, D.A., Vapalahti, M., Schutz, H., Langfitt, T.W.: CBF, $CMRO_2$ and intracranial pressure following a local cold injury to the cortex. In: Intracranial pressure, experimental and clinical aspects. Brock, M., Dietz, H. (eds.), pp. 85-89. Berlin, Heidelberg, New York: Springer 1972

6. Jatzkewitz, H.: Neurochemie, p. 36. Stuttgart: Thieme 1978

7. Kogure, K., Scheinberg, P., Kishikawa, H., Bustro, R.: The role of monoamines and cyclic AMP in ischemic brain edema. In: Dynamics of brain edema. Pappius, H.M., Feindel, W. (eds.), pp. 203-214. Berlin, Heidelberg, New York: Springer 1976

8. Lienert, G.A.: Verteilungsfreie Methoden in der Biostatistik, Bd. I, pp. 212-341. Meisenheim: Anton Hain KG 1973

9. Lowry, O.H.: Passonneau, J.V., Hasselberger, F.X., Schulz, D.W.: Effekt of ischemia on known substrates and cofactors of the glycolytic pathway in brain. Journal of biological chemistry 239/1, 18-29 (1964)

10. Reulen, H.J., Medzihradsky, F., Enzenbach, R., Marguth, F.: Elektrolytes, fluids and energy metabolism in human cerebral edema. Arch. Neurol. 21, 517-525 (1969)

11. Siesjö, B.K.: The bicarbonate/carbonic acid buffer system of the cerebral cortex of cats, as studied in tissue homogenates. Arch. Acta neurol. scand. 38, 98-120 (1962)

12. Sokoloff, L. et al.: The (^{14}C) deoxyglucose method for the measurement of local cerebral glucose utilization: theory, procedure and normal values in the conscious and anesthetized albino rat. Journ. of Neurochemistry 28, 897-916 (1977)

13. Wallenfang, Th., Bothe, H.W., Schürmann, K.: Experimental brain abscess in cats: Effect of antibiotherapy alone and in combination with dexamethasone on edema, regional metabolism and influence on antibody titer in serum. This paper will be read on the 7th International Congress of Neurological Surgery, München, July 1981

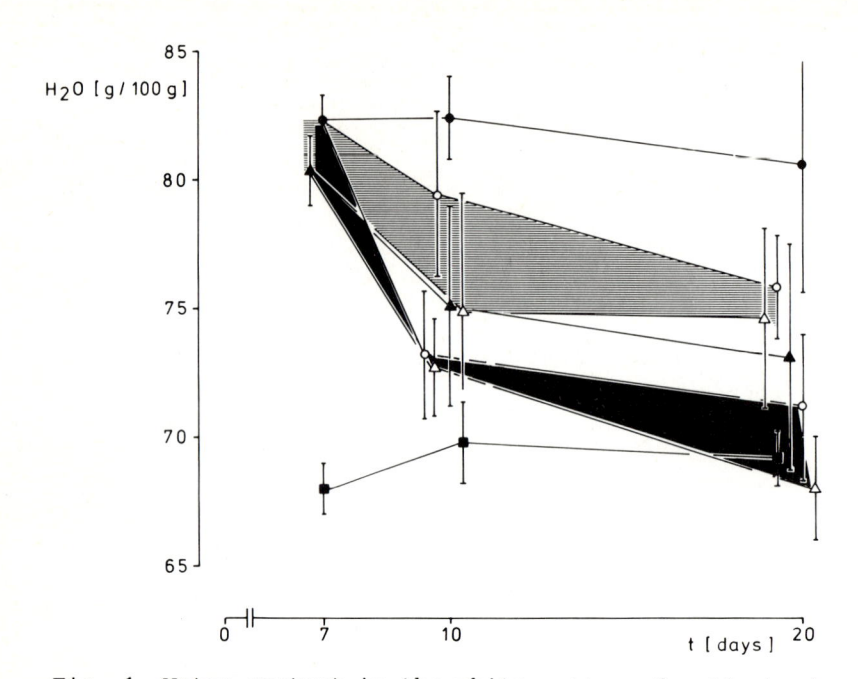

Fig. 1. Water content in the white matter of cat's brain adjacent, remote and contralateral to the abscess on the 7th, 10th and 20th day after inoculation with staphylococcus aureus A8. Antibiotherapy alone or combined therapy with glucocorticoids were instituted on 7th day after inoculation. Unit of ordinate: water content (g/100 g, wet weight). Mean and S.D. are given.
Black circle: adjacent to abscess - untreated; *black triangle:* remote to abscess - untreated; *black square:* contralateral to abscess - untreated; *white circle:* adjacent to abscess + grey area: antibiotic-therapy; *white triangle:* remote to abscess + grey area: antibiotic-therapy; *white circle:* adjacent to abscess + black area: antibiotics + glucocorticoids; *white triangle:* remote to abscess + black area: antibiotics + glucocorticoids

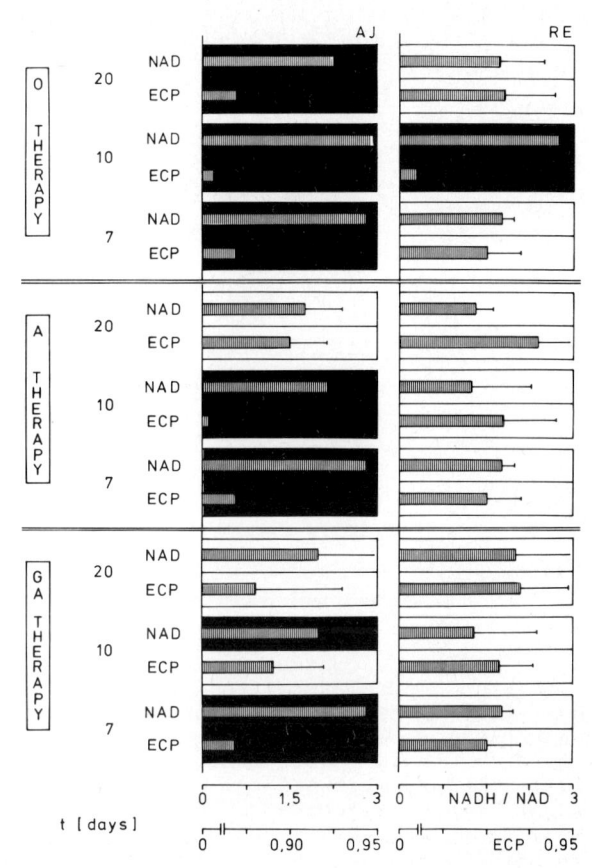

Fig. 2. NADH/NAD ratio and ECP in the white matter of cat's brain adjacent (AJ) and remote (RE) to the abscess on the 7th, 10th and 20th day after inoculation with staphylococcus aureus A8. Antibiotic-therapy alone or combined therapy with glucocorticoids were instituted on 7th day after inoculation. Mean and S.D. are given. *Black areas* represent pathologic values. *White areas* represent normal values

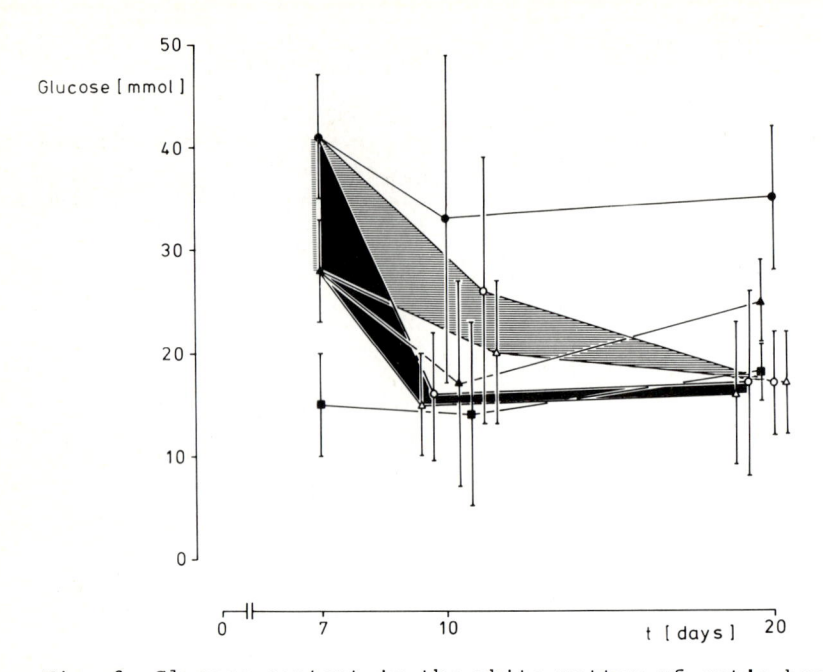

Fig. 3. Glucose content in the white matter of cat's brain adjacent, remote an contralateral to the abscess on the 7th, 10th and 20th day after inoculation with staphylococcus aureus A8. Antibiotictherapy alone or combined therapy with glucocorticoids were instituted on 7th day after inoculation. Unit of ordinate: glucose content (nmol/kg dry weight). Mean and S.D. are given.
Black circle: adjacent to abscess - untreated; *black triangle:* remote to the abscess - untreated; *black square:* contralateral to abscess - untreated; *white circle:* adjacent to abscess + grey area: antibiotictherapy; *white triangle:* remote to the abscess + grey area: antibiotictherapy; *white circle:* adjacent to abscess + black area: antibiotics + glucocorticoids; *white triangle:* remote to abscess + black area: antibiotics + glucocorticoids

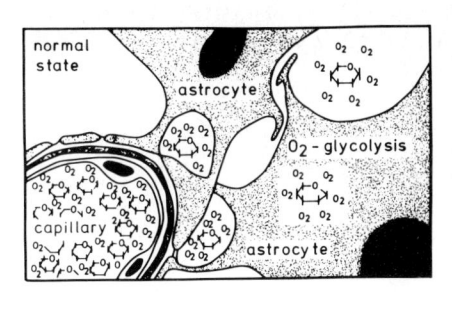

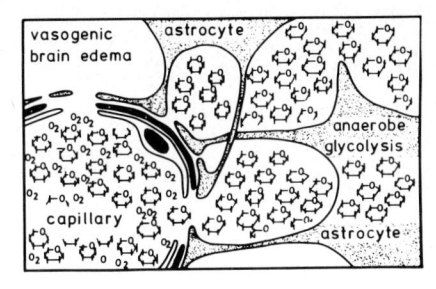

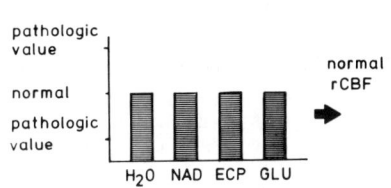

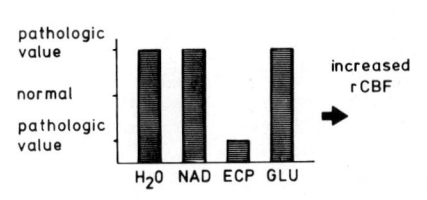

Fig. 4. Relationship of brain edema, energy metabolism, glucose content and rCBF. *Left:* normal state; *right:* vasogenic brain edema. H$_2$O = water content, NAD = NADH/NAD ratio, ECP = energy charge potential, GLU = glucose content, rCBF = regional cerebral blood flow

Circadian Rhythms of Catecholamines, Cortisol and Prolactin in Patients with Apallic Syndrome

D. Ratge, A. Hadjidimos, K. H. Holbach, and H. Wisser

Daily periodicity in man is controlled by selfsustained oscillators, which are independent from each other and possibly localized in the suprachiasmatic nuclei of the hypothalamus (3). These oscillators are influenced by exogenic periodic factors such as light-dark cycles or social cues (1). They cause a synchronization of the endogenous periodicity to a period of approximately 24 hours, which is in accordance with the period of the rotation of the earth (2). Patients, suffering from an apallic syndrome, who are in a state of "vegetative wakefulness" caused by a functional separation from brain cortex and stem or by an extensive destruction of the cortex, are protected against exogenous factors. The objective of this study was to investigate the degree of alteration of the circadian system by the apallic syndrome.

Six apallic patients with normal respiration, heart function and body temperature were studied. In four patients the apallic syndrome was of traumatic origin, in one patient it occurred through hypoxydosis and in one patient through multiple emboli. Besides anticonvulsants – and in the case of one patient additionally dexamethasone – the patients were given no further drugs. In each case more than ten days had elapsed between the incidence of the full stage of the apallic syndrome and the taking of the samples. Blood was withdrawn with the aid of an indwelling venous catheter over a period of 48 hours. Two-hour urine samples were also collected during this period. The control group consisted of four healthy volunteers (24 - 29 years of age), who were hospitalized during the whole period of investigation and were only allowed out of bed for urination.

Catecholamine determination was performed by a modified radioenzymatic assay (4), cortisol was determined by a competitive protein binding assay, and prolactin by a radioimmunoassay.

The results of the control group are summarized in Fig. 1, the absolute values being converted into percental deviations from the daily mean. A pronounced circadian rhythm could be seen in plasma and urinary norepinephrine during both experimental days with high concentrations in the morning and low concentrations in the night. The circadian rhythm of the urinary epinephrine excretion is more pronounced than that of plasma epinephrine concentration. This might be the result of the awakening of the subjects during the nocturnal withdrawals of blood which might produce a short-term elevation of epinephrine secretion. Dopamine in plasma showed no recognizable rhythmicity, whereas a little pronounced rhythm with peak values shortly before the awakening and minimum values in the evening and night hours. Serum prolactin also demonstrated a circadian rhythm with a maximum in the early morning.

Table 1. Catecholamine (norepinephrine, epinephrine, domapine), cortisol and prolactin concentrations in plasma as well as cortisol and catecholamine excretions in urine in the control group and the apallic patients. The values represent the means of 24 determinations (every 2 h over a 48 h period)

	Plasma (ng/l)			Urine (µg/24h)			Serum (µg/l)	Urine (µg/24 h)	Serum (µg/l)
	NA	A	DA	NA	A	DA	Cortisol	Cortisol	PRL
Control group mean (n = 4)	232	111	75	33.3	10.8	334	42.6	30.8	7.9
Range	200–276	98–119	61–85	27.6–37.1	7.5–13.6	298–426	31.3–47.4	29.0–35.3	6.1–10.6
Apallic patients									
Sch. W.	357	184	74	96.1	38.6	158	88.3	184.8	12.6
H. P.[a]	185	101	66	45.4	15.8	223	–	–	19.0
G. O.	397	151	46	76.9	45.6	246	157.5	258.1	12.3
T. H.	106	53	55	69.1	22.8	266	142.1	56.8	17.3
H. Th.	199	126	32	39.9	35.4	206	144.1	624.2	23.8
E. H.	–	–	–	26.6	19.9	255	85.1	106.4	22.3

[a]Dexamethasone-therapy

Only in one of the six apallic patients a circadian rhythm of catecholamines was detectable (Fig. 2). In this patient (H. Th.) the exclusion of exogenous factors led to a more pronounced catecholamine rhythm with a phase shift of 2 hours compared to the control group.

A circadian rhythm of urinary catecholamines could also be demonstrated in this patient only (Fig. 3).

Figure 4 shows the daily variation of cortisol and prolactin in the apallic patients. In all patients the prolactin rhythm was abolished. This is not surprising, because prolactin rhythm is coupled to the sleep-wake-cycle. Plasma and urinary cortisol rhythm is detectable in two patients, but with a diminished amplitude. It can be assumed that in these two patients the brain region which is responsible for the maintenance of circadian rhythms, is less damaged than in the other four patients. In the apallic patients the absolute concentrations of cortisol and prolactin as well as catecholamine excretion were clearly increased compared with the control group (Table 1).

The disappearance of the rhythms of cortisol, epinephrine and norepinephrine can be explained by the assumption that there is no accumulation of episodic secretion phases in the period shortly before and after the awakening, as can usually be seen. In the apallic patients the secretion seems to be uniformly distributed over the whole day. There are marked differences between the different patients concerning intensity and frequency of the still existing episodic secretion phases. It can be assumed, that intensity and frequency of the secretion phases decrease with increasing brain damage. In animal experiments a decreasing rhythmicity could be established with increasing lesions of different brain areas (5). The two patients with the little pronounced daily variations of hormone secretion (G.O., T.H.) died shortly after the end of this study, whereas the other patients with the greater daily variations survived. The number of patients in this study is too low to give a statement on the value of intensity and frequency of secretion phases as a prognostic parameter in apallic patients.

References

1. Aschoff, J., Wever, R.: Human circadian rhythms: a multioscillator system. Fed. Proc. 35, 2326-2332 (1976)
2. Halberg, F.: Physiologic 24-hour periodicity; general and procedural considerations with reference to the adrenal cycle. Z. Vitamin-, Hormon-, Fermentforsch. 10, 225-296 (1959)
3. Moore, R.Y., Eichler, V.B.: Loss of circadian adrenal corticosterone rhythm following suprachiasmatic lesion in the rat. Brain Res. 42, 201-206 (1972)
4. Peuler, J.D., Johnson, G.A.: Simultaneous single isotope radioenzymatic assay of plasma norepinephrine, epinephrine and dopamine. Life Sci. 21, 625-636 (1977)
5. Rusak, B., Zucker, I.: Neural regulation of circadian rhythms Physiological Reviews 59/3, 449-526 (1979)

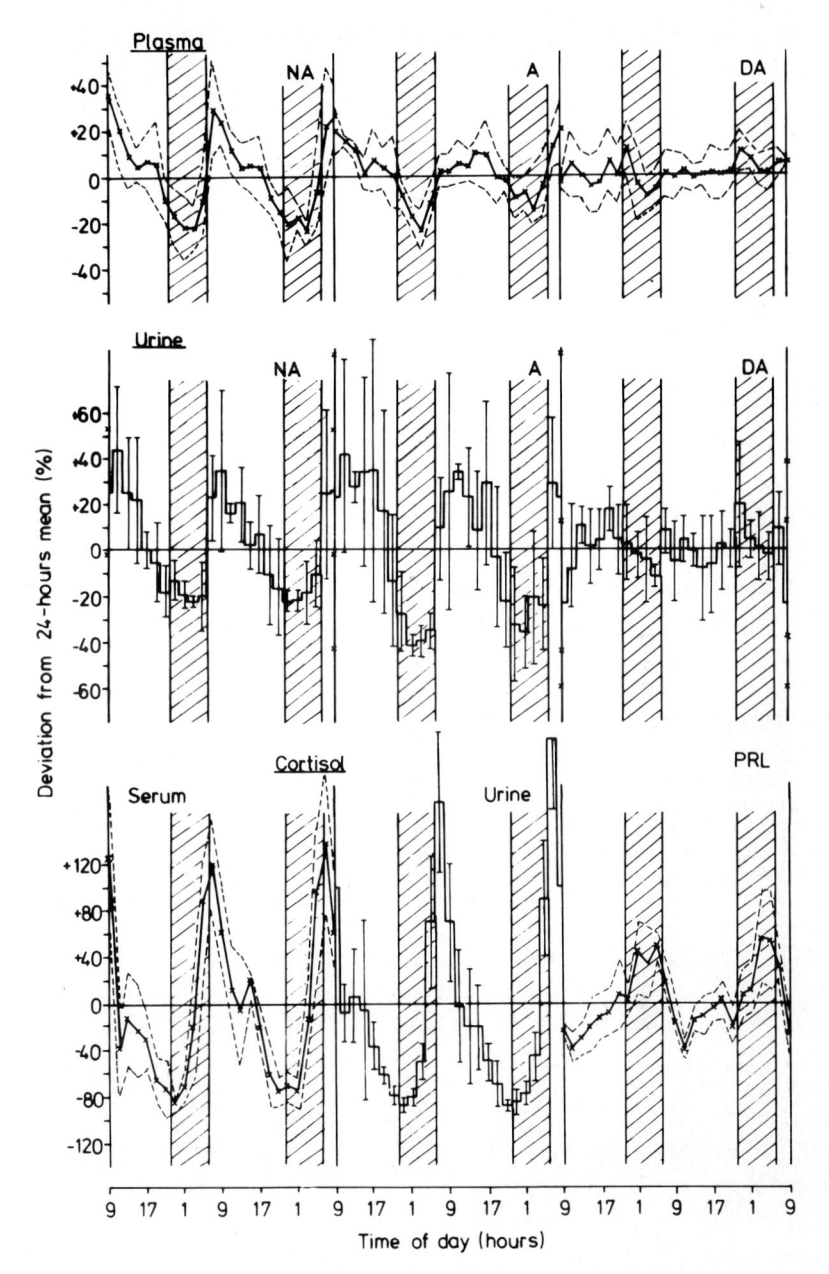

Fig. 1. Circadian rhythms of norepinephrine (NA), epinephrine (A), dopamine (DA), cortisol and prolactin (PRL) in four healthy volunteers. Values shown are means ± SD measured in 2-h intervals over 48 hours. Shaded bars represent sleep time

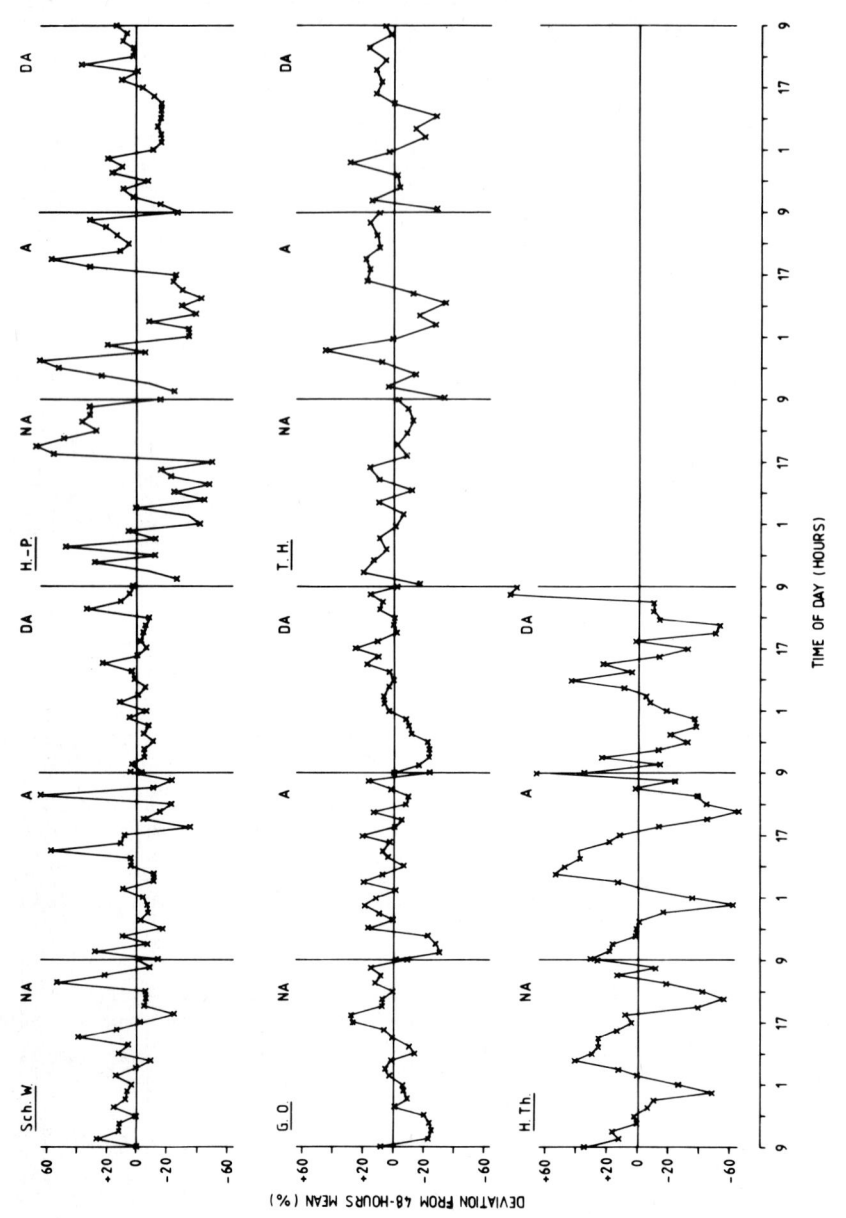

Fig. 2. Time course of norepinephrine (NA), epinephrine (A) and dopamine (DA) in serum over 48 hours in five patients with apallic syndrome

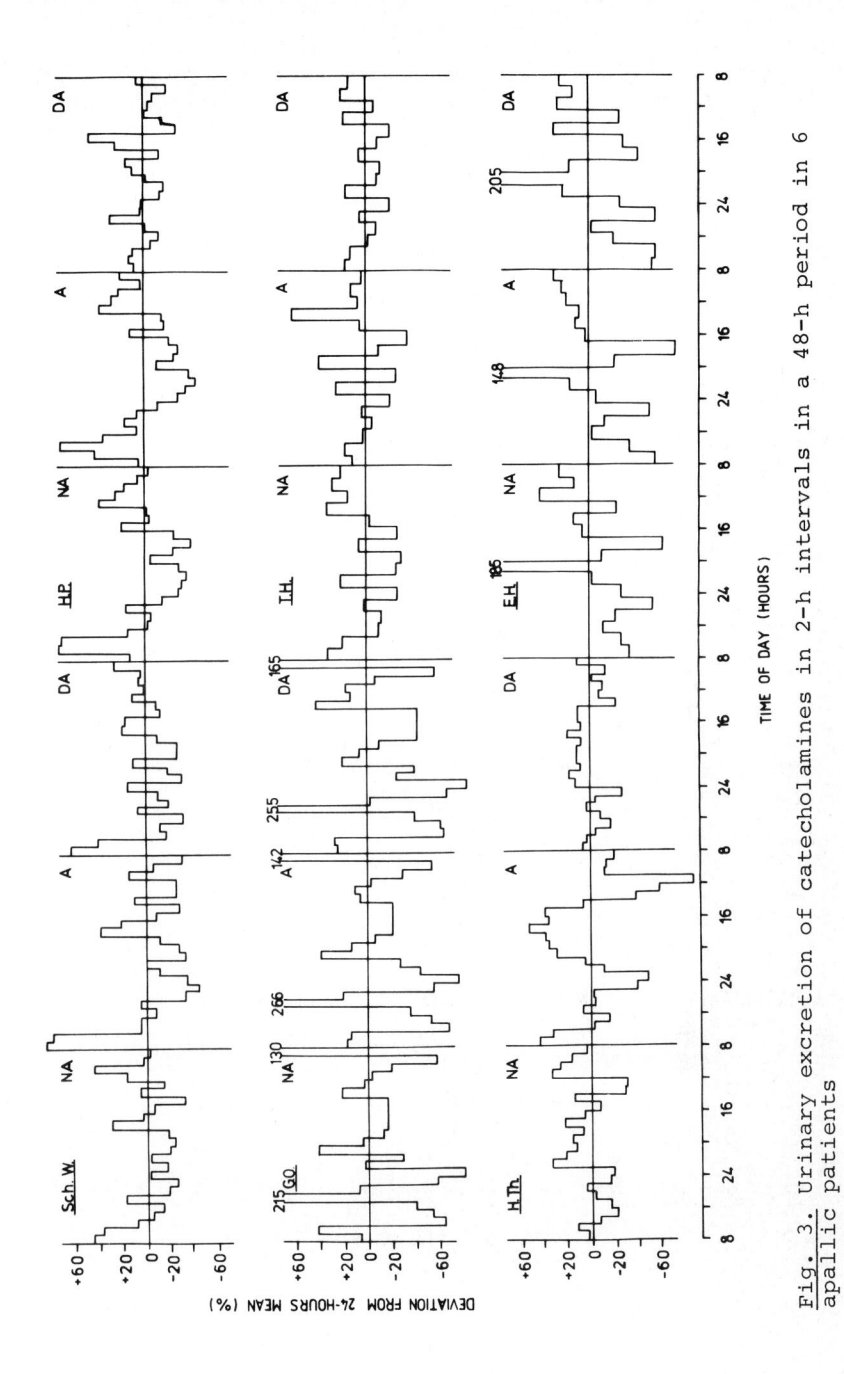

Fig. 3. Urinary excretion of catecholamines in 2-h intervals in a 48-h period in 6 apallic patients

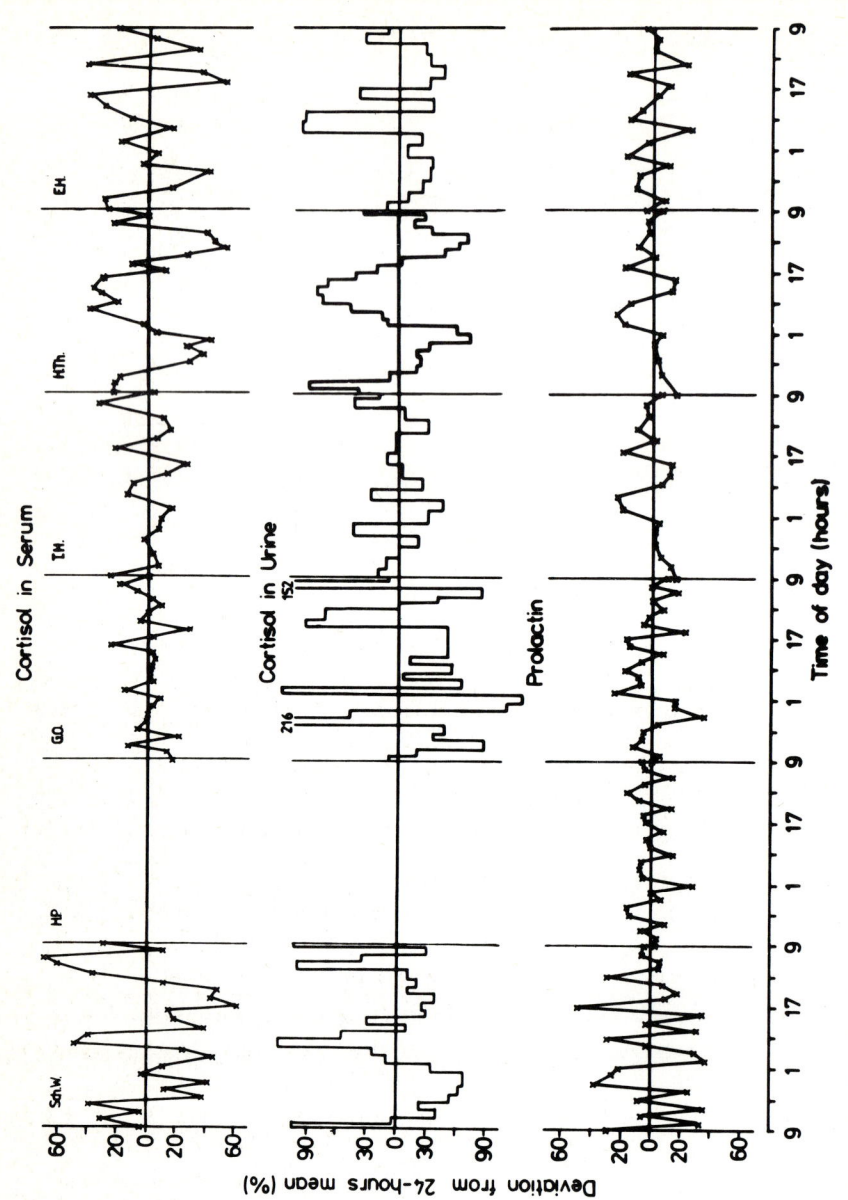

Fig. 4. Daily changes in serum concentrations of cortisol and prolactin as well as urinary excretion of cortisol over 48 hours in 6 apallic patients

Tissue Oxygen Supply Conditions in the Brain Cortex During Arterial Hypocapnia

R. SCHUBERT, K. ZIMMER, and J. GROTE

Pronounced hyperventilation induces a decrease of total and regional cerebral blood flow (CBF) (4, 6, 16, 18) and typical changes in brain metabolism (1, 7-9, 20, 24). The latter are characterized by increased tissue levels of lactate, pyruvate and NADH, as well as elevated lactate/pyruvate - and NADH/NAD$^+$ ratios. The metabolic alterations are in part the direct consequence of the decrease in brain tissue PCO_2. In addition it is assumed that brain tissue hypoxia secondary to severe arterial hypocapnia contributes to the above changes. However, since in previous studies measurements of the energy rich phosphate compounds in the brain cortex during marked hyperventilation resulted in normal values (7-9), this assumption has not as yet been substantiated.

The aim of the present study was to further investigate the tissue O_2 supply in the brain cortex of cats during arterial hypocapnia and to determine whether a severe decrease in $PaCO_2$ actually induces brain tissue hypoxia.

Methods

Twenty-two cats of both sexes weighing 2.8 to 4.5 kg, were premedicated with Ketamin-HCl (Ketanest, 10 - 20 mg/kg), anesthetized with sodium pentobarbital (Nembutal, 20 - 25 mg/kg i.v.) and immobilized with hexcarbacholinbromide (Imbretil, 1.6 to 2.0 mg at the beginning; 0.2 to 0.3 mg every 30 min during the experiments). Following tracheotomy the animals were artificially ventilated. Analyses of respiratory gas tensions and pH in arterial and cerebro-venous blood were performed using microelectrodes. Blood hemoglobin concentration was calculated taking into account the O_2 dissociation curve (2). To facilitate continuous blood pressure measurements and intermittent blood sampling, catheters were inserted into one femoral artery and into the superior sagittal sinus. After bilateral craniotomy and opening of the dura over the suprasylvian gyri regional blood flow (rCBF) was determined by means of the Kr^{85}-clearance technique following bolus injection into both lingual arteries (13, 19, 25) and tissue PO_2 measurements were performed employing multiwire surface microelectrodes (15, 21, 22). Regional cortical O_2 uptake ($rCMRO_2$) was calculated from the derived rCBF values and the arterio-venous differences in blood O_2 content.

To provide control data ten cats were studied under conditions of normoxic normocapnia. When the arterial PO_2, PCO_2 and pH reached constant values, two to four rCBF and about seventy tissue PO_2 measurements were performed in each hemisphere. The brain was subsequently frozen with liquid nitrogen and the areas under investigation were chiselled out to enzymatically assay tissue concentrations of glucose, lactate, pyruvate, ATP, ADP, AMP and phosphocreatine (3, 5, 11, 12, 14, 17). To exclude the presence of brain edema tissue water content of the gray and white matter was determined by drying the samples to a constant weight at 105° C.

Hyperventilation experiments were performed in twelve additional cats. After initial control measurements of rCBF and cortical tissue PO_2 the animals were hyperventilated first to a hypocapnic steady-state with an arterial CO_2 tension of approximately 2.5 kPa and secondly to 1.6 kPa at normal arterial O_2 tension. Both hypocapnic levels were maintained for 50 to 60 min during which the rCBF and tissue PO_2 measurements were repeated. Subsequently at a $PaCO_2$ of 1.6 kPa frozen tissue samples for metabolite assay were taken as described above.

Results

Hyperventilation induced in all experiments a reduction of mean regional blood flow in the investigated cortical regions (Table 1). The mean rCBF values, however, do not clearly describe the real cerebrovascular response to arterial hypocapnia as observed in the single studies. While the reduction of arterial CO_2 tension to 2.5 kPa caused a general fall of rCBF, the following lowering of $PaCO_2$ to 1.6 kPa induced different blood flow reactions with simultaneously further decreased as well as increased flow rates in the two compared brain regions (Fig. 1). The inhomogeneous blood flow pattern in the brain cortex under pronounced arterial hypocapnia was not static. Flow measurements, repeated over the same areas in short intervals showed in many cases that blood flow restriction was followed by a flow increase while after periods with relatively high flow rates rCBF decreased. Regional cortical O_2 uptake was reduced during severe arterial hypocapnia.

The tissue PO_2 measurements are summarized in frequency histograms (Fig. 2). During arterial normocapnia and normoxia the cortical O_2 tensions ranged from very low values (0 to 0.3 kPa) to values near the arterial O_2 tension. Under conditions of pronounced hypocapnia a marked displacement to low values was observed with a significant increase of O_2 tensions of 0 and near 0 kPa indicating the presence of insufficient tissue oxygenation in single cortical cells. The enzymatically determined tissue metabolite concentrations confirm the above findings. As compared with the control values a $PaCO_2$ reduction to 1.6 kPa induced significant decrease of the phosphocreatine concentration (Table 2). Cortical ATP was found to be normal while the glucose, ADP and AMP concentrations were increased.

Discussion

The mean cortical blood flow decrease as determined during arterial hypocapnia is in close agreement with the results of different previous investigations. It is assumed that the underlying increase in cerebrovascular resistance is mainly induced by the subsequent lowering of the brain extracellular H^+ concentration (4, 16, 18). The transitory vasodilatation observed in many experiments at pronounced hypocapnic levels seem to be due to the tissue hypoxia simultaneously found. An increase in the tissue adenosine concentration and a relative rise in the H^+ and K^+ concentrations of the perivascular space possibly mediate this effect (4, 10, 16, 23). The tissue PO_2 values, the metabolite concentrations as well as the regional cortical O_2 uptake rates provide conclusive evidence of the presence of insufficient

Table 1. Influence of moderate and marked hyperventilation on respiratory gas tensions and pH in arterial blood and on rCBF as well as rCMRO$_2$ in the brain cortex of cats. Mean values $\pm$ SE are given; n = 12

	Normoventilation	Moderate hyperventilation	Marked hyperventilation
PaO$_2$ [kPa]	13.32 $\pm$ 0.63	14.91 $\pm$ 0.81	14.87 $\pm$ 0.59
PaCO$_2$ [kPa]	3.93 $\pm$ 0.07	2.51 $\pm$ 0.05	1.62 $\pm$ 0.04
pHa	7.411 $\pm$ 0.013	7.509 $\pm$ 0.032	7.619 $\pm$ 0.031
rCBF [ml·100g^{-1}·min^{-1}]	129.2 $\pm$ 4.0	103.1 $\pm$ 3.4	97.6 $\pm$ 5.1
rCMRO$_2$ [ml·100g^{-1}·min^{-1}]	12.7 $\pm$ 0.7	12.9 $\pm$ 0.8	11.3 $\pm$ 0.7

Table 2. Influence of severe arterial hyperventilation (PaCO$_2$ = 1.6 kPa) on tissue metabolite concentrations in the brain cortex of cats. Mean values $\pm$ SE are given; normocapnic group n=10; hypocapnic group n=9

	Normoventilation	Marked hyperventilation
Glu [µmol·g w.wt.$^{-1}$]	4.88 $\pm$ 0.49	5.73 $\pm$ 0.59
La [µmol·g w.wt.$^{-1}$]	1.244 $\pm$ 0.141	5.915 $\pm$ 1.094
PCr [µmol·g w.wt.$^{-1}$]	4.59 $\pm$ 0.20	3.38 $\pm$ 0.25
ATP/ADP	7.6 $\pm$ 1.0	5.4 $\pm$ 0.6
La/Py	15.6 $\pm$ 2.9	26.6 $\pm$ 3.5

O_2 supply in small areas of the brain cortex during severe hypocapnia. The observed 10% decrease in $rCMRO_2$ is comparable to results of ALEXANDER and coworkers (1). Since the calculations of regional cortical metabolic rate of oxygen were based on the measured values for rCBF and the differences in O_2 concentrations between the arterial blood and the blood of the sinus sagittalis superior, the results are approximations only, possibly overestimating the real O_2 uptake.

The significantly increased tissue concentrations of lactate and pyruvate at low $PaCO_2$ are in line with the results of previous investigations of GRANHOLM and SIESJÖ (7-9), LEUSEN et al. (20) and WEYNE et al. (24). Since at the same time the lactate/pyruvate ratio was significantly increased and the tissue concentration of phosphocreatine was significantly decreased the observed hypocapnic effects on glycolytic activity must in part be the consequence of insufficient tissue oxygenation in the brain cortex.

In conclusion the results of the present experiments show that severe arterial hypocapnia at normal arterial oxygen tension leads to tissue hypoxia of the brain cortex. In the hypoxic regions the vasoconstrictive effects of hypocapnia seem to be reversed.

References

1. Alexander, S.C., Smith, T.C., Strobel, G., Stephen, G.W., Wollman, H.: Cerebral carbohydrate metabolism of man during respiratory and metabolic alkalosis. J. Appl. Physiol. 24, 66-72 (1968)
2. Bartels, H., Harms, H.: Sauerstoffdissoziationskurven des Blutes von Säugetieren (Mensch, Kaninchen, Hund, Katze, Schwein, Rind). Pflügers Arch. 268, 334-365 (1959)
3. Bergmeyer, H.U., Bernt, E., Schmidt, F., Stork, H.: D-Glucose. Bestimmung mit Hexokinase und Glucose-6-phosphat-Dehydrogenase. In: Methoden der enzymatischen Analyse. Bergmeyer, H.U. (ed.), pp. 1242-1246. Weinheim: Verlag Chemie 1974
4. Betz, E.: Cerebral blood flow: Its measurement and regulation. Physiol. Rev. 52, 595-630 (1972)
5. Czok, R., Lamprecht, W.: Pyruvat, Phosphoenolpyruvat und D-Glycerat-2-phosphat. In: Methoden der enzymatischen Analyse. Bergmeyer, H.U. (ed.), pp. 1491-1494. Weinheim: Verlag Chemie 1974
6. Gotoh, F., Meyer, J.S., Takagi, Y.: Cerebral effects of hyperventilation in man. Arch. Neurol. 12, 410-423 (1965)
7. Granholm, L., Siesjö, B.K.: The effects of hypercapnia and hypocapnia upon the cerebrospinal fluid lactate and pyruvate concentrations and upon the lactate, pyruvate, ATP, ADP, phosphocreatine and creatine concentrations of cat brain tissue. Acty physiol. scand. 75, 257-266 (1969)
8. Granholm, L., Lukjanova, L., Siesjö, B.K.: The effect of marked hyperventilation upon tissue levels of NADH, lactate, pyruvate, phosphocreatine and adenosine phosphates of the rat brain. Acta physiol. scand. 77, 179-190 (1969)
9. Granholm, L., Siesjö, B.K.: The effect of combined respiratory and nonrespiratory alkalosis on energy metabolites and acidbase parameters in the rat brain. Acta physiol. scand. 81, 307-314 (1971)

10. Grote, J.: Cerebral blood flow regulation under the conditions of arterial hypoxia. In: The arterial system. Bauer, R.D., Busse, R. (eds.), pp. 209-215. Berlin, Heidelberg, New York: Springer 1978

11. Gruber, W., Möllering, H., Bergmeyer, H.U.: Analytische Differenzierung von Purin- und Pyrimidin-Nuclotiden. Bestimmung von ADP, ATP sowie Summe GTP + ITP in biologischem Material. In: Methoden der enzymatischen Analyse. Bergmeyer, H.U. (ed.), pp. 2128-2137. Weinheim: Verlag Chemie 1974

12. Gutmann, I., Wahlefeld, A.W.: L- (+) - Lactat. Bestimmung mit Lactat-Dehydrogenase und NAD. In: Methoden der enzymatischen Analyse. Bergmeyer, H.U. (ed.), pp. 1510-1514. Weinheim: Verlag Chemie 1974

13. Hutten, H., Brock, M.: The two-minutes-flow-index (TMFI). In: Cerebral blood flow, clinical and experimental results. Brock, M., Fieschi, C., Ingvar, D.H., Lassen, N.A., Schürmann, K. (eds.), pp. 19-23. Berlin, Heidelberg, New York: Springer 1969

14. Jaworek, D., Gruber, W., Bergmeyer, H.U.: Adenosin-5'-diphosphat und Adenosin-5'-monophosphat. In: Methoden der enzymatischen Analyse. Bergmeyer, H.U. (ed.), pp. 2178-2181. Weinheim: Verlag Chemie 1974

15. Kessler, M., Grunewald, W.: Possibilities of measuring oxygen pressure fields in tissue by multiwire platinum electrodes. Progr. Resp. Res. 3, 147-152 (1969)

16. Kuschinsky, W., Wahl, M.: Local chemical and neurogenic regulation of cerebral vascular resistance. Physiol. Rev. 58, 656-689 (1978)

17. Lamprecht, W., Stein, P., Heinz, F., Weissner, H.: Creatinphosphat. Bestimmung mit Creatin-Kinase, Hexokinase und Glucose-6-phosphat-Dehydrogenase. In: Methoden der enzymatischen Analyse. Bergmeyer, H.U. (ed.), pp. 1825-1833. Weinheim: Verlag Chemie 1974

18. Lassen, N.A.: Brain extracellular pH: The main factor controlling cerebral blood flow. Scand. U. Clin. Lab. Invest. 22, 247-251 (1968)

19. Lassen, N.A., Ingvar, D.H.: The blood flow of the cerebral cortex determined by radioactive Krypton^{85}. Experientia 17, 42-43 (1961)

20. Leusen, I., Demeester, G.: Lactate and pyruvate in the brain of rats during hyperventilation. Arch. intern. Phys. Biochem. 74, 25-34 (1966)

21. Lübbers, D.W., Baumgärtl, H., Fabel, H., Huch, A., Kessler, M., Kunze, K., Riemann, H., Seiler, D., Schuchardt, S.: Principle and construction of various platinum electrodes. Progr. Resp. Res. 3, 136-146 (1969)

22. Lübbers, D.W.: Local tissue PO$_2$: Its measurement and meaning. In: Oxygen supply, theoretical and practical aspects of oxygen supply and microcirculation of tissue. Kessler, M., Bruley, D.F., Clark, L.C., Lübbers, D.W., Silver, I.A., Strauss, J. (eds.), pp. 151-155. München, Berlin, Wien: Urban & Schwarzenberg 1973

23. Rubio, R., Berne, R.M., Bockman, E.L., Curnish, R.R.: Relationship between adenosine concentration and oxygen supply in rat brain. Am. J. Physiol. 228, 1896-1902 (1975)

24. Weyne, J., Demeester, G., Leusen, J.: Effects of carbon dioxide, bicarbonate and pH on lactate and pyruvate in the brain of rats. Pflügers Arch. 314, 292-311 (1970)

25. Zierler, K.L.: Equations for measuring blood flow by external monitoring of radioisotopes. Circulation Res. 16, 309-321 (1965)

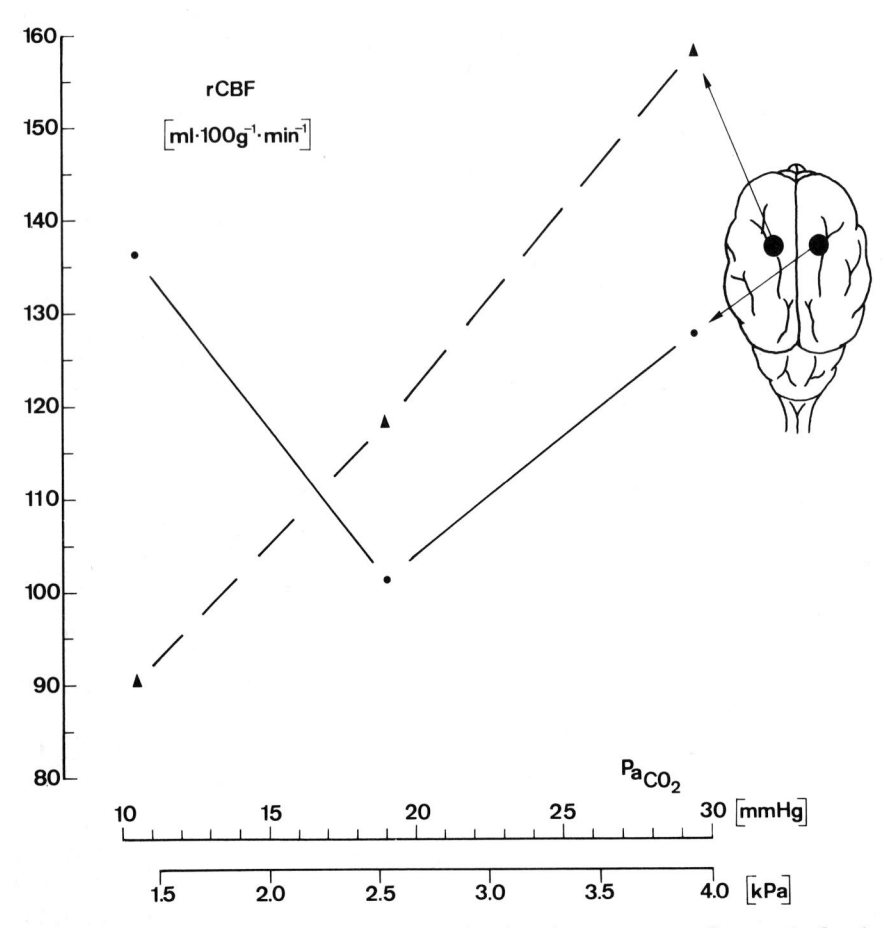

Fig. 1. Regional blood flow in the brain cortex of a cat during moderate and severe arterial hypocapnia

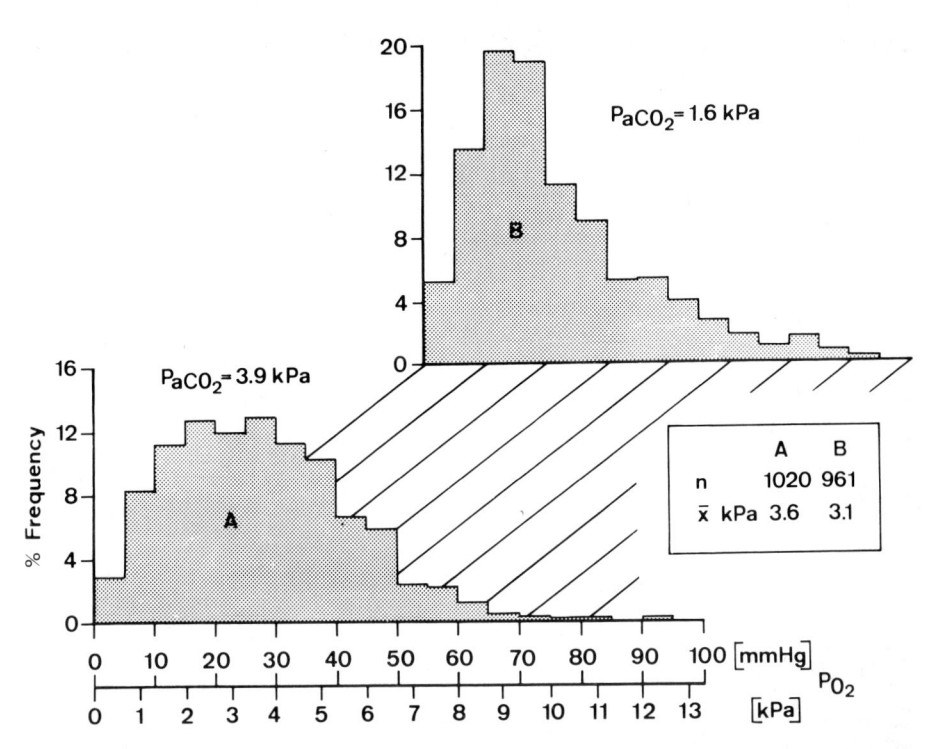

Fig. 2. Tissue PO$_2$ frequency histograms in the brain cortex of cats during arterial normocapnia and severe arterial hypocapnia

The Behavior of Sodium, Potassium, Magnesium and Zinc in the Brain with Special Attention to Cerebral Edema Following Experimentally Induced Burns

W. Heller, B. Domres, W. Hacker, and U. Oehler

Introduction

In the foreground of the pathogenesis of acute burn shock is a generalized increase in blood vessel permeability. This causes marked edema formation, not only in the immediate neighborhood of the thermally damaged skin, but in the entire organism as well. This generalized disturbance of permeability cannot be explained by the immediate effect of thermal energy on the blood vessels alone. Much more responsible for this disturbance are the histamines, prostaglandines, polypeptides, catecholamines and toxic burn products which are partially liberated from the burned tissue and partially from the organism by neurogenic and chemical stimulation. The functioning of all organs in the further course of the burn disease is hampered by this.

Clinical and scientific interest has been directed until now towards primarily the functional and pathological changes in kidneys, liver, lungs, the gastrointestinal tract, the endocrine glands and the reticuloendothelial system. Disturbances of the central nervous system, on the other hand, have hardly been studied, although severely injured patients regularly show neurological and psychological symptoms.

Autopsy showed cerebral edema in 24 of 30 mortalities from burns who died in the period from 1966 to 1975 in the Chirurgische Universitätsklinik in Tübingen. Of the 12 patients who died in the first 5 days, 11 died from cerebral edema.

Although burn patients in the clinic gain weight with calculated fluid administration during the first few days due to their tendency to edema, experimental animals who received no volume substitution showed a marked weight loss. Generous fluid replacement would probably increase the fluid content of the cerebrum beyond the amount found here.

The following questions are of interest in this connection:
1. Does cerebral edema occur regularly following a standardized burn trauma?
2. How do sodium, potassium, zinc and magnesium concentrations react in the blood and cerebral tissue?
3. Do disturbances in glucose or energy metabolism or a diminished supply of oxygen play a part in the pathogenesis of cerebral edema?

Methods and Materials

In a standardized burn model, 996 male SPF-Sprague Dawley rats received third degree burns over 20% of the body surface by means of an electrically heated copper stamp, which was heated to 250° C and applied for 30 seconds.

At 12, 24 and 48 hours as well as at 7 days, the brains were removed using the freeze-stop technique and the concentrations of the following parameters determined: H_2O content, sodium, potassium, zinc, magnesium and glucolytic metabolites, also adenosintriphosphate.

These last two parameters will not be discussed here. The statistical methods used were the F-test of FISHER, the t-test according to GROSSET, the aspin-test and the U-test according to WILCOXON, MANN and WHITNEY.

Results

Sodium. 12 hours subsequent to burn trauma there is a significant decline in sodium in the cerebral tissue (p = 0.036), which is again elevated following 24 hours (p = 0.033). The level which is reached at 24 hours changes only slightly following 48 hours. In the 7 day group, sodium concentration does not increase significantly again.

Potassium. The cerebral potassium concentration shows a significant increase (p = 0.001) 12 hours subsequent to experimentally induced burns and a decrease which is just as significant within 24 hours (p = 0.001). From 24 to 48 hours and from 48 hours to 7 days a slight, non-significant decrease occurs (Fig. 1).

Zinc (Fig. 2). 12 hours following administration of the burn trauma, the zinc level falls significantly in comparison with the control group. In 24 hours a significant climb back occurs, but the zinc level still lies significantly under that of the control group. At 48 hours no noticeable change occurs anymore, however the scatter range is then greater, so that no significant differences occur in comparison with the other group. On the other hand, the elevation of zinc levels after seven days is significant in comparison to the other burn groups. The seven day value is not different from that of the control group so that we may speak of a self-regulating mechanism in the burned animals with respect to the behaviour of zinc levels.

Magnesium (Fig. 3). Following experimental burning there is a significant elevation of the magnesium level in the brain which remains constant at 12, 24 and 48 hours. 7 days later occurs a significant decline in comparison with the other burned groups until the levels of the control group are attained. It is thus confirmed that both the magnesium and the zinc content in cerebral tissue attain their initial levels 7 days following experimental burning.

Fluid Content (Fig. 4). In comparison to the control group, all four groups show a significant increase in the fluid content of cerebral tissue following experimental burning. Even after only 12 hours, the moisture content is significantly increased (p = 0.023). From 12 to 24 hours no significant elevation of fluid content can be observed, but the transition period from 24 to 48 hours is again significant (p = 0.003). Against this, the decline from 48 hours to 7 days is not significant.

Mortality and Weight Loss. The highest mortality rate following experimental burning could be observed with the animals at the end of the second day p.c., which agrees with the observations of our other research groups who determined maximum mortality at 48 hours. This same maximum value occurs, remarkably enough, with the water content of the brain also.

Mortality and weight loss in the individual groups:

	12 hours	24 hours	48 hours	7 days
% Mortality	1.4	9.5	42.9	48.5
% Weight loss	0.3	2.7	10.9	19.3

Discussion

Our studies show a definite mortality maximum between 24 and 48 hours. The 192 animals who died in this period comprised 71.4% of the total number of animals who died. This is in agreement with an even more differentiated experimental series we have carried out in which 72% of the animals who died did so between the 46th to 50th hour.

If the increase in fluid content and mortality are compared, it can be clearly seen that both attain their maximum in the same time interval, between the 24th and 48th hour. Studies performed by our research group show that there is no ATP deficiency in the brain following burning. Likewise, an adequate blood supply to the brain seems guaranteed. This shows that cerebral edema is not due to failure of the sodium-potassium pump.

Symptomatology following burning modified according to HUGHS et al. (1973).

The increased moisture content cannot be attributed to the hypoglycemia-electrolyte mechanism, because, at this time, *hyper*glycemia is present and insulin values are not elevated (DOLECEK, 1971).

The cerebral edema following 48 hours can be effortlessly coordinated with the 48-hour mortality peak. This means that it is confirmed that cerebral edema is a co-factor in the cause of death. Likewise the incidence peak at 48 hours is in agreement with this. It could be shown that no failure of the sodium-potassium pump occurred.

The hypoglycemia-insulin-potassium mechanism could not be excluded as a factor (at 48 hours) although the values found for potassium in our studies do not indicate activity.

Conclusion

Changes in electrolyte concentrations, which usually occur at 12 hours and which then stabilize themselves more or less, could not be correlated with cerebral edema. Only the high potassium concentration at 12 hours might be a co-factor in the increased fluid content at this time. With the help of data from other studies (biochemical data and electron microscope studies), it could be shown that the electrolyte displacements were not due to failure of the sodium-potassium pumps.

The decline of zinc levels in the brain runs parallel to that in the blood. The cause lies in a permeability disturbance which ultimately leads to cerebral edema.

For magnesium an approximately antithetical mechanism in blood and cerebral tissue can be determined, with, however, normalization up to the 7th day. As cause for the magnesium increase, cell excretions for the purpose of balancing metabolic acidosis can be assumed.

References

1. Aleksandrowicz, J., Blicharski, J., Dzigowska, A., Lisiewicz, J.: Leuko- and oncogenesis in the light of studies on the metabolism of magnesium and its turnover in biogenesis. Acta med. po. 4, 289-302 (1970)

2. Brodribb, A.M., Rickets, C.R.: The effect of zinc in the healing of burns. Brit. J. Acid. Surg. 1, 24-29 (1971)

3. Broughton, A., Anderson, I.R.M., Bowden, C.H.: Mg-Deficiency syndrome in burns. Lancet 1156 (1968)

4. Clutier, C.T., Pearson, E., El-Zawahry, D., Rühimaki, H., Schwartz, M.S., Sorof, H.S., McAulay, A.C.: The effects of the administration of zinc sulfate on the healing of wounds in the burned patients. In: Res. burns. Matter, P. et al. (eds.), pp. 623-627. Bern: H. Huber 1971

5. Fodor, L., Dölp, R., Eschner, I., Ahnefeld, F.W.: Operationsbedingter Zinkverlust als limitierender Faktor im Zellstoffwechsel. Anästhesist 22, 393-399 (1973)

6. Fodor, L., Eschner, I., Dick, W., Ahnefeld, F.W.: Die klinische Bedeutung des Zinkmangelsyndroms. Anästhesist 21, 456-459 (1972)

7. Heller, W., Stolz, Chr.: Untersuchungen des Fettstoffwechsels bei schweren Verbrennungen unter dem Einfluß einer proteinaseninhibitorischen und vasoaktiven Therapie. Bücher des Päd. 70, 19-22 (1973)

8. Larson, D.L., Dobrkovsky, M., Abston, S., Lewis, S.R.: Zinc concentrations in plasma, red blood cells, wound exsudate and tissues of burned children. In: Res. burns. Matter, P. et al. (eds.), pp. 623-627. Bern: H. Huber 1971

9. Nielsen, S.P., Jemec, B.: Zinc metabolism in patients with severe burns. Scand. J. plast. reconstr. Surg. 2, 47 (1968)

10. Paschen, K., Fritz, G.: Neue vereinfachte Methoden zum empfindlichen und spezifischen Nachweis von Calcium, Magnesium und Zink im Serum mit der Atomabsorptions-Spektral-Photometrie. Ärztl. Forsch. 24, 202 (1970)

11. Quarantillo, E.P.: Effect of supplement zinc on wound healing in rats. Am. J. Surg. 121, 661 (1971)

12. Sandstead, H.H., Lanier, V.C., Shepard, G.H., Gillespie, D.D.: Zinc and wound healing. Effects of zinc deficiency and zinc supplementation. Am. J. clin. Nutr. 23, 514 (1970)

13. Savlov, E.D., Strain, W.H., Huegin, F.: Radiozinc studies in experimental wound healing. J. Speech. Res. 2, 209 (1962)

14. Seeling W., Ahnefeld, F.W., Dick, W., Fodor, L.: Die biologische Bedeutung des Zinks. Anästhesist 24, 329-343 (1975)

15. Strain, W.H., Pories, W.J., Hinshaw, R.: Zinc studies in skin repair. Surg. Forum 11, 291 (1960)

16. Thorén, L.: Magnesium metabolism. A revue of the problems related to surgical practice. Progr. Surg. 9, 131-156 (1971)

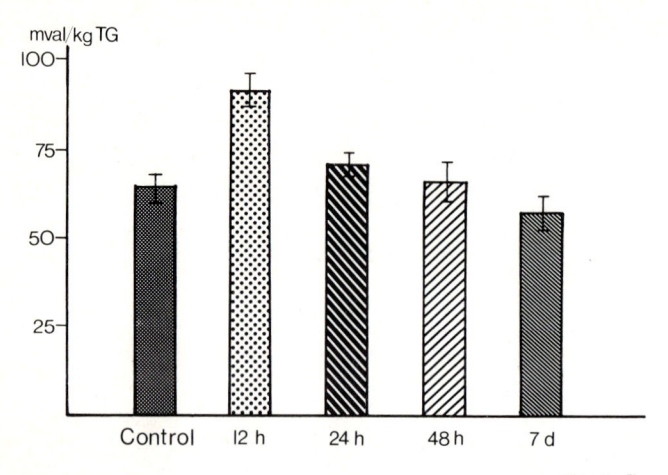

	Control	12h	24h	48h	7d
$\bar{x}$	63.96	91.03	70.95	66.25	57.04
s	12.16	12.34	9.67	15.58	13.53
$s_{\bar{x}}$	3.65	4.37	2.92	5.57	4.51
n	10	8	11	8	9

	12h	24h	48h	7d
Control	0.000	n.s.	n.s.	n.s.
12h		0.000	0.001	0.000
24h			n.s.	0.015
48h				n.s.

Fig. 1. Potassium content in the brain after experimental burn in comparison to that in a control group

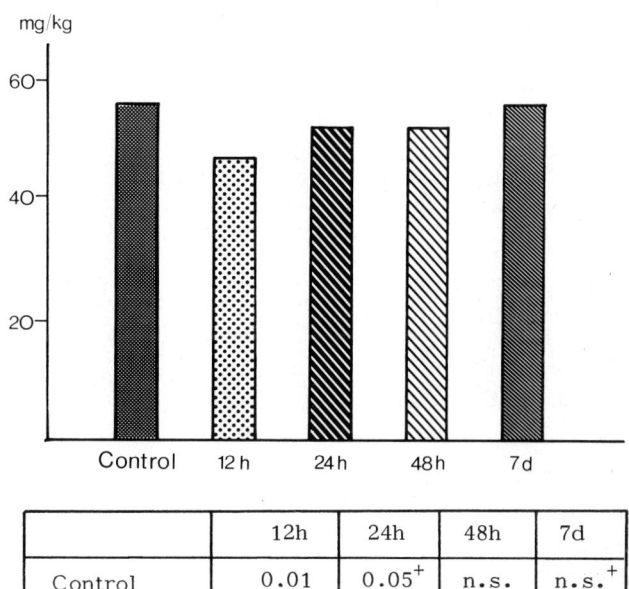

	12h	24h	48h	7d
Control	0.01	0.05[+]	n.s.	n.s.[+]
12h		0,05	n.s.	0,01
24h			n.s.[+]	0.01
48h				0.05[+]

Fig. 2. Zinc content in the brain after experimental burn in comparison to that in a control group

	12h	24h	48h	7d
Control	0.05	0.05	0.05	n.s.
12h		n.s.	n.s.	0.01
24h			n.s.	0.05[+]
48h				0.05[+]

Fig. 3. Magnesium content in the brain after experimental burn in comparison to that in a control group

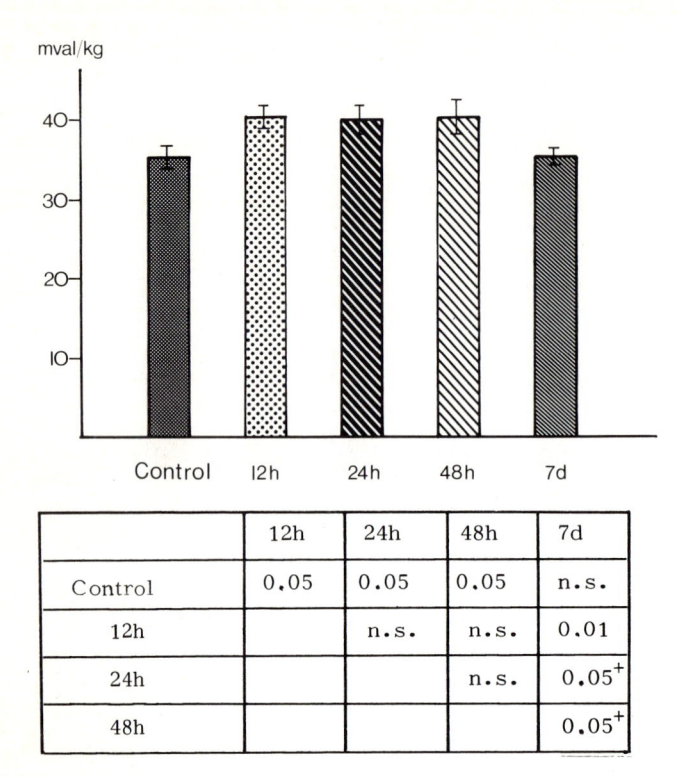

	Control	12h	24h	48h	7d
$\bar{x}$	76.17	76.66	76.74	77.38	77.27
s	0.68	0.29	0.51	0.41	0.34
$s_{\bar{x}}$	0.18	0.08	0.14	0.13	0,10
n	14	13	13	10	12

	12h	24h	48h	7d
Control	0.023	0.021	0.000	0,000
12h		n.s.	0.000	0.000
24h			0.003	0.005
48h				n.s.

Fig. 4. Fluid content in the brain after experimental burn in comparison to that in a control group

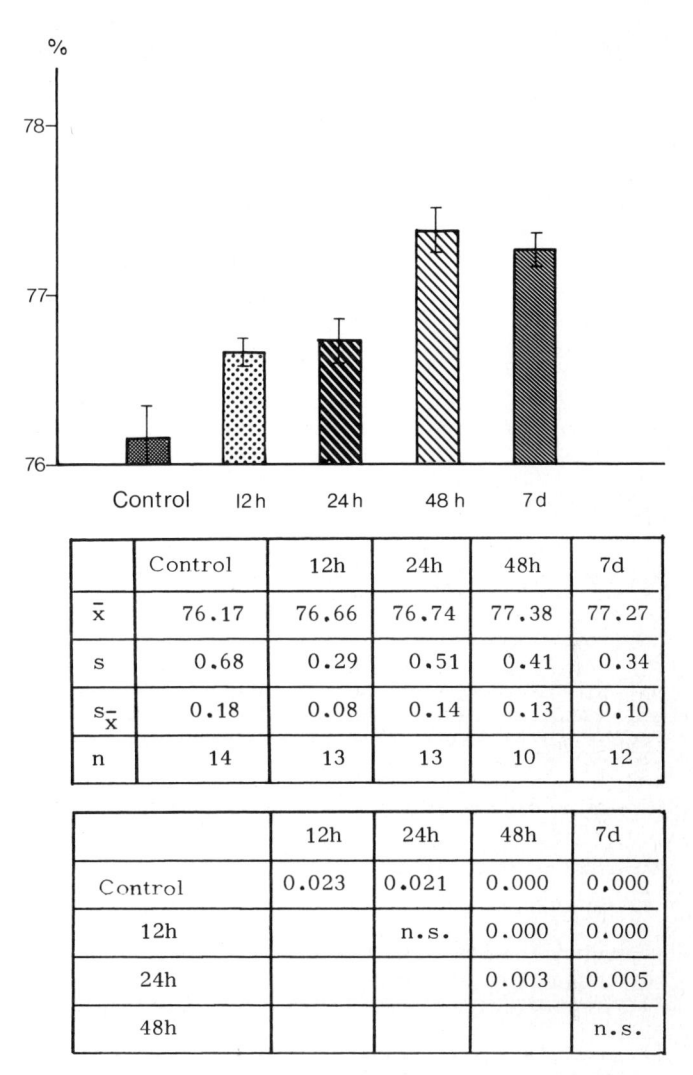

Determination of Dexamethasone with Radioimmunassay in Case of Head Injury

D. P. LIM, D. REINHARDT, and W. J. BOCK*

Besides controlled respiration, administration of saluretics or osmodiuretics, most authors recommend high doses of dexamethasone in the basic therapy of the traumatic cerebral edema. Moreover, different doses of dexamethasone are prescribed in the treatment of perifocal edemas in the neighbourhood of cerebral tumors, and after operations for cerebral tumors. Although this therapy is generally accepted, the half-life, the bioavailability, the therapeutic serum levels and other pharmacokinetic parameters are unknown so far. Hence, the use of dexamethasone and its dosage in neurosurgery, are mainly based on clinical experiences and observations. After the introduction of different radioimmunassays for the determination of endogenous glucocorticoids, the radioimmunologic determination of dexamethasone and other synthetic steroids has recently been described. Endeavouring to put the therapy of cerebral edema with dexamethasone on a more rational basis we have measured in the course of the therapy, the serum levels in several cases of head injuries. The determination that will be continued in several groups of patients aims at establishing a dosage scheme and pharmacokinetic data of dexamethasone.

Method

Patients having suffered head injuries of different severity (degree I to IV) were given immediately after the accident, a high dose of dexamethasone by bolus injection i.e. (1 mg/kg). Hereafter, a continuous maintenance therapy (6 x 8 mg of dexamethasone daily) was carried out for at least 4 to 5 days, dependent upon the severity of the clinical picture as well as upon the CT- and the EEG-findings.

During the entire course of the treatment, serum samples were taken at various moments spread over 72 hours, before the injections of dexamethasone. The samples were frozen, and the dexamethasone concentrations of the plasma were determined, by a specific radioimmunassay.

Assay

Tritium-labelled dexamethasone was added to "stripped" plasma containing different concentrations of dexamethasone, and to the plasma of the patients itself; hereafter, antibodies were added. After cold incubation of 12 hours duration and separation on coal, the concentrations of dexamethasone were determined by a liquid scintillation counter.

---

*We thank Prof. VECSEI and Dr. HAAK (Institut of Pharmacology, University of Heidelberg) for technical instructions

Results and Discussion

An intravenous bolus injection of dexamethasone (1 mg/kg) produced a plasma level of 10 µg/100 ml (Fig. 1).

Despite injections of 8 mg of dexamethasone every 4 hours, the dexamethasone concentrations decreased within the first 24 hours to 8 - 10 µg/100 ml. In the further course of the treatment (6 x 8 mg per day) a steady-state was reached at approx. 8 - 9 µg/100 ml, that means an equilibrium between the blood compartment and the tissue compartment (Fig. 1).

CT-controls made in one patient before the first administration of dexamethasone, and in the further course of the treatment, displayed a generalized swelling of the brain, the external space of the cerebrospinal fluid being effaced, and the lateral ventricles being narrowed (Fig. 2). On the third day of the treatment with dexamethasone, the cerebral edema had considerably subsided, an involution of the liquor spaces had occurred, and the ventricular system was dilated again (Fig. 3).

Investigations made by HAACK, LICHTWALD and VECSE in healthy volunteers to clarify the pharmacokinetics of dexamethasone after a single injection of the drug have revealed a half-life of dexamethasone in the plasma of approx. 4 hours. The present experiences show that an initial dose of 1 mg/kg followed by a maintenance therapy (6 x 8 mg of dexamethasone daily) ensures a continuous blood level of about 8 - 10 µg/100 ml. The investigations have shown furthermore the specific radioimmunassay that offers no technical difficulties to be well suited for the control of dexamethasone levels. However, in order to develop optimal dosage schemes, the exact pharmacokinetics of dexamethasone must be elucidated.

Furthermore, the clinical data and the serum level of dexamethasone must be compared in further studies in order to find out which "therapeutic window" must be reached for the purpose of optimizing the therapeutic results.

References

1. Cooper, P.R., Moody, S., Clark, W., Kirkpatrick, J., Maravilla, K., Gould, A.L., Drane, W.: Dexamethasone and severe head injury. J. Neurosurg. 51, 307-316 (1979)
2. Faupel, G., Reulen, H.J., Müller, D., Schürmann, K.: Clinical double-blind-study on the effects of dexamethasone on severe closed head injuries. In: Advances in neurosurgery, Vol. 4. Wüllenweber, R., Brock, M., Hamer, J., Klinger, M., Spoerri, O. (eds.), pp. 200-203. Berlin, Heidelberg, New York: Springer 1977
3. Feil, P.J.: Kinetic studies of cortisol and synthetic corticosteroids in man. Clin. Endocrinol. 1, 65-72 (1972)
4. Gaab, M., Herrmann, F., Kerscher, J., Rausch, K., Lochner, J., Pflughaupt, K.W.: Comparison of the effects of dexamethasone, barbiturate and tham on experimental brain oedema. Acta Neurochirurgia 28, 493-497 (1979)
5. Gobiet, W.: Die Behandlung des akuten traumatischen Hirnödems. Notfallmedizin 2, 98-103 (1976)

6. Gobiet, W., Bock, W.J., Liesegang, J., Grote, W.: Treatment of acute cerebral edema with high dose of dexamethasone. In: Intracranial pressure III. Beks, J.W.F., Bosch, D.A., Brock, M. (eds.), pp. 231-235. Berlin, Heidelberg, New York: Springer 1976
7. Haack, D., Vescei, P., Lichtwald, K., Klee, H.R., Gless, K.H., Weber, M.: Some experiences on radioimmunoassays of synthetic glucocorticoids. Allergologie 5, 259-267 (1980)
8. Tsuei, S.E., Moore, R., Ashley, J.J., McBride, W.G.: Disposition of synthetic glucocorticoids. I. Pharmacokinetics of dexamethasone in healthy adults. J. Pharmacokinetics and Biopharmaceutics 3, 249-264 (1979)

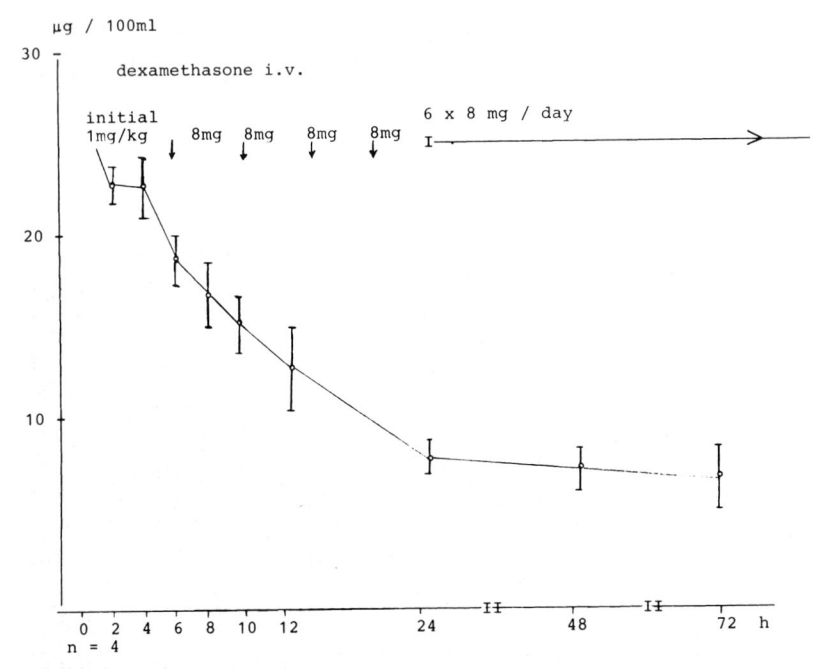

Fig. 1. Dexamethasone plasma concentrations of 4 patients in case of head injury during 72 hours after intravenous injection

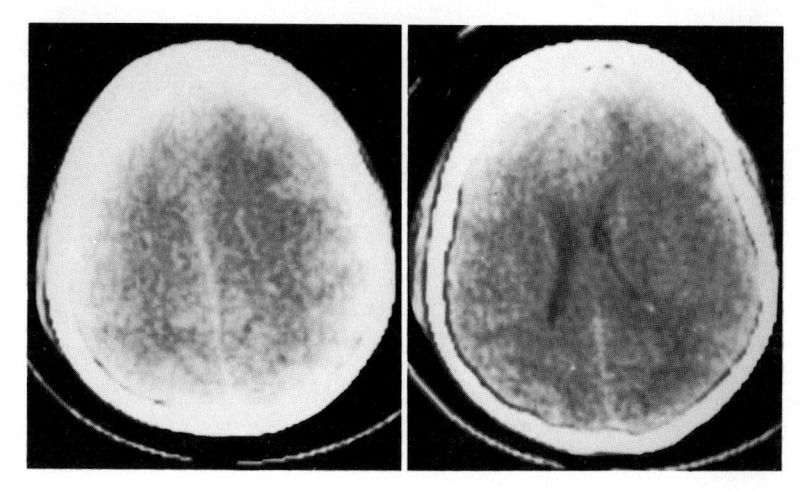

Fig. 2. Initial CT-scans (patient M. H.) in case of acute cerebral edema before treatment with high dose of dexamethasone

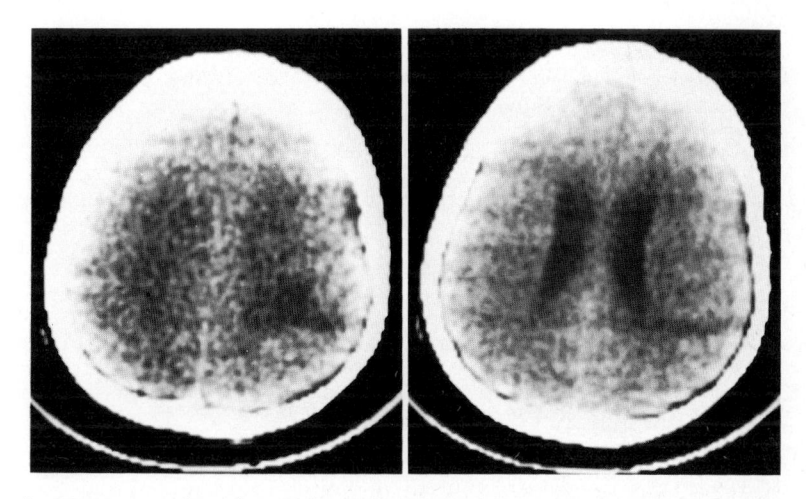

Fig. 3. Control CT-scans (patient M. H.) after treatment with dexamethasone

Investigations of the Effects of Dexamethasone on Surgical Stress in Neurosurgical Patients, on the Basis of Radioimmunological Hormone Determinations (LH, FSH, GH, ACTH, Cortisol, Testosterone)

M. BRANDT, H. WAGNER, K. H. KRÄHLING, and H.-J. KÖNIG

Introduction

Very few of the numerous publications (1, 7, 8, 9) dealing with the treatment of cerebral oedema by dexamethasone, also examine the effects of this substance on hormonal balance (2, 3). Using radioimmunological methods, we therefore investigated the effects of dexamethasone on the plasma levels of the following hormones:
Cortisol, ACTH, GH, LH, FSH and testosterone.
We were particularly concerned to find answers to the following questions:

1. Does dexamethasone bring about any changes in the hormone plasma levels?
2. How do the basal hormone plasma levels of brain-tumour patients compare with those of patients operated on for intervertebral disc prolapse?
3. Does the surgical stress lead to changes in plasma hormone concentrations?
4. Is the hormonal stress reaction influenced by the administration of dexamethasone?

Materials and Methods

Pre- and post-operative radioimmunological hormone determinations were performed under defined conditions in 61 neurosurgical patients operated on either for brain tumour or intervertebral disc prolapse. Twenty-six brain tumour patients and 18 prolapse patients were treated with dexamethasone. Seventeen prolapse patients were treated with dexamethasone. Seventeen prolapse patients to whom no dexamethasone was administered, served as a control group.

Dexamethasone was administered in the following dosage:

In the prolapse patients for three days prior to the operation and for four days after the operation, a daily dose of 2 x 8 mg per patient. On the 5th and 6th postoperative day, the dose was reduced to 2 x 4 mg dexamethasone. In the case of the brain-tumour patients, the dose regiman was, for therapeutic clinical reasons, modified as follows: on the day of the operation 4 x 8 mg and 3 x 8 mg on the first post-operative day. Otherwise, the regimen was the same as for the prolapse patients.

Hormone determinations were carried out at 8 a.m. in the fasting patient, and again at 4 p.m. in accordance with the following time schedule: on the day prior to the administration of dexamethasone, on the second day after starting the patient on dexamethasone, on the day of the operation prior to and after surgery, on the first and sixth post-operative days and, finally, 2 days after taking the patients off dexamethasone.

The statistical evaluation was performed using the T-test after STUDENT, WELSCH or GOSSET, with the WILCOXON test and the correlation analysis after PEARSON.

Results

Cortisol. The circulating cortisol level manifests a daily rhythm, being higher in the morning and lower in the evening. This daily rhythm was established in all the patients prior to the start of treatment with dexamethasone. The administration of dexamethasone brought about a drop in the level of cortisol both in brain-tumour and in prolapse patients. Following the operation, the cortisol levels rose again in response to the stresses of surgery, the rise being greater in the brain-tumour patients. All in all, the levels in particular in the prolapse patients, remained low under dexamethasone medication, and increased to normal levels only when dexamethasone medication was stopped (Fig. 1).

This is compatible with a rapid recovery of the adrenal cortex after a short-term inhibition of its secretory activity by dexamethasone.

ACTH. ACTH also manifests a daily rhythm, the concentration being higher in the morning and lower in the evening. This daily rhythm can be recognized in the basal ACTH plasma levels of the prolapse patients. Following administration of dexamethasone, a marked drop in the plasma ACTH level was observed. After surgery, the brain-tumour patients showed a considerable increase in the plasma ACTH concentrations. The daily rhythm was now reversed. After termination of dexamethasone treatment, a slight increase in the plasma ACTH levels was observed.

GH. The basal GH plasma level of the prolapse patients, with and without the administration of dexamethasone, are lower than those of the brain-tumour patients. Under dexamethasone, the GH level drops, both in the brain-tumour and in the prolapse patients. Post-operatively, the plasma GH levels increase in all three groups of patients. The GH increase in most marked in the prolapse patients not receiving dexamethasone, which may be considered the manifestation of an unattenuated stress reaction.

LH. The basal plasma levels for the luteinizing hormone are lower in the brain-tumour patients than in the prolapse patients (Fig. 2). After the administration of dexamethasone, the plasma LH level increases both in the brain-tumour and in the prolapse patients. After surgery, all plasma LH levels first drop, the decrease being greatest in the patients not treated with dexamethasone. In the other two groups, the surgery-induced drop is apparently attenuated by the prior administration of dexamethasone. When the patients are taken off dexamethasone, the corresponding plasma levels drop again.

Testosterone. The basal plasma testosterone levels are lower in the brain-tumour patients than in the prolapse patients (Fig. 3). Dexamethasone leads to a reduction in the level of testosterone both in the brain-tumour and in the prolapse patients. In all three groups of patients, the levels decrease further after surgery, and remain low until the 6th post-operative day. The mean values remain low even when the administration of dexamethasone is discontinued.

FSH. Both dexamethasone and the stress of surgery brought about a drop in the plasma FSH levels, which was, however, not significant.

Discussion and Conclusions

Since the majority of the hormones investigated are subjected to daily and short-term fluctuations, and also react very sensitively to external stress factors, the interpretation of the changes in the hormone levels determined, presents something of a problem even when statistical methods are employed. Simplifying, however, the following points may be established:

1. Differences in basal plasma levels were found between brain-tumour and prolapse patients for the following hormones:
   LH and testosterone were significantly lower, and GH significantly higher, in brain-tumour patients than in prolapse patients.
2. Surgical stress results in an increase in cortisol, ACTH, GH levels and a drop in LH, testosterone and FSH levels (10, 11). The increase in plasma cortisol was twice as large after brain-tumour surgery than after operations for intervertebral disc prolapse. This is interpreted as a greater stress response in brain-tumour operations (2, 5).
3. The investigations show that dexamethasone reduces the postoperative stress reaction for the hormones corticol, ACTH, GH and LH, but enhances it for the hormones testosterone and FSH (Fig. 4) (4, 6). Thus, an antistress effect can be attributed to dexamethasone for some of the hormones studied. This investigation should be considered an initial attempt to obtain an insight into the complicated hormonal reactions in neurosurgical operations, and treatment with dexamethasone. Further studies are necessary to check the results and their significance.

References

1. Baethmann, A., Schmiedek, P.: Pathophysiology of cerebral edema. In: Advances in neurosurgery, Vol. 1. Schürmann, K., Brock, M., Reulen, H.-J., Voth, D. (eds.), pp. 5-18. Berlin, Heidelberg, New York: Springer 1973
2. Bouzarth, W.F., Shenkin, H.A., Gutterman, P.: Adrenal cortical response to neurosurgical problems, noting the effects of exogenous steroids. In: Steroids and brain edema. Reulen, H.-J., Schürmann, K. (eds.), pp. 183-193. Berlin, Heidelberg, New York: Springer 1972
3. Brandt, M., Wagner, H., Walter, W.: Wachstumshormon, LH und FSH unter funktionsdynamischen Bedingungen im Serum sowie basale Kortisol- und Testosteron-Serumspiegel bei Schädelhirnverletzten unter Dexamethasonbehandlung. Neurochirurgia 20, 79-83 (1977)
4. Doerr, P., Pirke, K.: Response of plasma testosterone and luteinizing hormone to cortisol or dexamethasone. Acta endocr. suppl. 199, 228-232 (1975)
5. Gutterman, P., Bouzarth, W.F.: The adrenocortical response to craniotomy for brain tumor. J. Neurosurg. 34, 657-664 (1971)
6. Hierholzer, K., Neubert, D.: Endokrinologie. München: Urban und Schwarzenberg 1977

7. Klatzo, I.: Pathophysiological aspects of brain edema. In: Steroids and brain edema. Reulen, H.-J., Schürmann, K. (eds.), pp. 1-8. Berlin, Heidelberg, New York: Springer 1972

8. Reulen, H.-J., Hadjidimos, A., Schürmann, K.: The effect of dexamethasone on water and electrolyte content and on rCBF in perifocal brain edema in man. In: Steroids and brain edema. Reulen, H.-J., Schürmann, K. (eds.), pp. 239-252. Berlin, Heidelberg, New York: Springer 1972

9. Reulen, H.-J., Hadjidimos, A., Hase, U.: Steroids in the treatment of brain edema. In: Advances in neurosurgery, Vol. 1. Schürmann, K., Brock, M., Reulen, H.-J., Voth, D. (eds.), pp. 92-105. Berlin, Heidelberg, New York: Springer 1973

10. Wendt, F.: Die postoperative Streß-Reaktion nach neurochirurgischen Eingriffen im Vergleich zum Standardverhalten. Langenbecks Arch. klin. Chir. 321(2), 114-125 (1968)

11. Wagner, H., Böckel, K., Hrubesch, M., Hauss, W.: Einwirkung von Glukokortikoidgaben auf die Spiegel von ACTH, TSH, LH und FSH im menschlichen Serum. Verh. Dtsch. Ges. Rheumatologie 3, 271 (1974)

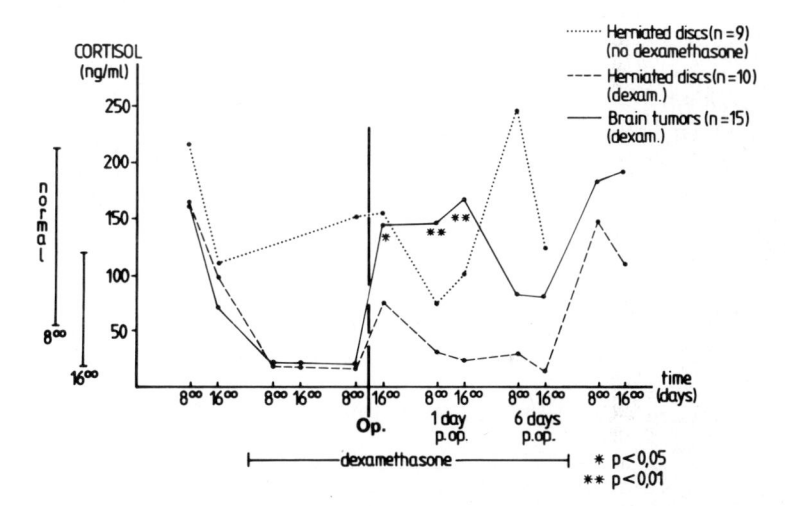

Fig. 1. Pre- and post-operative plasma cortisol levels in neurosurgical patients with and without the administration of dexamethasone

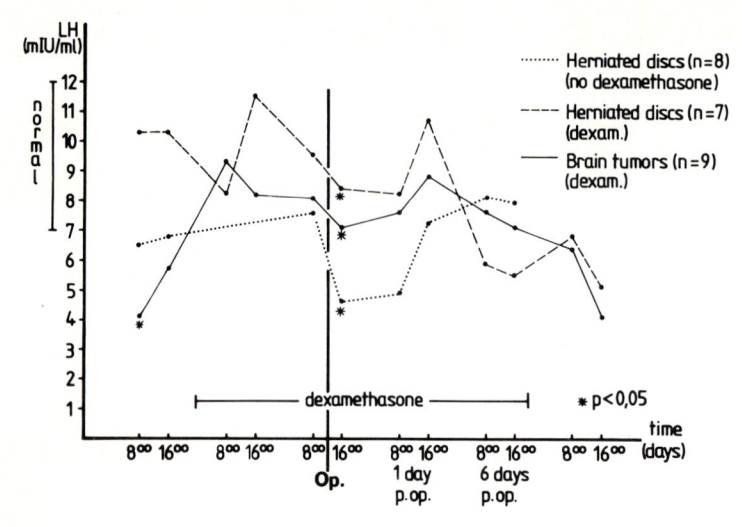

Fig. 2. Pre- and post-operative plasma LH levels in neurosurgical patients with and without the administration of dexamethasone

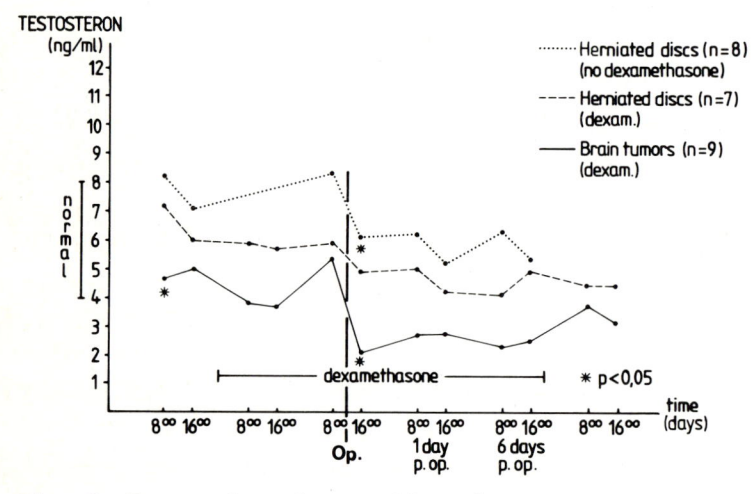

Fig. 3. Pre- and post-operative plasma testosterone levels in neurosurgical patients with and without the administration of dexamethasone

	ACTH	CORTISOL	GH(STH)	LH	TESTOSTERONE	FSH
Dexamethasone:	↓	↓	↓	↑	↓	(↓)
Operation:	↑	↑	↑	↓	↓	(↓)

Fig. 4. Changes in the plasma hormone levels in neurosurgical patients induced by dexamethasone and surgery (schematic)

An in Vitro Model of Cytotoxic Brain Edema: Cell Volume and Metabolism of Cultivated Glial- and Nerve-Cells*

O. Kempski, U. Gross, and A. Baethmann**

Introduction

Cytotoxic brain edema, i.e. swelling of nerve- and glial elements is a common result of cerebral ischemia, metabolic disorders, intoxications, and develops secondarily in vasogenic edema. Contrary to vasogenic brain edema, the mechanisms causing cytotoxic edema are far from being understood. Studies of this edema type under in-vivo conditions are obscured by the multitude of simultaneous changes occurring in brain after a cytotoxic insult, e.g. breakdown of intra-extracellular ion gradients, release of metabolites and eventually toxic substances into the extracellular space (ECS), dysregulation of neurotransmitter homeostasis, and abnormalities of the extracellular pH and PO_2. Since it is impossible to monitor or even control these factors simultaneously in-vivo, we have developed an in-vitro model to examine the mechanisms of cytotoxic cell swelling under strictly controlled conditions. For that purpose, measurements of cell volume of cultured nerve- and glial cells were performed together with parameters of cell metabolism, as e.g. O_2-consumption.

In a first experimental series, the system was tested in studies on the effect of glutamic acid, a potential cytotoxic brain edema factor ([10]) on cultured glial cells. Glutamate has been shown to cause cytotoxic brain edema under in-vivo conditions ([12]) and by measurements of cerebral impedance ([7]). In the current experiments cell volume and oxygen consumption of suspended glial cells were measured during exposure to glutamic acid.

Material and Methods

The established cell lines of C_6M glioblastoma and F-115 neuroblastoma cells were used as model cells. The cells were suspended either after mechanical (F 115) or enzymatical harvesting with trypsin (C_6M) in Dulbecco's modified minimum essential medium (MEM). The experiments were carried out in a gas-tight test chamber (content: 10 ml) which was furnished with PO_2-, pH- and temperature probes. A porous plastic tube provided oxygen to the chamber and was used to ventilate the medium with any gas-mixture desired. Alterations of the pH were controlled by modification of the CO_2 supply.

The oxygen consumption per single cell was determined from the slope of the PO_2, which fell during a transitory interruption of the oxygen

---

*Supported by Deutsche Forschungsgemeinschaft, Ba 452/5
**The excellent technical assistance of ULRIKE GOERKE, ANGELIKA MÜLLER and SYLVIA SCHNEIDER is gratefully acknowledged

supply to the chamber. For cell volume determination, suspended cells were retrieved from the chamber via stainless steel cannulas inserted into the chamber. The cell volume was analyzed electrically by an advanced Coulter method (6) using hydrodynamic particle focussing. Two different concentrations of Na^+-glutamate were used. Oxygen consumption of glial cells was measured during exposure to 2 mM glutamate, whereas cell volume was determined upon exposure to 15 mM glutamate. Cell viability was tested by exclusion of trypan blue prior to and after termination of the experiment.

Results

Suspension in 2 mM glutamate led to a significant increase in O_2-uptake of C_6M glioblastoma cells, while the O_2-uptake of F 115 neuroblastoma cells was not influenced (Table 1). However, cell viability was found to decrease for 15% in neuroblastoma cells during exposure to glutamate, whereas viability of glial cells remained almost unchanged.

Only glial cells were used to study cell volume response during suspension in 15 mM glutamate (Table 2). Suspension in medium containing 15 mM glutamate was found to increase cell volume for about 6%, which was already significant 8 minutes after exposure. Cell viability decreased in 15 mM glutamate from 92.1% at the beginnqng to 81.4% at termination of the experiment.

Table 1. Oxygen consumption of suspended glio- and neuroblastoma cells in 2 mM glutamate

Time after exposure [min]	Oxygen consumption [$\mu l \cdot 10^{-5}$/cell·h+SEM] C_6M		F 115	
0 (= control)	0.914 ± 0.125	(5)	0.852 ± 0.116	(5)
8	0.939 ± 0.071	(4)	0.916 ± 0.141	(5)
27	1.151 ± 0.201	(5)	0.817 ± 0.087	(5)
46	1.200 ± 0.123	(4)	0.855 ± 0.128	(5)
66	1.258 ± 0.179	(4)	0.823 ± 0.107	(5)
72	1.302 ± 0.193	(3)	0.981 ± 0.111	(5)

Table 2. Cell volume changes after incubation with 15 mM glutamate (C_6M-glioblastoma)

Time after exposure [min]		Mean cell volume % control	SEM	p^a
Control	(6)	100.0		
2	(6)	103.1	1.2	n.s.
8	(6)	105.3	0.9	<0.05
15	(6)	106.0	0.4	<0.05
25	(5)	106.7	1.5	<0.01
37	(4)	107.8	1.4	n.s.
59	(4)	106.2	0.6	<0.05
75	(6)	106.8	1.5	<0.05
110	(6)	106.4	1.9	n.s.
168	(4)	103.6	4.2	n.s.

[a] Arc-sin-transformation, paired t-test

Discussion

The model presented has two important advantages to study the mechanisms of cytotoxic brain edema:
1. Pertinent parameters such as PO_2, pH, temperature, concentrations of pharmacological and toxicological relevant compounds, the osmolarity and electrolyte composition can be strictly controlled.
2. Due to the large medium to cell volume ratio being almost infinite, metabolic waste discharge into the medium from the suspended cells or other kinds of cell response can be considered to be attenuated down to ineffective concentrations. Hence, the experimental conditions remain largely unchanged.

For experimental reasons, two different concentrations of glutamate, i.e. 2, and 15 mM were used. Determination of cellular O_2-uptake required to conduct the experiment with a constant number of suspended cells. Addition of higher concentrations of glutamate than 2 mM would have made it necessary to remove some of the suspension fluid, which would have caused a decrease in total cell count. On the other hand, the determination of cell volume did not require the presence of a constant number of suspended cells in the test chamber. As seen, exposure of glial cells to 2 mM glutamate led to a significant increase in cellular oxygen consumption. This may have resulted from enhancement of the aminoacid on membrane permeability to Na^+-ions. Based on other experimental studies it is supposed that addition of glutamate led to an enhanced influx of Na^+-ions together with chloride and water into the suspended glial cells, which in turn led to an increase in oxydative energy metabolism to provide the active Na^+-pumps with additional metabolic energy. This phenomenon is reflected by the increase of O_2-uptake of the suspended cells. Moreover, it has been shown (2, 4, 9), that glial cells have high-affinity uptake systems for glutamate, which under in-vivo conditions are considered to clear the extracellular fluid space from the transmitter after synaptic excitation. The increase in oxygen consumption therefore may result also from stimulation of such specific, energy dependent uptake systems.

Preliminary experiments on growth kinetics of C_6M glial cells (unpublished) have shown that glutamate concentrations of 15 mM retard markedly growth of these cells under the culture condition employed in our laboratory, whereas concentrations of 2 mM were found ineffective. Therefore concentrations of 15 mM were used to study cell volume response of C_6M glial cells. Respective experiments using concentrations of 2 mM glutamate are in progress.

As shown in Table 2, 15 mM glutamate induced a significant increase in cell volume immediately after addition of the amino acid to the suspension medium. However, the swelling of glial cells upon exposure to glutamate has a tendency to recover within 100 - 200 minutes. Several mechanisms may be considered to result in swelling of glial cells secondary to glutamate exposure.

If glutamate is taken up by glial cells via the high-affinity uptake and transport system, 1 Mol of glutamic acid is accompanied by 2 Mols of Na^+-ions (9). This would increase the intracellular osmolarity which in turn causes a net fluid shift from the extra- into the intracellular compartment, resulting in cell swelling (11, 3). Increasing the membrane permeability for Na^+-ions, with or without specific binding to a glutamate receptor on the cell surface is also conceivable which also would lead to an uptake of Na^+- and Cl^--ions, which are accompanied by water again leading to an increase of cell volume.

An increase of membrane permeability for Na^+-ions by glutamate has been frequently shown (1, 5). It is not clear yet, why and how glial cells exposed to glutamate have a tendency to recover spontaneously. Since the final concentrations of glutamate present in the suspension fluid cannot be assumed to change markedly because of the large medium to cell volume-ratio, recovery of cell volume cannot be attributed to an effective decrease in extracellular glutamate concentration due to intracellular uptake of the amino acids. Desensitization of glial cells to the amino acid as a mechanism explaining recovery or normalization of cell volume although the extracellular glutamate concentration remains high, may be considered as alternate mechanism. Desensitization to glutamate has been reported (8). The present studies further support the concept that glutamate is a brain edema promoting mediator compound. Extracellular concentrations of only 2 mM of glutamate were found to enhance substantially the oxidative metabolism of glial cells. Stimulation of the metabolic turnover may be considered detrimental in conditions as e.g. traumatic tissue damage or ischemia, where glutamate is likely to become released into the interstitial fluid compartment. Stimulation of O_2-consumption increases conceivably the O_2-debt of the tissue thus enhancing anoxic tissue injury. The measurement of cell volume during exposure to glutamate clearly demonstrates that glutamate induces cell swelling. Until now this has been concluded indirectly from in-vivo experiments using impedance measurements during ventriculo-cisternal perfusion with glutamate (7). The demonstration of glial cell swelling under in-vitro conditions render this model suitable to investigate in detail not only the mechanisms involved, but also measures which prevent or interfere with glutamate induced cell swelling.

Conclusions

An in-vitro method is presented which allows the study of mechanisms of cell swelling under controlled conditions. Further evidence is provided supporting the role of glutamic acid as mediator compound for secondary tissue damage. Glutamic acid is shown not only to increase oxydative cell metabolism, but also to induce swelling of C_6M glioblastoma cells under in-vitro conditions. The model presented can also be used to test specific methods which interfere with the biochemical mechanisms of secondary mediator compounds. This would finally benefit the development of a more specific treatment of brain edema.

References

1. Ames III, A., Tsukuda, Y., Nesbett, B.: Intracellular Cl^-, Na^+, K^+, Ca^{++}, Mg^{++}, and P in nervous tissue, response to glutamate and to changes in extracellular Ca^{++}. J. Neurochemistry 14, 145-159 (1967)

2. Balcar, N.F., Borg, F., Mandel, P.: High affinity uptake of l-glutamate and l-aspartate by glial cells. J. Neurochemistry 28, 87-93 (1977)

3. Chan, P., Fishman, R.A., Lee, J., Candelise, L.: Effects of excitatory neurotransmitter amino acids on swelling of rat brain cortical slices. J. Neurochem. 33, 1309-1315 (1979)

4. Hertz, L., Schousboe, A., Boechler, N., Mukerji, S., Fedoroff, S.: Kinetic characteristics of the glutamate uptake into normal astrocytes in cultures. Neurochem. Res. 3, 1-14 (1978)

5. Hösli, L., Andres, P.F., Hösli, E.: Ionic mechanisms associated with depolarisation by glutamate and aspartate on human and rat spinal neurones in tissue culture. Pflügers Arch. 363, 43-48 (1976)
6. Kachel, V.: Basic principles of electrical sizing of cells and particles and their realization in the new instrument "Metricell". J. Histochem. Cytochem. 24, 211-230 (1976)
7. Kempski, O.: Thesis, University Munich (1981)
8. Van Harreveld, A., Fifkova, E.: Effects of amino acids on the isolated chicken retina and its response to glutamate-stimulation. J. Neurochem. 20, 947-962 (1973)
9. Wheeler, D.D., Hollingsworth, R.G.: A model of high-affinity glutamatic acid transport by cortical synaptosomes from the long-evans rat. J. Neurochem. 30, 1311-1319 (1978)

Books

10. Baethmann, A., Öttinger, W., Rothenfußer, W., Kempski, O., Unterberg, A., Geiger, R.: Brain edema factors. Current state with particular referen-e to plasma constituents and glutamate. In: Advances in neurology, Vol. 28. Cervos-Navarro, J., Ferszt, R. (eds.), pp. 171-195. New York: Raven Press 1980
11. Van Harreveld, A.: Brain tissue electrolytes. Molecular Biology and medicine series. London: Butterworths 1966
12. Van Harreveld, A., Fifkova, E.: Light- and electron-microscopic changes in central nervous tissue after electrophoretic injection of glutamate. Exptl. and Molec. Pathol. 15, G 1-81 (1971)

Barbiturate Influence on Subcellular Organelles in Experimental Cold Lesion

D. STOLKE and H. DIETZ

The sedative and anesthetic effect of barbiturates is well known since the introduction of these drugs into therapy. In the early seventies MICHENFELDER (19) and NILSON (21) opened discussion on barbiturates once more because of their beneficial effect in experimental brain ischemia and hypoxia.

In the following years this field was thoroughly studied (2, 3, 13, 14, 26, 27, 32).

Clear improvements and less neurological deficits were documented by all the authors when animals were treated with barbiturates during brain ischemia.

MARSHALL et al. (16-18) could decrease the ICP of severely brain injured patients with barbiturates and could so improve the outcome and reduce mortality rate. In Pittsburgh SAFAT (23) and his co-workers could prolong survival time of the brain, as well after experimental as after circulatory arrest (15), brain ischemia and hypoxia.

While the reports on the experimental and clinical effect are very similar, the site and place of barbiturate effectivness are still under discussion. Primarily they assumed the effect to be a consequence of the reduction in cerebral metabolic rate (4, 19, 21).

Some authors could demonstrate by their studies that the protective effect of barbiturates surpassed the reduction effect in cerebral metabolic rate (22).

Reports were continued that barbiturates ameliorated ischemic brain damage with the improvement and normalisation of CBF, with improved brain glucose availability and utilisation. Anaerobic glucose utilisation was suppressed and oxygen utilisation coefficient improved (20).

ASTRUP suggested that there is a cell membrane stabilizing effect by barbiturate therapy (1).

Because of these reports with our studies we tried to answer if there is an influence of pentobarbital on lysosomal membrane stability in the white and grey matter of the brain tissue of the cat after experimental cold lesion.

We postulate such a membrane stabilizing effect on subcellular organelles, because of our studies (28-30) on the membrane stabilizing effect of barbiturate anesthesia on lysosomal membranes of the brain tissue of the cat. Some of these results were presented last year, in 1980, in Erlangen, at the annual meeting of the Deutsche Gesellschaft für Neurochirurgie.

Lysosomes are small subcellular organelles or particles found in all animal cells. They are surrounded by a lipoprotein membrane and contain a large collection of acid hydrolytic enzymes. These lysosomes are sites of intracellular digestion.

Uncontrolled released lysosomal enzymes may catalyze destructive damage throughout the cell and the surrounding tissue.

We studied the long acting barbiturate pentobarbital. The lysosomal enzyme β-glucuronidase was assayed to indicate lysosomal membrane stability.

De DUVE et al. (6, 7) defined the grade of stability of the lysosomal membranes as the relation of the share of free activity to total activity of the lysosomal enzymes after the destruction of the membranes by polyethylene-glycol-monoether (Triton x-100). I.e. a decrease of the share of free activity means an increase in lysosomal membrane stability.

Material and Methods

We had three groups of 8 adult cats each, both sexes, 2 - 4 kg bodyweight, which underwent the following procedures:

The first group served as a control and was sacrificed under ketamine anesthesia (30 mg/kg i.m.), the second underwent a cold lesion of the right supra-sylvian gyrus of the right hemisphere according to the KLATZO method under ketamine anesthesia (30 mg/kg i.m.), the third had the same procedure as second group but under pentobarbital anesthesia (60 mg/kg i.p.).

Both groups were sacrificed 24 hours later. The brain was removed and the grey and white matter were separated as well as the right and the left hemisphere. Homogenates were prepared in a 0.25 mol sucrose medium. The share of free activity of β-glucuronidase was assayed in a 10% homogenate. After destruction of the lysosomal membranes by Triton x-100 total activity was assayed.

Results

Our results (Tables 1, 2 and Figs. 1, 2) indicate that under barbiturate anesthesia in the white matter of the right (injured) and of the left (uninjured) hemisphere the share of free activity of β-glucuronidase is significantly decreased compared to the control group and especially compared to the group injured under ketamine anesthesia:

Control group: white matter - 55.1% mean value (mv), 49.7 - 60.5% confidence interval (ci).
Experimental group under ketamine anesthesia: white matter of the left hemisphere - 50.4% mv, 39.6 - 61.1% ci, of the right - 64.6% mv, 55.2 - 70.0% ci.
Experimental group under pentobarbital anesthesia: white matter of the left hemisphere - 40.8% mv, 32.2 - 49.4% ci, of the right - 48.0% mv, 43.3 - 52.6% ci.

Table 1. Results comparing the control group and the experimental groups, the one under ketamine anesthesia and the other under pentobarbital anesthesia. The values of the white matter assays are presented

	Right	Left	
Control ketamine	55.10 49.69 - 60.51 5.61		mv 95% ci ta u/g·100
Ketamine	64.58 55.16 - 74.00 2.79	50.36 39.60 - 61.12 4.02	mv 95% ci ta u/g·100
Pentobarbital	48.00 43.41 - 52.59 3.54	40.83 32.25 - 49.41 4.76	mv 95% ci ta u/g·100
p <	0.001	0.05	Significant

mv = mean value; ci = confidence interval; ta u/g·100 – total activity in units per gramm · 100

Table 2. Results of the grey matter assays

	Right	Left	
Control ketamine	58.05 54.95 - 61.16 6.57		mv 95% ci ta u/g·100
Ketamine	62.60 52.64 - 72.56 4.20	60.54 53.77 - 67.31 4.95	mv 95% ci ta u/g·100
Pentobarbital	49.47 44.29 - 54.65 4.99	50.41 45.96 - 54.86 5.88	mv 95% ci ta u/g·100
p <	0.05	0.05	Significant

The results of the grey matter are as follows:

Control group: 58.1% mv, 54.9 - 61.2% ci.
Experimental group under ketamine anesthesia:
- right-hemisphere 62.6% mv, 52.6 - 72.6% ci,
- left hemisphere 60.5% mv, 53.8 - 67.3% ci,
Experimental group under pentobarbital anesthesia:
- right hemisphere 49.5% mv, 44.3 - 54.6% ci,
- left hemisphere 50.4% mv, 46.0 - 54.9% ci.

The results of both hemispheres as well in grey matter as in white matter are significant, i.e. the decrease of the share of free activity of the lysosomal enzyme β-glucuronidase under pentobarbital anesthesia and experimental cold lesion means an increase in lysosomal membrane stability.

Conclusion

From our results we conclude that the protective effect of barbiturates can at least partly be deduced from a membrane stabilizing effect. Because of the lipid soluble properties of barbiturates we suggest that their effect takes place in the membrane itself.

From our studies we are not able to determine which of the hypotheses - WEISSMANN (29) who found that steroids cause stabilization by condensing or restricting the fluidity of the phospholipid chains - or - FLAMM and co-workers (8, 10) who suggest that barbiturates control or prevent free radical reactions - is more likely to explain the membrane stabilizing barbiturate effect.

As a matter of fact the increased membrane stability prevents the release of acid hydrolytic lysosomal enzymes throughout the cell and into the surrounding tissue. Therefore greater damage i.e. more severe neurological deficits can be inhibited by barbiturate therapy in experimental brain injury.

References

1. Astrup. J., Nordström, L.-H., Dehncrona, S.: Rate of rise in extracellular potassium in the ischemic rat brain and the effect of preischemic metabolic rate: evidence for a specific effect of phenobarbitone. Acta Neurol. Scand. 56, Suppl. 64, 148-149 (1977)

2. Bleyaert, A.L., Nemoto, E.M., Safar, P., Stezoski, S.W., Moossy, J., Rao, G.R., Mickell, J.: Thiopental amelioration of post-ischemic encephalopathy in monkeys. Acta Neurol. Scand. 56, Suppl. 64, 144-145 (1977)

3. Breivik, H., Fabritius, R., Lind, B., Lust, P., Mullie, A., Orr, M., Renck, H., Safar, P., Snyder, J.: Brain resuscitation clinical feasability trials with barbiturate. Crit. Care Med. 6, 93 (1978)

4. Cucchiara, R.F., Michenfelder, J.D.: The effect of interruption of the reticular activations system on metabolism in canine cerebral hemispheres before and after thiopental. Anesthesiology 39, 3-12 (1973)

5. Clubb, R.J., Maxwell, R.E., Chou, S.N.: Experimental brain injury in the dog. The pharmacological effects of pentobarbital and sodium nitroprusside. J. Neurosurg. 52, 189-196 (1980)

6. De Duve, C.: The role of lysosomes in the pathology of disease. Scand. J. Rheum. Suppl. 12, 63-66 (1975)

7. De Duve, C., Pressman, B.C., Gianetto, R., Wattiaux, R., Appelmans, E.: Tissue fractionation studies. Intracellular distribution patterns of enzymes in cat liver tissue. Biochem. J. 60, 604-612 (1955)

8. Demopoulos, H.B., Flamm, E.S., Seligman, M.L., Jorgensen, E., Ransohoff, J.: Antioxidant effects of barbiturates in model membranes undergoing free radical damge. Acta Neurol. Scand. 56, Suppl. 64, 152-153 (1977)

9. Fink, B.R., Haschke, R.H.: Anesthetic effects on cerebral metabolism. Anesthesiology 39, 199-215 (1972)

10. Flamm, E.S., Demopoulos, H.B., Seligman, M.C., Mitamura, J.A., Ransohoff, J.: Barbiturates and free radicals. In: Neural trauma. Popp, A.J., Bourke, R.S., Nelson, L.A., Kimmelberg, H.K. (eds.), pp. 289-296. New York: Raven-Press 1979

11. Furth, A.J., Robinson, D.: Specificity and multiple forms of β-galactosidase in the rat. Biochem. J. 97, 59-66 (1965)

12. Guttman, R.: Stabilization of spider crab nerve membranes by alkaline earths, as manifested in resting potential measurement. J. Gen. Physiol. 23, 346-369 (1940)

13. Hoff, J.-T., Pitts, L.H., Spetzler, R., Wilson, C.B.: Barbiturates for protection from cerebral ischemia in aneurysm surgery. Acta Neurol. Scand. 56, Suppl. 64, 158-159 (1977)

14. Hoff, J.-T., Smith, A.L., Hankinson, H.L., Nielson, S.L.: Barbiturate protection from cerebral infarction in primates. Stroke 6, 28-33 (1975)

15. Hoffmann, L., Gethmann, J.-W., Schmidt, D., Schwarz, M., Rating, D.: Hochdosierte Thiopentalgabe zur Therapie der postischämischen Anoxie des Gehirns. Anästhesist 28, 339-342 (1979)

16. Marshall, L.F., Bruce, D.A., Bruno, L., Schut, L.: Role of intracranial pressure monitoring and barbiturate therapy in malignant intracranial hypertension. J. Neurosurg. 47, 481-484 (1977)

17. Marshall, L.F., Shapiro, H.M.: Barbiturate control of intracranial hypertension in head injury and other conditions: iatrogenic coma. Acta Neurol. Scand. 56, Suppl. 64, 156-157 (1977)

18. Marshall, L.F., Shapiro, H.M., Smith, R.W.: Barbiturate treatment of intracranial hypertensive states. In: Neural trauma. Popp, A.J., Bourke, R.S., Nelson, L.A., Kimmelberg, H.K. (eds.), pp. 347-351. New York: Raven Press 1979

19. Michenfelder, J.D., Theye, R.A.: Cerebral protection by thiopental during hypoxia. Anesthesiology 39, 510-517 (1973)

20. Nemoto, E.M., Kofke, W.A., Wessler, P., Hossma-n, K.-A., Stezoski, W.S., Safar, P.: Studies on the pathogenesis of ischemic brain damage and the mechanism of its amelioration by thiopental. Acta Neurol. Scand. 56, Suppl. 64, 142-143 (1977)

21. Nilson, L.: The influence of barbiturate anesthesia upon energy state and upon acid-base parameters of the brain in arterial hypotension and in asphyxia. Acta Neurol. Scand. 47, 233-253 (1971)

22. Nordström, C.-H., Calderini, G., Rehncrona, S., Siesjö, B.K.: Effects of pentobarbital anesthesia on postischemic cerebral blood flow and oxygen consumption in the rat. Acta Neurol. Scand. 56, Suppl. 64, 146-147 (1977)

23. Safar, P.: Cardiopulmonary-cerebral resuscitation (CPCR). In: Advances in cardiopulmonary resuscitation. Safar, P. (ed.), pp. 195-207. New York, Heidelberg, Berlin: Springer 1977

24. Sellinger, O.Z., Hiatt, R.A.: Cerebral lysosomes IV. The regional and intracellular distribution of arylsulfatase and evidence for two populations of lysosomes in rat brain. Brain Research 7, 191-200 (1968)

25. Seeman, P.: The membrane actions of anethetics and tranquillizers. Pharmacol. Rev. 24, 583 (1972)

26. Simeone, F.A., Frazer, G., Lawner, B.S., Lawner, P.: Ischemic brain edema, comparative effects of barbiturates and hypothermia. Stroke 10, 8-12 (1979)
27. Smith, A.L., Hoff, J.T., Nielson, S.L., Larson, P.: Barbiturate protection in acute focal ischemia. Stroke 5, 1-7 (1974)
28. Stolke, D.: The influence of barbiturate treatment on the stability of lysosomal membranes in the cat brain. Acta Neurochirurgia 52, 142 (1980)
29. Stolke, D., Weidner, A., Dietz, H.: The protective effect of steroid treatment on lysosomal enzymes after cold lesion of the cat brain. Neurochirurgia 22, 220-224 (1979)
30. Stolke, D., Seidel, B.U., Hartmann, N.: Barbiturate treatment and membrane stability of subcellular organelles. Anaesthesist 29, 539-541 (1980)
31. Weissmann, G.: Corticosteroide and membrane stabilization. Circulation 53, Suppl. 1, 171-172 (1976)
32. Yatsu, F.U., Diamond, J., Graziano, C., Lindquist, P.: Experimental brain ischemia protecting from irreversible damage with a rapid-acting barbiturate (methohexital). Stroke 3, 726-732 (1972)

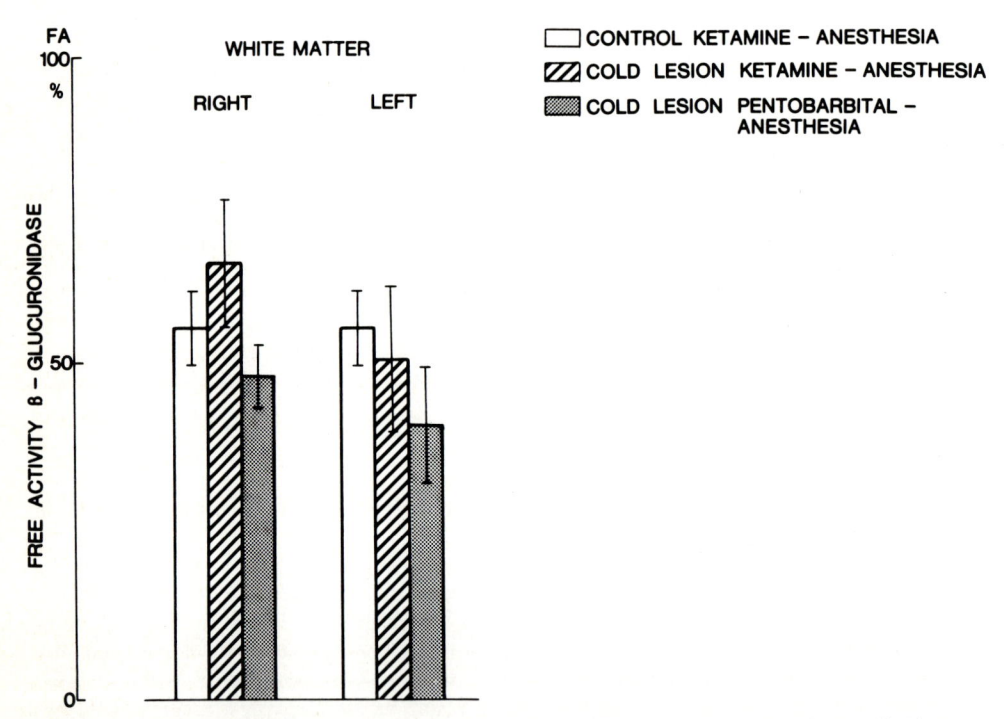

Fig. 1. Graphic presentation and comparison of the results of the white matter assays

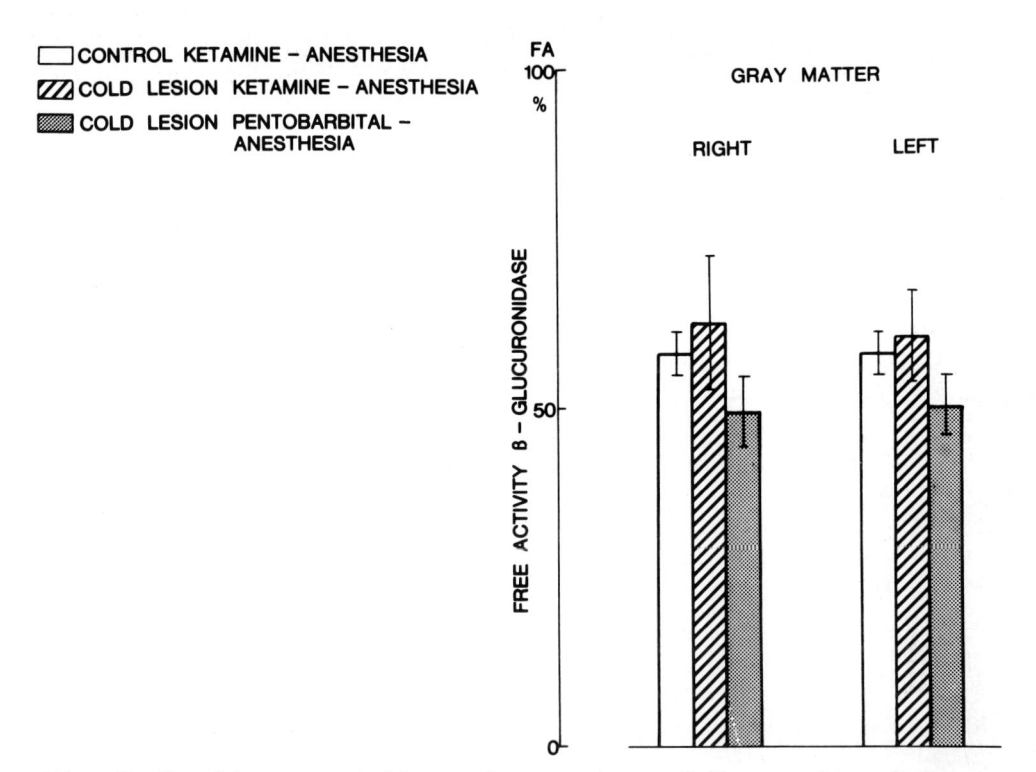

Fig. 2. Graphic presentation and comparison of the results of the grey matter assays

Dead Space Ventilation and Intracranial Volume Capacity

K. E. RICHARD and T. HASHIMOTO

For many years ventilation by means of a tube used to magnify dead space has been practised for post-operative and posttraumatic prophylaxis of atelectasis (1). A deepening of respiration with unfolding of the alveoli aimed at by an increase in arterial carbon dioxide tension ($PaCO_2$).

There is a linear relation between the cerebral blood volume (CBV) and the change in $PaCO_2$, as GRUBB et al. (1974) (2) pointed out at all.

The change in $PaCO_2$ leads to an increase of intracranial pressure dependent upon the intracranial space reserve (3).

Material and Method

In 111 patients with intracranial space-occupying lesions it was possible to examine the post-operative and post-traumatic behaviour of the intracranial pressure (ICP) during dead space ventilation (DSV).

The additional dead space volume was 500 ml in adults, the time of application with simultaneous supply of oxygen being 3 - 5 min.

DSV was ended, if ICP passed a level of 40 mm Hg or the pulse rate rose above 120 per min.

Results

Increases in $PaCO_2$ of 5 - 15 mm Hg with an average of 7 mm Hg, were measured during DSV. Taking into consideration this scattering, it can be expected according to the GRUBB-formula (CBV = 0.041 $PaCO_2$+2.0) that the CBV will increase by 2.2 - 2.6 ml, with an average of 2.4 ml per 100 g of brain tissue.

This relative large test volume corresponds to the quantity of the additional CBV that would be expected in patients during daily treatment, for example in horizontal positioning of upper part of the body and the head during bed-making or during measurement of the central venous pressure (see Figure 5 in (5)).

Individual measurements show that the alteration of $PaCO_2$ and of ICP are simultaneous and nearly parallel: The upper curve in Figs. 1 and 2 represents the $PaCO_2$-values before, during and after DSV. The square symbols represent the simultaneously measured $PaCO_2$, the lower curve the ICP-values.

The values in Fig. 1 were measured in a 22-year-old patient, 2 days after severe head injury. At this point the patient was in a coma with extensor reactions. The normal ICP increased from 8 to 13 mm Hg during DSV with a supply of 9 l oxygen (Fig. 1a). The repetition of the test on the same day again showed a pressure increase of 5 mm Hg with an increase in $PaCO_2$ of about 3 - 5 mm Hg in the normal range (Fig. 1a). On the 3rd day a higher initial pressure was registered in the still comatous patient. It increases by about 5 mm Hg during DSV at the most (Fig. 1b). In the afternoon of the same day there was an increase in ICP of 8 mm Hg (Fig. 1b).

The 4th post-operative day showed no neurological changes. During DSV there was no ICP increase greater than 5 mm Hg (Fig. 1c). The patient recovered in the course of time and became capable of reaction on the 8th day.

On the first day after extirpation of an infratentorial meningioma in a 69-year-old woman, $PaCO_2$ and ICP increased by 5 mm Hg during DSV with normal air within the normal pressure range (Fig. 2a). In the afternoon of the same day, an increase in $PaCO_2$ by 12 mm Hg led to an increase of ICP of 7 in values over 40 mm Hg (Fig. 2). On the 2nd day, after additional supply of oxygen there was an increase in $PaCO_2$ of 15 mm Hg, an increase in ICP from 7 to 35 mm Hg, i.e. 28 mm Hg (Fig. 2b).

On the 4th day, ICP again increased parallel to $PaCO_2$, but now only by 13 mm Hg (Fig. 2b).

During the following days the patient became mobile very quickly. The patient was discharged at the end of the 3rd post-operative week.

If the effect of DSV on ICP is regarded in a *prognostic* light, the results gained from 238 individual tests show that, independent of the kind of the process or the degree of the brain function disturbance, recognizable by the state of consciousness, the ICP shows an average fewer significant increases in patients with favourable development than in patients with a primary or secondary lethal course (Fig. 3).

Our measurements up until now give evidence that increases in ICP during DSV by more than 5 mm Hg show a distinct, dangerous restriction of the intracranial volume capacity.

If the increase is greater than 15 mm Hg, this restriction can be fatal.

Discussion

The increase in the CBV during DSV takes place within a few minutes. This volume test, however, does not register brain elasticity, as shown by MILLER's volume-pressure test (4), but the quantity of intracranial volume compensation, especially because of the time-consuming CSF-shifting.

The examination of the intracranial volume reserve by means of DSV only allows a qualitative or semi-quantitative assessment, but avoids risk of infection and is also applicable to patients with inaccessible slit ventricles.

Conclusion

Our findings show that ventilation through a dead-space tube makes monitoring of intracranial space reserve possible. ICP increases during DSV of mor than 5 mm Hg indicate to a significant, and if more than 15 mm Hg, a vitally threatening restriction of the intracranial volume capacity.

The advantage of this method, as opposed to the elasticity testing by addition of a fluid bolus, is that the patients are not submitted to any higher risk of infection and that the test is applicable in patients with brain swelling and slit ventricles.

References

1. Giebel, O.: Ventilation, Gasaustausch und Kreislauf unter künstlicher Totraumvergrößerung. Anaesthesiologie und Wiederbelebung. Berlin: Springer 1969
2. Grubb, R.L., Raichle, M.E., Eichling, J.O., Ter-Pogossian, M.M.: The effect of changes in PaCO$_2$ on cerebral blood volume, blood flow, and vascular mean transit time. Stroke $\underline{5}$, 630-639 (1974)
3. North, J.B., Jennet, S.: Cerebrovascular response pattern during CO$_2$ rebreathing. In: Cerebral circulation and metabolism. Langfitt, Th. W. (ed.), pp. 249-286. Berlin, Heidelberg, New York: Springer 1975
4. Miller, J.D., Pickard, J.D.: Intracranial volume/pressure studies in patients with head injury. Injury $\underline{5}$, 265-268 (1974)
5. Richard, K.E.: Liquorventrikeldruckmessung mit Mikrokatheter und druckkontrollierte externe Liquordrainage. Acta Neurochir. $\underline{38}$, 73-87 (1977)

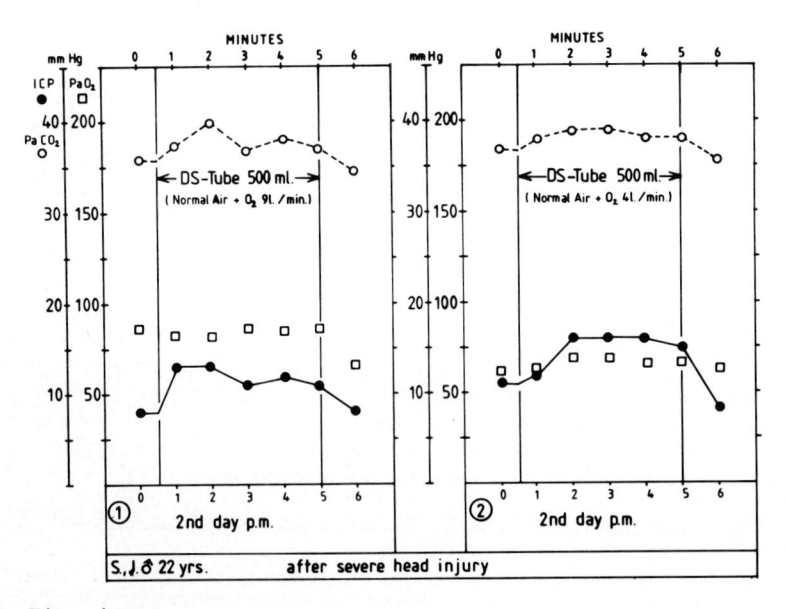

Fig. 1 a

Fig. 1 b

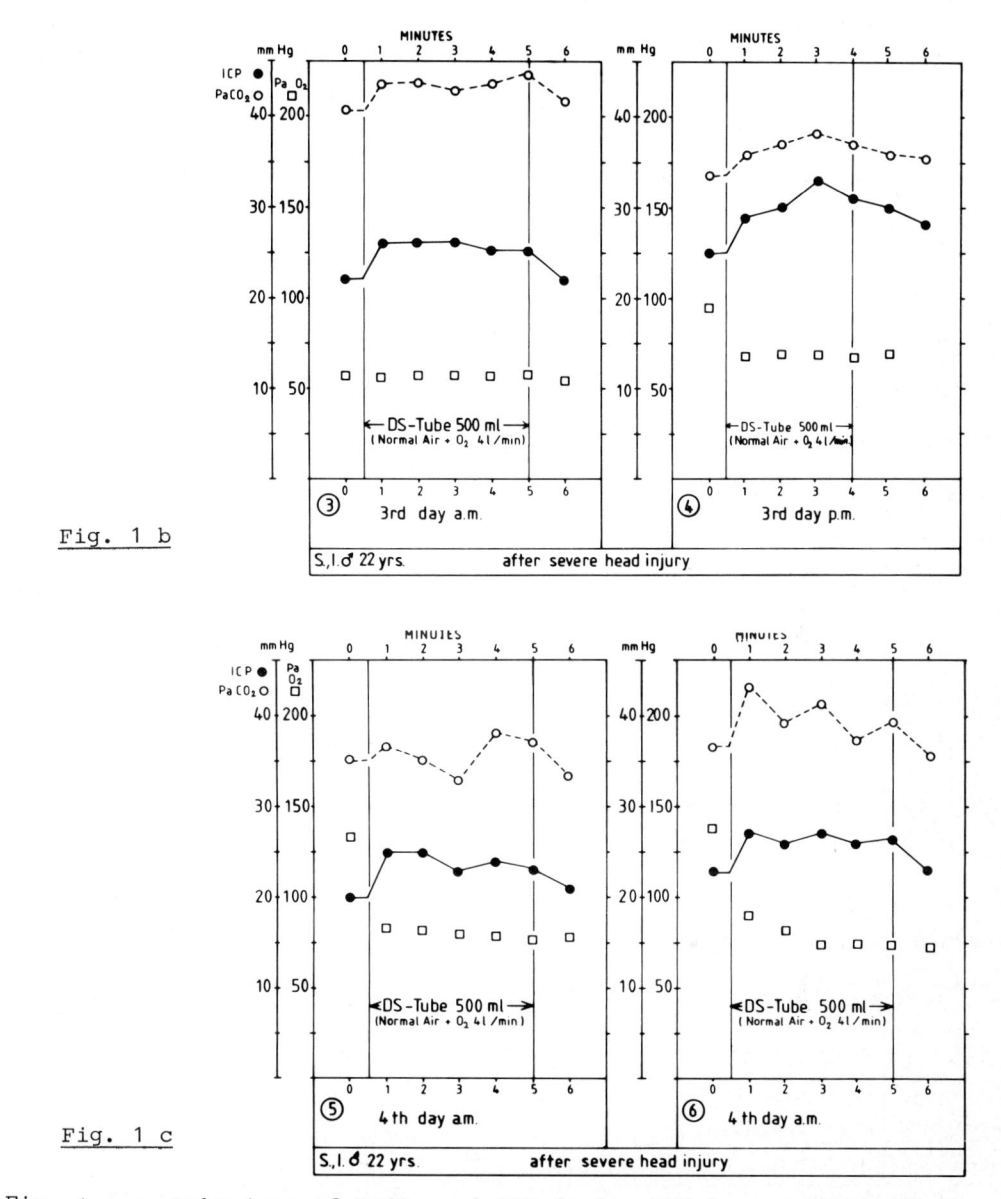

Fig. 1 c

Fig. 1 a-c. Behaviour of PaCO$_2$ and ICP during DSV in a patient after severe head injury on the 2nd (a), on the 3rd (b), on the 4th posttraumatic day (c). The highest increase of ICP was 8 mm Hg on the 3rd day p.m. (c). Despite of the lasting coma with extensor reactions the patient recovered

Fig. 2 a

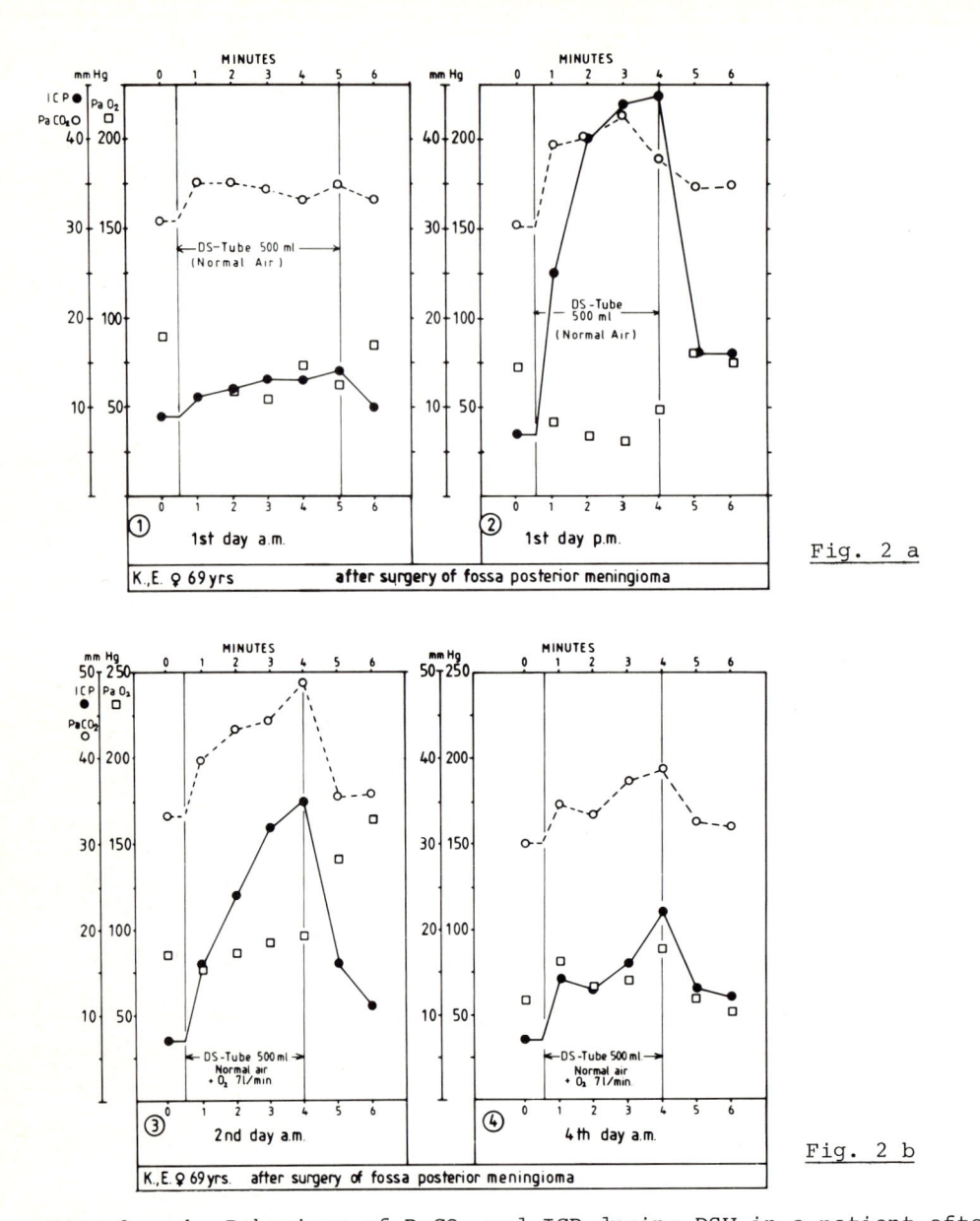

Fig. 2 b

Fig. 2 a, b. Behaviour of $PaCO_2$ and ICP during DSV in a patient after extirpation of an intracranial meningioma. a On the 1st day and b on the 2nd and the 4th post-operative day. The highest increases of ICP were 35 mm Hg on the 1st day p.m., and 28 mm Hg on the 2nd day p.m. After external fluid drainage, however, recovery in the course of time

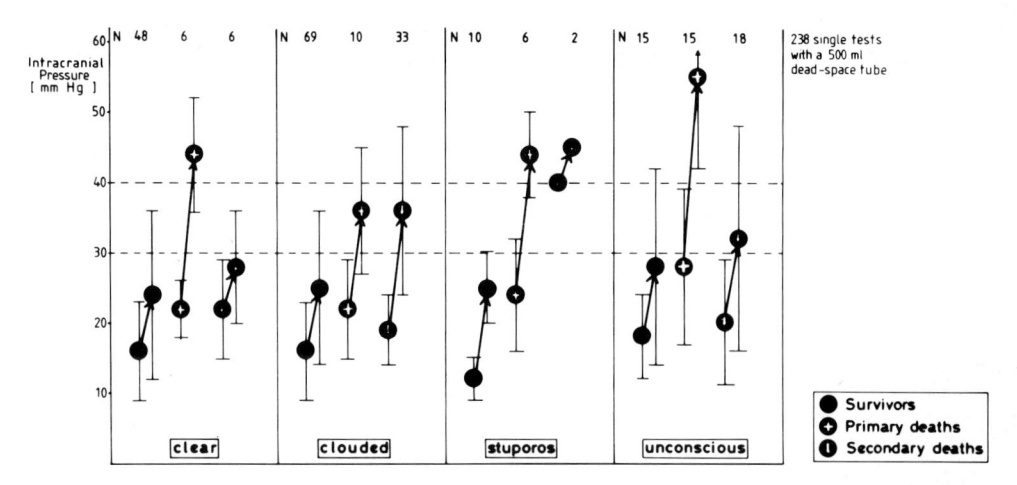

Fig. 3. Dead space ventilation and intracranial pressure. In survivors the mean ICP increases were between 5 and 10 mm Hg, independent of the brain function (state of consciousness). But in patients with fatal outcome the mean ICP increases were more than 15 mm Hg

Spinal Injuries

Injuries of the Spinal Cord and Their Prognosis
W. DRIESEN

The vertebral column is more and more seen to be afflicted by trauma through traffic accidents and by injuries which occur in professional life. Despite the introduction of seat belts in cars designed to protect the body to a certain extent and application of various precautionary measures at places of work subluxations, tears of ligaments and fractures following accidental crashes often finally determine the fate of disability of the patient. Additional complications are severe posttraumatic haemorrhages in the region of the spinal cord.

Depending on the location of the injury the duration and extent of neurological deficit vary within a wide range. Bone injuries alone may cause severe complications when the cervical part of the spine is afflicted. Whiplash injuries at the same location often are the reason for pain and neurological deficits in the patient's arm and hands which can last for several years. Additional injuries of the spinal cord itself or of the cauda equina aggravate the patient's situation and reduce the probability of his rehabilitation.

Dislocation of vertebrae through fracture and subluxation forces may cause haemorrhages or traumatic infarction of parts of the spinal cord followed by neurologically manifest paraparesis or paraplegia. The outlook of patients with this type of vertebral injury is poor particularly when the thoracic part of the spine has been injured since the spinal canal leaves only little room to the nervous structures due to its smallest diameter in this area.

Contusion of the thoracic part of the spinal cord usually results in irreversible destruction of nervous tissue. So the prognosis of recovery usually is bad and the injured patient will be dependent on a wheelchair.

Injuries of the lumbar part of the (vertebral column and) spine are seen to have a better prognosis as the cauda equina is more resistant to contusions than upper parts of the spinal cord. Possibly only single fibres may be injured resulting in physical disability or discomfort. Complete paralysis is not seen in cases representing this type of lesions.

Depending on the extent and seriousness of the neurological deficit surgery is indicated. Patients developing a paraparesis due to extradural or intradural bleedings without pathological findings initially have to be operated on as further aggravation can be prevented and restitution of normal functions is possible.

Surgery is not indicated in cases with initial atonic paraplegia. These patients are to get conservative treatment and do not cause neurosurgical problems. Myelography and computer tomography are adequate means of easy and immediate neuroradiological investigation of the extent of lesions helpful in determinating the indication for a neurosurgical procedure.

Indications for the Operative Treatment of Spinal Injuries and Technical Problems in Stabilizing the Spine

B. Hübner, K. Leyendecker, and A. Pihera

To this day, indications for operative treatment of spinal injuries are subject to various disputes. For example the late Sir LUDWIG, GUTTMANN and PAESLACK, head of the department for paraplegics in Heidelberg, consider operative treatment of spinal cord injuries, especially in paraplegia, only indicated in very exceptional cases. According to their conviction, operative treatment of such injuries must be considered as a mistake, as the frequent instability following decompression laminectomy is harmful to the patient and may prolong or essentially hinder his rehabilitation. GUTTMANN and PAESLACK claim that on the other hand instability without preceding operation is extremely rare.

As far as we are concerened, we do not think that those arguments are unjustified. Instability following decompression laminectomy without any or unskilled stabilisation is not too rare, but it also can be seen after conservative treatment of serious spinal injuries. For this reason, our paper is dedicated to this problem in particular as the risk of possible instability should not be an obstacle to operation for important indications.

We consider operative treatment not only indicated in open injuries, but also for dislocation and gross deformation of the spine which cannot be reduced, as well as in all cases of immediate or late manifestation of instability. Every late manifestation of instability is easily recognized by the complaints of the patient and X-ray diagnosis, especially the so-called functional X-rays. The diagnosis of immediate instability is far more difficult. This is particularly true in comminuted fracture with disruption of the interposed intervertebral disk, which frequently consolidates with cufflike callus formation only after a long period of immobilization or, especially with insufficient immobilization, will remain unstable. In extreme cases the X-ray will show impressively the so-called elephant foot pseudo-arthrosis. In those cases, according to our opinion, early operative stabilization is indicated. Operative intervention is also indicated in some cases of radicular syndromes and other painful conditions arising from changes in the anatomical situation, for instance in the very rare picture of genuine traumatic herniation of intervertebral disk (Table 1).

Much more problematic and, of course more controversial, are indications for operative treatment of spinal column injuries with damage to the spinal cord. Here again, without any doubt, open injuries require operative treatment. But their stabilization can be particularly difficult. Also paraplegic symptoms after a symptom-free interval or following diagnostic procedures such as myelography may call for operative measures like evacuation of an epidural haematoma (Table 2).

Table 1. Indications for operative treatment of spinal injuries *without* injury of the spinal cord

1. Open injuries
2. Unreducable luxations and dislocations of considerable extent
3. Gross early or late instability
4. Radicular symptoms and other severe pain, for instance following traumatic disc prolapse

Table 2. Indications for operative treatment of spinal injuries *with* spinal cord injury

1. Open injuries
2. Paraplegic symptoms after free interval
3. Aggravation of paraplegic syndrome following
   - Oedema, haemorrhage
   - Space constraint (prolapse, fragments)
   - Pronounced instability of the spine
4. Gross luxations and fracture dislocations in incomplete paraplegia
5. Insufficient restitution or severe pain in incomplete paraplegic syndrome and anatomical malalignment of the spine or constraint of the spinal canel

Decisions for operative intervention are far more difficult to make in cases of progression in incomplete paraplegia due to oedema or hemorrhage, or due to space constraint as a consequence of herniation of the intervertebral disk or by bone fragments, or, as we said before, due to marked instability of the vertebral column which will show symptoms of spinal cord irritation or progression or neurological symptoms after the slightest change of position of the patient. Of course, in those case diagnostic and operative measures have to be executed with utmost care. Very similar care and precautions are required in cases of pronounced dislocation and fracture dislocations with incomplete paraplegia, because of the immanent danger of finally destroying the already severely damaged spinal cord.

All these indications require stabilization and correction of the anatomical situation as conservative measures like immobilization of the patient in plaster bed or application of a plaster corset are practically never sufficient. In contradistinction to the cervical spine where due to anatomical and functional particularities relatively good reduction and stabilization can be achieved with relatively minor intervention, to mention only the methods of CLOWARD and ROBINSON, conditions in the area of thoracic and lumbar spinal column are quite different. Possibilities and results of operative reduction and stabilization in these areas are markedly less favorable due to anatomical and functional particularities. We are confronted with a very strong soft tissue, particulary of muscles and tendons, and the spinal column is deeply embedded in the body. Good visualization of the anatomical structures, especially by the ventral approach can only be accomplished by a major operative intervention with consequences to the supportive apparatus and the entire organism. The effect of enormous muscles tension has to be considered in addition.

Insufficient alleviation of neurological symptoms or severe pain in incomplete paraplegia as well as gross anatomical deformation of the spine or constraint of the spinal canal can be further indications for operative measures. The extent of clearing of the area depends on the type of damage. In quite a few cases reduction, removal of lacerated intervertebral disk tissue and stabilization are sufficient measures. In many other cases however, additional extensive decompression by laminectomy is indicated. In very special cases the dura has to be opened for removal of a haematoma or for excision of scar tissue which may cause pain or constraint in the spinal neural canal (Table 3).

For stabilization various methods and the application of most varied materials have been suggested. It would certainly go beyond the compass of this paper to discuss all the different methods of stabilization possible, from their historical origin and development. One has to keep in mind that all alloplastic material such as screws, plates, wires, springs or rods can only temporarily hold in position and immobilize the lacerated area until sufficient stabilization is achieved by the healing process. But since, as a consequence of already mentioned factors like the strong muscular tension effect, loosening of all alloplastic material and hence instability can easily occur, it is necessary to stimulate the healing process and even to speed it by implantation of autologous bone grafts such as shaped bone material as recommended by HARMON, CLOWARD or ROBINSON, or more or less extensive implantation of bone chips. The implantation of bone alone which is often possible at the cervical spine, will only be manageable in exceptional cases at the thoracic and lumbar spine (Table 4).

Table 3. Technical possibilities of operative interventions

---
1. Sufficient denudation of injured area of the spine, reduction and stabilisation without extensive exposition of the spinal cord, eventual removal of sequestered disc tissue.
2. Same interventions as 1. with additional extensive decompression of the spinal cord and laminectomy
3. Same intervention as 1. and 2. with additional opening of the dura, myelolysis evacuation of haematoma in case of haematomyelosis eventually plastic closure of the dura
---

Table 4. Possibilities of operative stabilization of the injured spine

---
1. With autologous and homologous grafts
    - As recommended by HARMON, CLOWARD or ROBINSON
    - Implantation of cortical bone "chip-rods"
2. With alloplastic material
    - Metal: screws, plates, rods, wire and springs
    - Plastic material
3. Combinations of 1. and 2.

On the other hand, for reason of space constraint alone, immobilization with considerable quantities of metal or plastic material, very often does not lead to bone consolidation in a tolerable span of time. If a combination of alloplastic materials and bone chips is applied, preference should be given to the method, which, according to our experience, leads to sufficient early stability with a little alloplastic material as possible, in order to permit healing of the bone and assimilation of autologous material as quick and undisturbed as possible, and, most important, that by later removal of alloplastic material the recently achieved osseous stability will not be disturbed again.

At the Frankfurt Accident Clinic more than 40 cases were operated upon during the last 18 years and all attempts with plates, screws, wiring have lead to little satisfactory results in general. We will discuss this type of operation more extensively in another paper. Even after years, sintering and loss of correction was observed, especially if it was tried, to shorten the average duration of strict bed rest of 8 - 12 - 16 weeks and to start with early mobilization.

After the disappointing results of the past, about two years ago we have started treating the instability of the spine by using the HARRINGTON instrumentation. Compression with rods is generally not indicated, because it is mostly unfeasable or even impossible , whereas good correction and fixation could be achieved with distraction rods in quite a number of cases. Following this presentation, my colleague will discuss this particular topic.

We are dealing with preliminary results, which certainly can be improved when more experience with the new method has been gained. Since distraction basically will delay healing of fractures, the application of as much autologous bone material as possible and sufficiently long immobilization are important pre-requisites for the success of such measures. The loss of time for rehabilitation can be compensated sufficiently by systematic and skillfully applied physiotherapy especially isometry.

Summary

With modern methods of stabilization of the spine, indication for operative treatment of spinal injuries should be carefully and correctly considered but should not be too restricted because of fear of instability. Besides correct reconstruction of anatomical structures with decompression of the damaged neural tissue a reliable method of fixation of the spine is necessary pre-condition for the operative treatment. After various attempts in the past, distraction fixation with generous implantation of cancellous bone, the HARRINGTON method, seems to be a very promising operative technique which we continually try to improve in order to obtain even better results.

Preliminary Results with Surgery in Trauma to the Thoracic and Lumbar Spine, Using the Harrington Method

K. LEYENDECKER, B. HÜBNER, and A. PIHERA

In the large clinical BG Accident Unit Frankfurt/Main, there were among 569 injuries to the vertebral column 179 fragment fractures and fracture dislocations. To this group, 233 compression fractures with involvement of the inter-vertebral disc are added and so 412 cases of vertebral column trauma are to be considered, which are unstable and a threat to the spinal cord.

In most cases the well-tried, active conservative management, proves satisfactory in order to achieve a good or acceptable result. Problems arise when the posterior disc-ligament complex has ruptured as complications of treatment to the spinal movement segment can be expected when the following factors contribute:

- loss of stability,
- loss of intervertebral distance,
- segmental dislocation.

Disregarding these factors, unstable healing, statically relevant deformity, as well as early and late spinal cord and root damage threaten and may supervene.

The indications for advising surgical treatment to disimpact and stabilise fractures of the vertebral column have been discussed in the previous chapter. We have in the last 2 years, 1979/80, in the BG Accident Unit Frankfurt/Main, operated upon 21 patients with severe fracture dislocations, which LOB calls complete lesions of the vertebral column. The injuries were mostly due to falls. Analysis of the mechanism of trauma reveals that flexion compression injuries in young patients, especially at the thoracolumbar junction was the most frequent type of fracture dislocation. It was surprising how few suffered a complete transverse neurological lesion.

At operation (Table 1) a torn dura was frequently encountered and in 6 cases the cauda equina were found extruded. In only a few cases was the intervertebral disc found to be implicated in contra-distinction to the posterior portions of the adjacent vertebral bodies.

Return of neurological function was evaluated (Fig. 1) using the schema after FRÄNKEL. As expected, operation did not influence the outcome in 3 cases with a complete transverse lesion. However, in 6 out of 12 cases with total motor loss but some sensory sparing, motor recovery occurred to a functional level where the limb could be lifted against gravity.

We have been particularly critical in assessing the results of bony healing (Fig. 2). Scoliosis or glissement was not the problem, but late collapse of the vertebral spongiosa and loss of alignment with marked kyphosis.

Table 1. Intraoperative situs (HARRINGTON-operation) (n = 21)

Rough lesions of the *dura*	9
Herniation/incarceration of *Cauda* substance	6
obvious laceration	5
Prominence of the dorsal vertebral wall	19
Space occupying disk ruptures	2

The primary reduction after use of the HARRINGTON "distraction instrument" was always good, since the normal vertebrae with intact laminae above and below the fracture present a perfect fulcrum for the re-alignment of the vertebral column. The problem was, how could the reduction be maintained under weight-bearing? Secondary collapse of the spongiosa of the vertebral bodies has to be recorded in 11 cases with a loss of correction of 10 degrees (Table 2).

It has to be remembered here that in every case of kyphosis, healing of bone in dorsal spondylodesis has to occur not under pressure but actually under a distraction force (Figs. 3, 4). We therefore decided to use strips of bone as grafts along the line of the interpedicular joints. But even in these cases post-operative loss of correction had to be accepted, in view of plastic deformation of the bone grafts at the level of the kyphosis. This confirms the experience of other orthopaedic surgeons when attempting to correct severe kyphosis: We know for example that after the calculations of FOURRIER, a kyphotic angle of $10°$ at the 2nd lumbar vertebra requires an additional effort of the erector spinae of 180 kp. We therefore finally decided that at operation spongiosa bone chips were to be inserted into the fractured vertebral bodies vertically and the intervening intervertebral space. We achieved our best results with this procedure (Figs. 5, 6).

To summarize. The aim is to achieve stable healing without statically relevant deformity in severe fragment-fracture dislocations at the thoraco-lumbar region, and to provide the best chance for any neurological recovery. Pure decompressive laminectomy is no longer compatible with these aims and is only indicated when neurological deterioration or a so-called free interval had been observed.

In 21 cases of severe fragment-fracture dislocations with neurological deficit, stabilising operations using the HARRINGTON distraction method were performed. Initial reduction with 2 rigid rods inserted between intact laminae was always satisfactory. Occasionally impacted laminae had to be resected.

Table 2. Complications after stabilizing operations (HARRINGTON-operation) (n = 21)

Premature loosening of rods	2
after 4 months	7
Infections	2

The chances for any neurological recovery were increased, since not only neurolysis was achieved but also realignment of the involved posterior edge which encroached upon the space within the neural canal.

The method does not gain time in early mobilisation, as any dorsal spondylodesis means bone healing not under pressure but a distraction force.

Late vertebral spongiosa collapse and consequent loss of alignment are as unsatisfactory as before. The problem is not that of scoliosis or glissement, but marked kyphotic angulation. Even dorsal grafts gave under weight-bearing and could not prevent this complication.

Comparing different methods: if the posterior edges of the vertebrae are intact, then the use of the WEISS-Feder(pen) combined with the distracting KNODT-rod is also a promising method. If, however, the posterior limits of the vertebrae are fractured and the intervening disc is involved, we submit the surgical method described as the treatment of choice. We continue to strive to improve it.

		Final check				
		A	B	C	D	E
		3				
Admission	A	3				
	B	12		1	5	6
	C	6+		2	3	
	D					
	E					

Fig. 1. Scheme of neurological remission according to FRÄNKEL (n=21).
+ = one of them died (polytrauma)

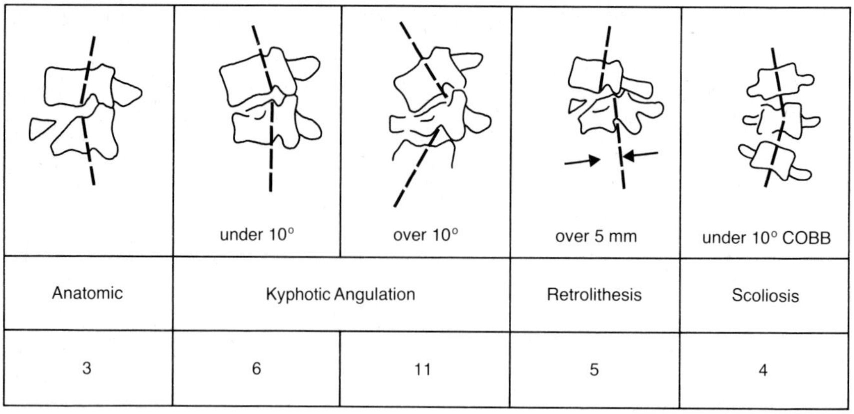

	under 10°	over 10°	over 5 mm	under 10° COBB
Anatomic	Kyphotic Angulation		Retrolithesis	Scoliosis
3	6	11	5	4

Fig. 2. Results of the stabilizing operations (HARRINGTON distraction instrumentarium)

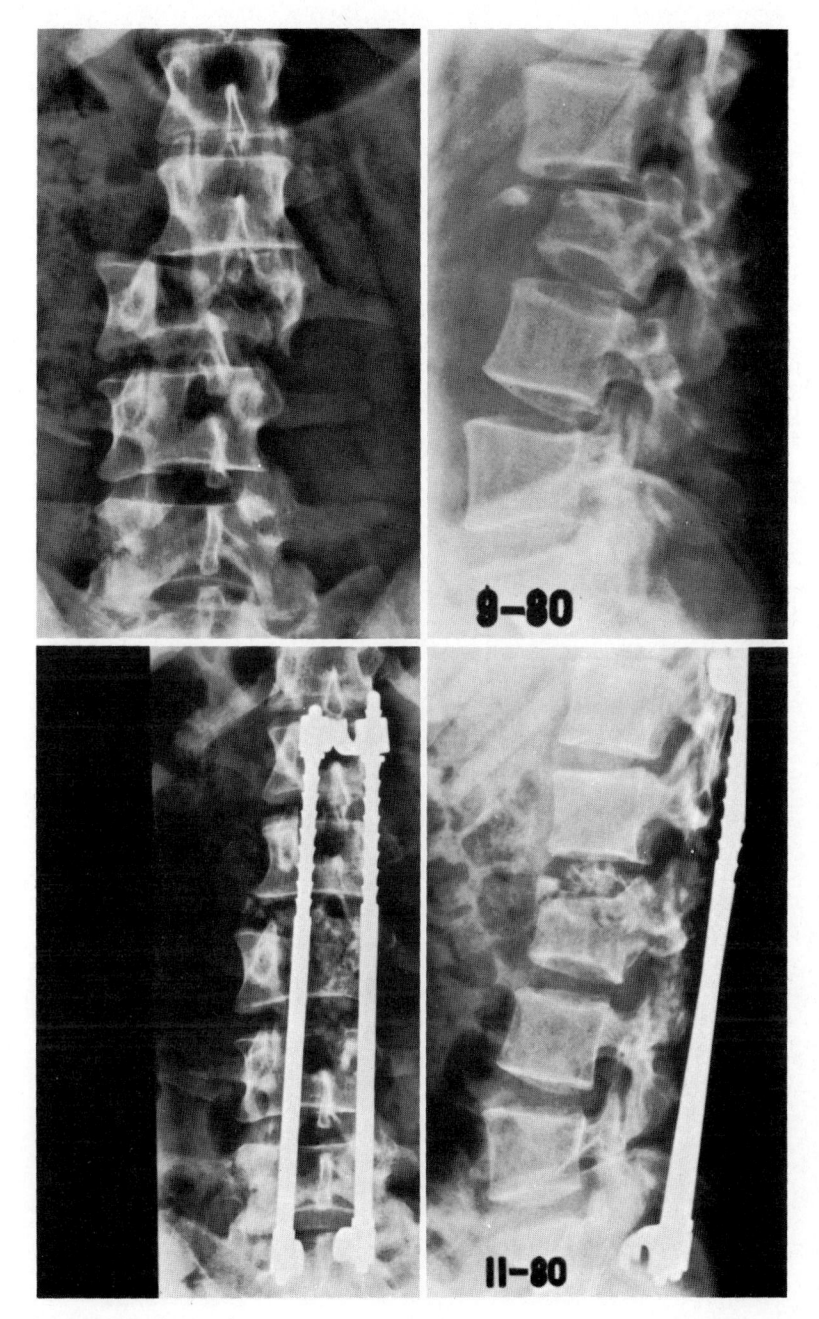

Fig. 3 *(above)* and 4 *(below)*. Rough luxation piece fracture L 3. Note widening of pedicle distance. Fine erection after stabilizing. Ventral deposition of spongiosa within the disk gap and debris

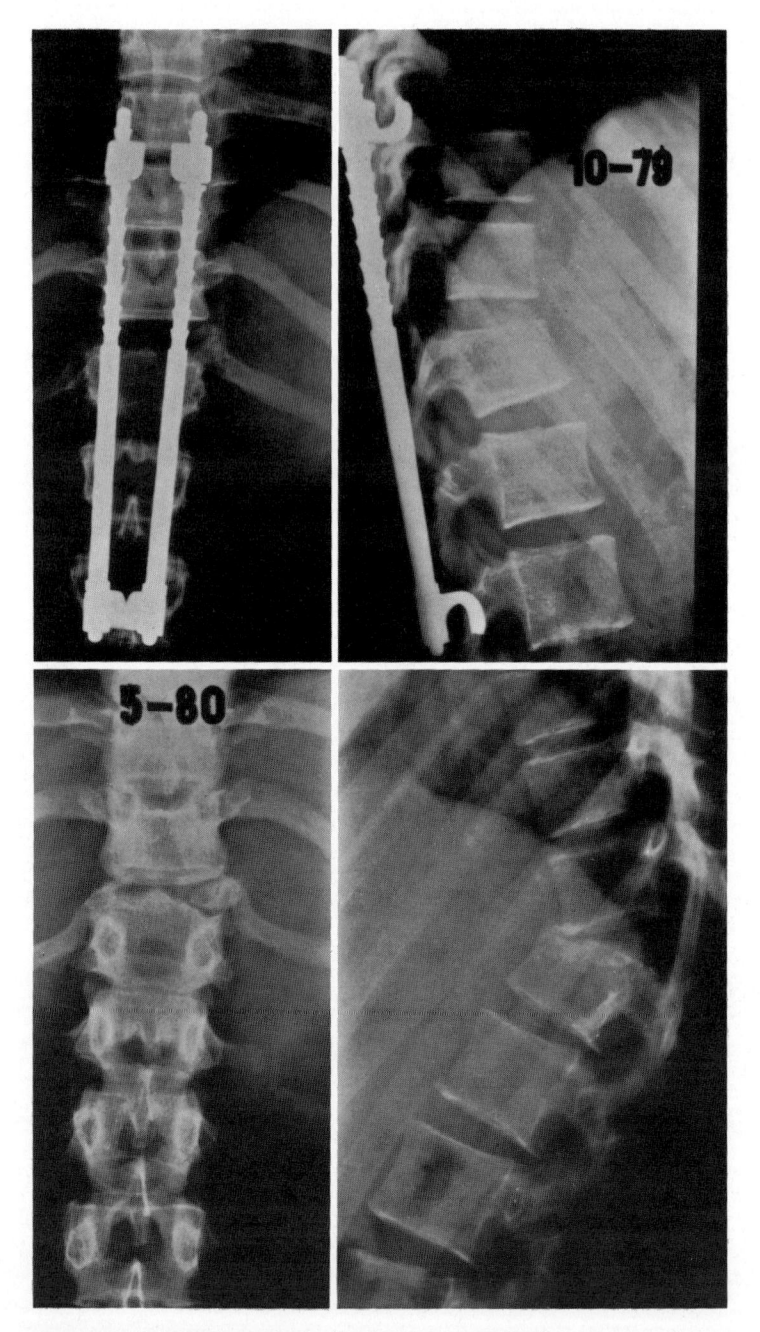

Fig. 5 (*above*) and 6 (*below*). Rough luxation fracture Th 12. Primary good reposition. No deposition of bone chips. Removal of the rods after 7 months. Late kyphotic angulation because of missing osseous consolidation

Transoral Fusion of the First and Second Cervical Vertebra

W. ELIES and H. KRETSCHMER

Because of their special topography lesions of the clivus as well as dislocations of the cranio-cervical region and the upper cervical spine are of particular surgical interest. These bony malformations and dislocations are hidden in the depth of the skull base and close behind the roof or the posterior wall of the epi- and mesopharynx. Teamwork is essential in dealing with these special problems. Successful surgery is only possible by using the most suitable approach and meticulous microsurgical techniques. This avoids damage to the structures of the central nervous system.

Compressive lesions of the brain stem as well as of the upper spinal cord can be caused by the elevated dens axis in cases of the anterior form of the cranio-cervical dysplasia and also in cases of dislocation between the vertebrae of the upper cervical spine. The successful treatment of these disorders is only possible by using the ventral, transoral approach. If one use a combination of neursurgical and otolaryngological operative techniques for the transoral approach the operative risks are minimal (1-18).

In 1930 GERMAN proved that the anterior approach was possible by using it on dogs. Orthopedic surgeons and otolaryngologists used this route for the drainage and treatment of inflammatory processes and also for the stabilisation of dislocations in the cranio-cervical region (1-18). In 1951 SCOVILLE and SHERMAN emphasized the possibility as well as the necessity of the transoral resection of the dense in cases of basilar impression. FANG and ONG reported on their results with the transoral route for the surgical treatment in atlanto-axial disorders in 1962.

GREENBERG et al. described two cases of atlanto-axial disorders treated by the transoral route in 1968. In 1965 ROBERTS and in 1971 GROTE et al. resected the odontoid process in cases of cranio-cervical dysplasia. The reported functional results were fairly good and no severe complications were mentioned. In 1974 the French surgeons PECH et al. reported on four cases of transorally treated patients having a chordoma of the clivus, a tumor of the foramen magnum, a metastasis of the axis and a basilar impression. Surgery was described as very simple and no complications were mentioned. In 1980 MENEZES reported on 17 patients having cranio-cervical dysplasia or atlanto-axial dislocations. Depending on the stability of the cranio-cervical region or the spine as well as the anterior or the posterior form of spinal cord compression the surgical approach is different.

If one reviews the literature it is evident that complications were seen only in the early stages of transoral surgery. FANG and ONG as well as MULLAN et al. described secondary infections and bleeding from the vertebral artery. Publications during the following years did not reveal intra- or postoperative complications. It is also of particular interest that postoperative dislocations of the upper cervical joints has been never seen. Because of the above mentioned literature we decided to use the transoral approach in a case having a severe atlanto-axial dislocation with neurological signs.

Case Report

A 19-years-old female was suffering from rheumatoid arthritis for 5 years. In September 1980 a progressive tetraparesis developed. The neurological examination made at the second week of December showed the following neurological findings:
paresis of the right soft palate, a spastic tetraparesis of the distal type and a hypaesthesia beginning at the level of D_2. The lateral plain X-rays and midline tomograms showed a severe atlanto-axial dislocation (Fig. 1). The apex of the odontoid process was hypoplastic and there was no bony connection between the apex and the base of the dense. The axis was dislocated posteriorly for 8 mm. The diameter of the spinal canal was 6 mm at the level of C_2 measured in the lateral projection. The dislocated axis and particularly the base of the odontoid process compressed the spinal cord and were responsible for the neurological findings.

On the 22nd of December the patient was operated on. A special preoperative preparation was not necessary. The performance of a tracheostomy was not needed and no preoperative antibiotic treatment was required. General anaesthesia was used and the patient was in the supine position with his head hyperextended. The surgeon stands at the head end of the patient. Fluoroscopic control was essential and the equipment had to be in position for the lateral fluoroscopy of the cranio-cervical region. Nearly the whole operative procedure was done with the operating microscope and appropriate microsurgical instruments had to be used. The uvula and the soft palate were held upward by holding sutures going out through the nose (Fig. 2). After the insertion of a self-retaining mouth gag the posterior wall of the epi- and mesopharynx became visible. The operation field had to be disinfected. A midline incision was than made over the anterior surface of the distal end of the clivus, anterior arch of the atlas and the axis. Mucosa, submucosal tissue and the prevertebral muscles were separated in the midline (Fig. 3). Two self-retaining CUSHING specula of different length were inserted crosswise to retain the tissue of the posterior wall of the pharynx as well as the tongue and the palate. The arch of the atlas and the body of the axis were exposed. By using a cutting drill the anterior arch of the atlas was partly drilled out from below. By using a diamond drill the upper layer of the base of the odontoid process was drilled away also. Then the upper posterior part of the base of the dense - the hypomochlion for the spinal cord - was grounded out by the diamond drill. Every important step of the operative procedure was controlled by lateral fluoroscopy. After hemostasis a piece of individual formed heterologous bone was inserted between the arch of the atlas and the base of the odontoid process. Then a halo ring was fixed and brought under traction by the use of weights.

Lateral plain X-rays of the atlanto-axial region made at the end of the procedure showed a good position of the axis. Two days later the halo ring was fixed on a thoracic plaster cast. Several days later the patient was allowed to get out of bed. The neurological signs disappeared rapidly and the patient recovered completely from the tetraparesis. Six weeks after surgery the halo cast had been removed and replaced by a stiff neck support. Some days later an X-ray follow-up of the atlanto-axial region was made. Lateral plain X-rays and midline tomography showed beginning of bony fusion between the atlas and the axis. The diameter of the spinal canal was 1.5 cm at the level of C_2 (Fig. 4). Because of the stability of the atlanto-axial region the indication for the posterior fusion will depend on the further course.

For the surgical management of the clivus, the cranio-cervical region and the upper cervical spine the transoral approach has to be used. A tracheotomy or a speical preoperative treatment are not needed. The use of lateral fluoroscopy, the operating microscope and microsurgical instruments is essential. The operative risks are low, the procedure rather simple and severe complications are not to be expected.

References

1. Alonso, W., Black, P.: Transoral-transpalatal approach for resection of clivus chordome. Laryngoscope 81, 1626-1691 (1971)
2. Bhatia, M.L., Yadav, Y.C.: Chordoma (retropharynageal) Case report. J. Laryngol. 79, 656-661 (1965)
3. De Rougemont, J., Abada, M., Barge, M.: Les possibilitès de la voie d'abord antérieure dans les lésions de trois premières vertêbres cervicales. Neuro-Chirurgie 13, 559-570 (1967)
4. Elies, W.: Surgery for compressive lesions of the brain stem paper presented at the first meeting on skull base surgery. New Haven: Connecticut 1980
5. Fang, H.S.Y., Ong, G.B.: Direct anterior approach to the upper cervical spine. J. Bone Jt. Surgery 44, 1588-1604 (1962)
6. German, W.J.: In: Transoral decompression of atlanto-axial dislocation due to the odontoid hypoplasia. Greenberg, A.D. et al. (eds.). J. Neurosurg. 28, 266-269 (1968)
7. Greenberg, A.D., Scoville, W.B.: Transoral decompression of atlanto-acial dislocation due to the odontoid hypoplasia. J. Neurosurg. 28, 266-269 (1968)
8. Grison, C.: Abord chirurgical direct par voie buccale des trois premierś vertêbres cervicales. J. franc. Otorhino-laryng. 16/4, 271-273 (1967)
9. Grote, W., Roemer, F., Bettag, W.: Der ventrale Zugang zum Dens epistropheus. Langenbecks Arch. Chir. 331, 15-22 (1972)
10. Menezes, A.H., Van Gilder, B.S.J., Graf, C.J., Mc Donnell, D.E.: Craniocervical abnormalities. J. Neurosurg. 53, 444-455 (1980)
11. Mullan, S., Nauton, R., Kehman-Panam, J., Vailati, G.: The use of an anterior approach to ventrally placed tumors in the foramen magnum and vertebral column. J. Neurosurg. 24, 536-543 (1966)
12. Nissen, R., Klingler, M.: Klivustumoren: Operative Möglichkeiten Schweizer Arch. Neurol. Neurochir. et Psych. 94-122 (1964)
13. Pech, A., Cannoni, M., Magnan, J., Appaix, M., Gitenet, P., Vigouroux, R.P., Pellet, W., Guillerman, P., Alliês, B.: Les voies trans-orales en oto-neuro-chirurgie. Ann. Oto-Laryng. (Paris) 91, 281-292 (1974)

14. Roberts, L.: Discussion of the paper by Stevenson et al. Proc. 3rd Internat. Congr. Neurol. Surg., Kopenhagen 1965. Excerpta med. (Amsterdam) Intern. Congr. Series 110, 514 (1966)
15. Rougerie, J., Guiot, G., Bouche, J., Trigo, J.: Les voies d'abord des chordomes du clivus. Neuro-chirurgie 13, 559-570 (1967)
16. Scoville, W.B., Sherman, I.J.: Platybasia: Report of ten cases with comments on familial tendency, a special diagnostic sign, and the end results of operation. Ann. Surg. 133, 496-502 (1951)
17. Southwick, W.O., Robinson, R.A.: Surgical approaches to the vertebral bodies in the cervical and lumbar regions. J. Bone Jt. Surgery 39A, 631-644 (1957)
18. Thompson, H.: Transpharyngeal fusion of the upper cervical spine. Proc. Roy. Soc. Med. 63, 893-896 (1970)

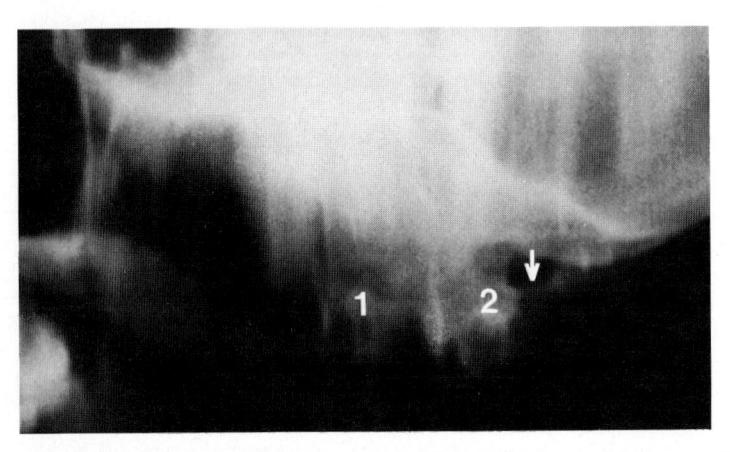

Fig. 1. Lateral midline tomogram of the upper cervical spine. Anterior arch of the atlas (1), axis (2), narrowed spinal canal (arrow). By courtesy of Prof. VOIGT, Head of the Neuroradiological Department, University of Tübingen

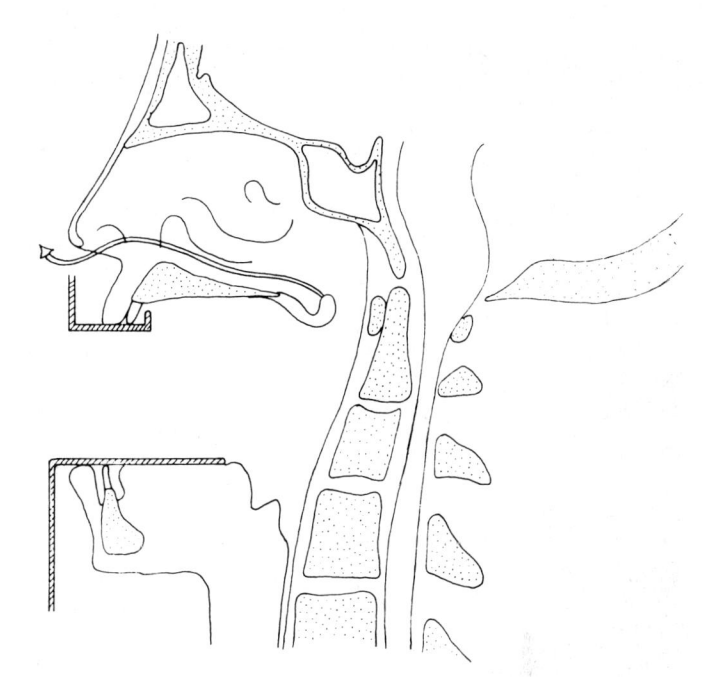

Fig. 2. Exposure of the posterior wall of the pharynx after insertion of a mouth-gag and retaining sutures for the soft palate (schematic drawing)

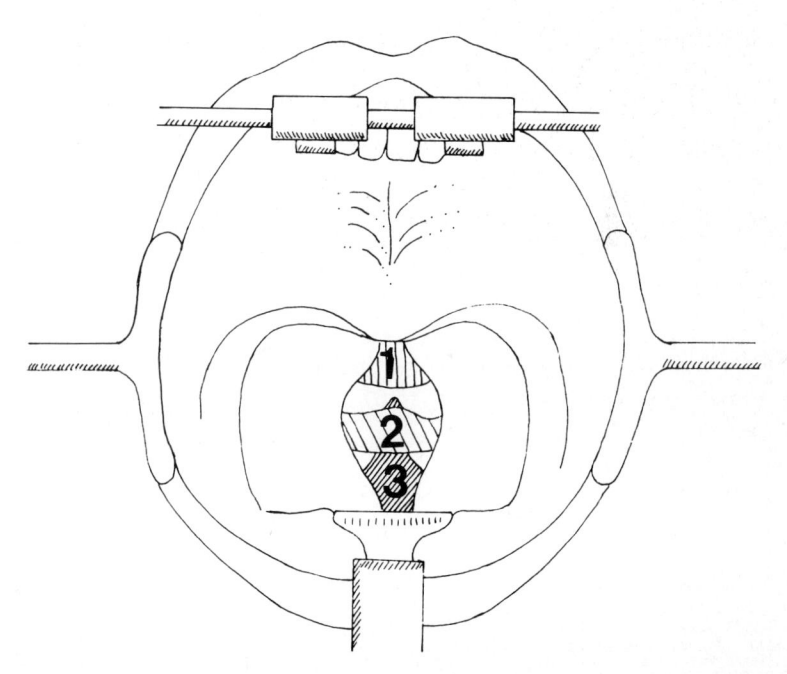

Fig. 3. Situation after midline incision and soft tissue preparation. Clivus (1), anterior arch of the atlas (2), axis (3)

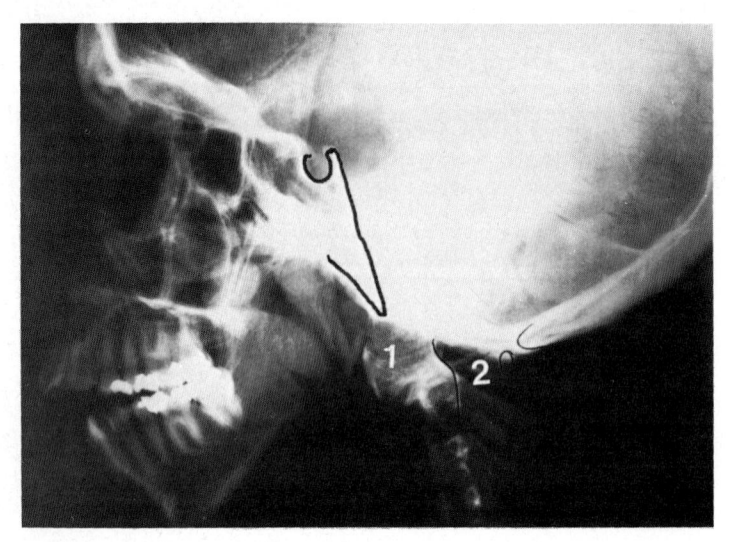

Fig. 4. Lateral plain X-ray of the upper cervical spine 8 weeks after surgery. Atlanto-axial fusion (1), enlarged spinal canal (2). By courtesy of Prof. VOIGT, Head of the Neuroradiological Department, University of Tübingen

Spinal Epidural Hematoma

B. N. Rana and O. Orio-Glaunec

Spontaneous epidural hematoma are extremely rare. Since the first case reported by JACKSON 1869 (16), we find in German literature for the first time the report from WEIGERT 1961 (34), and the last reported cases from SCHWARTZ et al. (32). In the meanwhile we find about 130 reported cases in English, American and German literature (22, 33). Out of these cases we observe so far including our own only 9 cases among youths under 16 years (27).

Because this disease is extremely rare, it is not often considered in differential diagnosis; especially, when no obvious causes are known, such as trauma - with or without fracture of the spine (12, 14, 18, 26) - or disturbances of blood coagulation due to either a disease (25) or anticoagulant therapy (1, 2-4, 5, 6, 8, 9, 23, 30, 34-36) or vascular malformation (10, 11, 33). If clinical signs appear without any previously known origin, we speak of spontaneous spinal epidural hematoma, which may appear at any age, patients, between 50 - 70 years are particularly afflicted (17, 19-21); more in men than in women. It can even appear in infants of 14 months as found by JACKSON (15). That is why one must always keep in mind, that in so-called acute myelitis either spontaneous or chronic spinal epidural hematoma could be the cause.

Material

From this point of view we once again try to emphasize the importance of this disease by referring to our own 6 cases, which were treated in our department from Oct. 1976 to March 1980 (Table 1).

Because of the limited space and because of exceptional rarity of the case, we will report only on the 13 years old girl.

Case 2 (413/77). 13-year-old female suddenly felt severe pain of her back especially between the scapulae on 9.5.1977 whilst on a school-outing. On the afternoon of the same day she felt numbness and weakness in both legs. She was then admitted to a neuro-pediatric department. The X-ray of the spine and lumbar puncture showed no abnormalities. On 12.8.1977 she developed a flaccid paraplegia with lack of knee and ankle reflexes of both legs, complete loss of sensation from T3 downwards, bowel and bladder disfunction, and on 13.8.1977 she was transferred to our department. The lumbar puncture showed a clear and clourless CSF and a positive Queckenstedt test. The myelography (by lumbar injection of 7 ml Duroliopaque) showed a complete block at T3 (Figs. 1, 2). She was taken immediately to the operation-room. A laminectomy was performed from T2 to T4 and a partly fluid and partly clotted epidural hematoma was removed. The histological examination revealed a venous malformation. Postoperatively, she slowly

Table 1

Case No.	Age (years)	Sex	Etiology	Surgical findings	Duration of symptoms	Results
1	48	M	Unknown	C4-6 clot	2 days, Brown-Sequard with hemiparesis of the right side and sensory loss from T5 downwards	Slight weakness of the right leg
2	13	F	Unknown	T2-4 partly fluied and partly clotted	4 days of increasing flaccid paraplegia with absent knee and ankle reflexes of both legs, complete loss of sensation from T3 downwards, bowel and bladder dysfunction	Complete recovery after 5 months
3	63	F	Unknown	C3-6 clot	9 hours, immediate triparesis after onset pain in neck and scapular region with absent biceps- and triceps reflexes right, hyperreflexes on both legs, bilaterally positive Babinski sign, bowel and bladder dysfunction	Complete recovery after many months
4	64	M	Trauma (without a fracture)	C5-T2 clot	Developed 6 hours after the trauma a flaccid paraplegia with loss of all spinal cord function below T2	Minimal recovery of paraplegia, died after 4 weeks of pneumonia
5	58	M	Anticoagulant therapie	T1-4 clot	Cervicodorsal discomfort of 6 days duration, followed by increasing paraplegia of both legs with loss of spinal cord function below the level of T7	Spastic paresis of left leg with bowel and bladder dysfunction
6	55	F	Anticoagulant therapy	C5-T4 clot	Pain in upper-thoracic and neck region for 5 days, followed by quadriparesis and anesthesia below C6 10 hours before the operation	Slight weakness of right hand (C7 and 8)

regained the sensory and motor functions and after 5 months she showed no neurological abnormalities.

In all these cases, we hold in accordance with the great quantity of other literature the opinion, that a locus minoris resistentiae is to be assumed that through anticoagulants, minor traumas or through increased intraabdominal intrathoracic pressure-growth will be put out of balance.

Our experience with these six cases emphasizes, that following speedy diagnosis and laminectomy, the time factor prior to operation and its site are of decisive importance for the restoration of neurological function.

References

1. Alderman, D.B.: Extradural spinal-cord hematoma: report of a case due to dicumarol and review of the literature. New Engl. J. Med. 255, 839-842 (1956)

2. Angstwurm, H., Frick, E.: Neurologische Komplikationen der Antikoagulationstherapie. Münch. med. Wschr. 109, 1103 (1967)

3. Arieff, A.J., Pyzik, S.W.: Paraphlegia following or associated with excessive dicumarol therapy. Quart. Bull. Northw. Univ. med. Sch. 28, 221 (1954)

4. Askey, J.M.: Hemorrhage during long-time anticoagulant therapy. Caliv. Med. 104, 6-10 (1966)

5. Brandt, M.: Spontaneous intramedullary haematoma as a complication of anticoagulant therapy. Acta Neurochirurgica 52, 73-77 (1980)

6. Brandt, R.A.: Chronic spinal subdural haematoma. Surg. Neurol. 13, 121-123 (1980)

7. Busse, O., Hamer, J., Paal, G., Piotrowski, W.: Spontane epidurale Hämatome während und nach Antikoagulantienmedikation. Nervenarzt 43, 318-322 (1972)

8. Fischer, M.: Therapie mit Antikoagulantien (I.). Med. Welt 13, 534-539 (1970)

9. Fischer, M.: Therapie mit Antikoagulantien (II.). Med. Welt 14, 620-626 (1970)

10. Foo, D., Ghang, Y.C., Rossier, A.B.: Spontaneous cervical epidural hemorrhage, anterior cord syndroma, and familial vascular malformation: case report. Neurology 30, 308-311 (1980)

11. Guthkelch, A.N.: Hemangiomas involving spinal epidural space. J. neurol. neurosurg. 5 Psychiat. 11, 199-210 (1948)

12. Helperin, S.W., Cohen, D.D.: Hematoma following epidural anesthesia: report of a case. Anesthesiology 35, 641-644 (1971)

13. Herrmann, E., Lorenz, R., Vogelsang, H.: Zur Diagnostik der spinalen epiduralen Hämatome und Abszesse. Radiologie 5, 504-508 (1965)

14. Hurt, R.W., Shaw, M.D.M., Russell, J.A.: Spinal subdural hematoma: an unusual complication of lumbar puncture. Surg. Neurol. 18, 296-297 (1977)

15. Jackson, F.E.: Spontaneous spinal epidural hematoma coincident with whooping cough: case report. J. Neurosurg. 20, 715-717 (1963)

16. Jackson, R.: Case of spinal apoplexy. Lancet 2, 5-6 (1869)

17. Jellinger, K.: Spinal epidural hematoma. In: Traumatic vascular disease of the spinal cord. Handbook of clinical neurology, Vol. 12. Vinken, P.J., Bruyn, G.W. (eds.). Amsterdam: North Holland Publ. Comp. 1971

18. Jonas, A.F.: Spinal fractures: opinions based on observation of sixteen operations. JAMA 57, 859-865 (1911)

19. Levy, A., Klingler, M.: Das spontane epidurale Hämatom. Acta neurochir. 11, 530-544 (1964)

20. Lowrey, J.J.: Spinal epidural hematomas: Experiences with three patients. J. Neurosurg. 16, 508-513 (1959)

21. Markham, J.W., Lynge, H.N., Stahlman, G.E.B.: The syndrome of spontaneous spinal epidural hematoma. Report of three cases. J. Neurosurg. 26, 334-342 (1967)

22. Mraček, Z.: Spontaneous spinal epidural hematoma: Experiences with four patients and a review of the literature. Zbl. Neurochirurgie 41, 19-30 (1980)

23. Oldenkott, H.P., Driessen, W.: Spontanes epidurales Hämatom im Brustwirbelkanal während Antikoagulantien-Langzeitbehandlung. Med. Welt 305-307 (1966)

24. Pendl, G., Ganglberger, J.A., Horcajada, J.: Spinal extradural hematoma. Acta Neurochir. (Wien) 24, 207-212 (1971)

25. Priest, W.M.: Epidural hemorrhage due to hemophilia causing compression of spinal cord. Lancet 2, 1289-1291 (1935)

26. Reid, J., Kennedy, J.: Extradural spinal meningeal hemorrhage without gross injury to spinal column. Br. Med. J. 2, 946 (1925)

27. Robertson, W.C. Jr., Lee, Y.E., Edmonson, M.B.: Spontaneous spinal epidural hematoma in the young. Neurology 29, 120-122 (1979)

28. Russman, B.S., Kazi, K.H.: Spinal epidural hematoma and the Brown-Sequard syndrome. Neurology (Minncap.) 21, 1066-1068 (1971)

29. Scharfetter, F.: Das spontane spinale epidurale Hämatom in der Differentialdiagnose des akuten spinalen Insultes. Dtsch. med. Wschr. 97, 13-16 (1972)

30. Schicke, R., Seitz, D.: Spinales epidurales Hämatom unter Antikoagulationstherapie. Dtsch. med. Wschr. 95, 275-277 (1970)

31. Schultz, E.C., Johnson, A.C., Brown, C.A. et al.: Paraplegia caused by spontaneous spinal epidural hemorrhage. J. Neurosurg. 10, 608-616 (1953)

32. Schwartz, R.B., Müke, R., Lüdecke, D.: Spontanes spinales epidurales Hämatom. In: Spinale raumfordernde Prozesse. Schiefer, W., Wieck, H.H. (eds.), pp. 55-56. Erlangen: Verlag Dr. D. Straube (1976)

33. Solero, G.L., Fornari, M., Savoiardo, M.: Spontaneous spinal epidural haematoma arising from ruptured vascular malformation. Acta Neurochirurgia 53, 169-174 (1980)

34. Weigert, M.: Akutes spinales epidurales Hämatom als Folge von Behandlung mit Antikoagulantien. Der Nervenarzt 32, 85-89 (1961)
35. Whaley, R.L., Lindner, D.W.: Spontaneous spinal epidural hemorrhage associated with anticoagulant therapy. Grace Hosp. Bull. (Detroit) 40, 27 (1962)
36. Winer, B.S., Horenstein, S., Starr, A.M.: Spinal epidural hematoma during anticoagulant therapy. Circulation 19, 735 (1959)

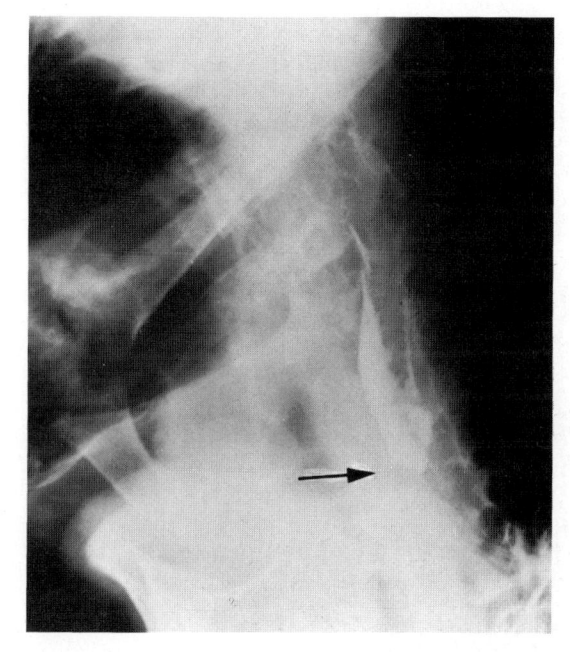

Fig. 1. Sagittal view of myelogram with an elevated arm complete block at T3 *(arrow)*

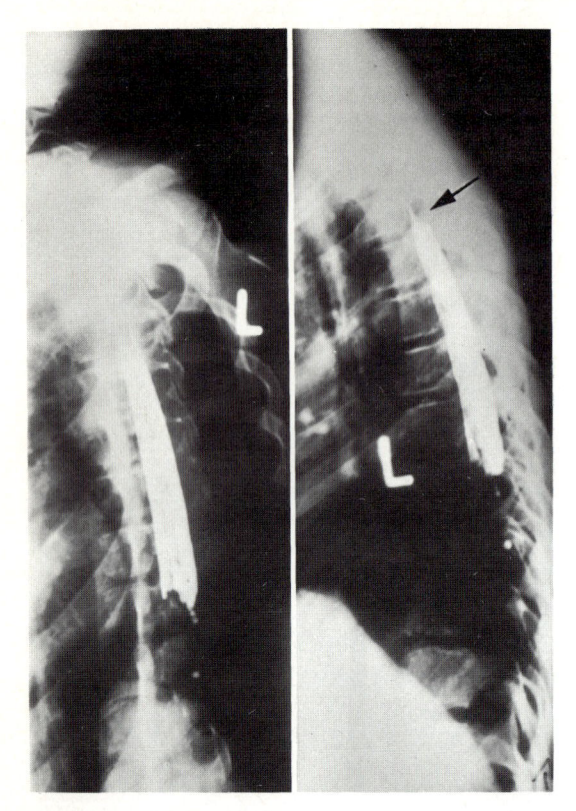

Fig. 2. Sagittal view of myelogram *(arrow)* complete block at T3

30 Cases of Traumatic Central Cervical Spinal Cord Injury

J. Lemke, F. Koschorek, U. Larkamp, and H.-P. Jensen

Introduction

The syndromes of both acute central and acute anterior spinal cord injuries have been described by SCHNEIDER et al. in 1954 and 1955.

Characteristic for the first syndrome is a disproportionately greater motor impairment of the upper extremities rather than the lower ones. Usually there is urinary retention as well as varying degrees of sensory impairment below the level of the lesion.

In the case of an acute anterior spinal cord injury there usually is not only an immediate complete paralysis in the cervical level, depending on the location of the lesion, but also hypesthesia and hypalgesia. However, sensitivity to touch, motion, position and vibratory senses are preserved.

Later examinations and observations made clear however, that a strict differentiation between these clinical syndromes usually cannot be made. This type of injury usually occurs through severe hyperextension traumas of the cervical spine which can be accompanied by a simultaneous posterior and anterior pinching and squeezing of the spinal cord. Such spinal cord injuries may occur without major injuries to the spine having been caused by an inward bulge of the ligamentum flavum during hyperextension or by a herniated disk during hyperflexion of the neck. However, this syndrome may also be associated with certain cervical compression fractures and with typical hyperextension or flexion fracture-dislocations of the cervical spine.

KARIMI (1978) and MAYNARD et al. (1979) however stressed that there are no neurological impairments with fractures of the cervical spine in 10 to 20% of the cases.

It seems surprising that even in recent clinical surveys, some of them with numerous case histories, the clinical syndrome of acute central cervical spinal cord injuries is very rarely mentioned.

Most studies group the neurological impairments as complete tetraplegia, incomplete tetraplegia and radicular signs.

We, therefore, have examined our own case histories of the past 10 years with injuries of the cervical vertebral column.

Material and Results

X-ray and clinical findings of 542 cases are shown in Table 1. 97 patients (18%) showed fractures with or without dislocations in their radiological findings.

15 of these patients with fractures showed no neurological findings.

Apart from the injuries, identified radiologically, 107 of our patients (20%) had definite neurological deficits.

In 32 cases it was tetraplegia, in 39 tetraparesis, in 6 cases radicular impairments, and in 30 cases symptoms of acute central cervical spinal cord damage was found, which means, that they constitute 28% of the damages which can be definitely established as injuries of the nervous system and 5.5% of the total 542 cases.

Table 2 shows the neurological signs of the cases with central cervical spinal cord injuries. In 6 cases only, there were slight neurological signs also in the legs.

The most frequent combination was that of sensory and motor impairments at the upper extremities only, mainly in the lower arm or hand (Table 3).

The main symptom was burning pain in the arms, mostly distal but also proximal in the region of the shoulder, frequently with a strong sensitivity to touch, usually in combination with hypesthesia.

Furthermore there was weakness in the hands when forming a fist and less frequently in the elbow and shoulder joint. In this acute stage dissociate sensory loss of hot and cold stimula but a retained touch stimulus were only rarely identifiable.

Tests of the cerebral spinal fluid were done in 16 cases and showed pathological values in 8 of them.

Seventeen of the injuries were caused by car accidents, 6 by sport accidents and 7 by various other accidents.

In 19 cases the symptoms receded completely, in 10 of these within a week, and in the other 9 within 4 weeks. After half a year 8 patients still retained paresthesia, sensory loss, or trophic impairments. In 3 cases irreversible damage had occurred.

In all cases treatment consisted of the non-operative approach.

Three additional patients with complete tetraplegia died. In the post mortem examination they have had typical cervical hematomyelia or hemorrhagic necrosis.

Discussion

In contrast to complete and incomplete tetraplegia with rupture of the long pathway by contusion or severance, injuries of the central cervical spinal cord usually are reversible, mainly in the area of the grey matter at the level of the lesion. The distribution of the fibre bundles in the white matter with outward fibres for the distal supply areas explains the slight involvement of the lower extremities with a respective extension of central functional disorders.

Table 1. Acute cervical spine injuries 1970 – 1980

Clinical signs/ X-ray findings	Fracture with dislocation	Fracture	Stretching position/ functional impairment	No traumatic disorders	No. of cases
Complete tetraplegia	22	9	0	1	32
Incomplete tetraplegia	20	17	1	1	39
Radicular signs	0	1	5	0	6
Central cervical spinal cord syndrome	6	7	5	12	30
Cervical syndrome	0	0	215	0	215
No neurological deficits	2	13	184	21	220
No. of cases	50	47	410	35	542

Table 2. Neurological signs

	Motor deficits	Sensory disturbances	Motor/sensory disturbances	No. of cases	Mainly unilateral	Bilateral
Solely upper limbs	–	7	17	24	8	16
Upper and to a lesser degree lower limbs	–	–	6	6	–	6
No. of cases	–	7	23	30	8	22

Table 3. Localisation of neurological signs

	Motor signs	Sensory signs
Mainly upper arm	7	7
Mainly lower arm/hand	18	23
Total	25	30

Only if the findings are caused by a central cord distruction with bleeding, hematomyelia, there may be caudal or cephalad extension of the lesion with further progression of symptoms, perhaps culminating in complete tetraplegia or death.

Several factors play an important role for the origin of pathomorphological developments.

BRIHAYE et al. as well as others furthermore lay stress on the significance of a congenitally narrow spinal canal or on the development of spondylosis or spondylarthritis. Thus, the importance of biomechanic factors varies from case to case.

JELLINGER pointed out that the lower brainstem and the spinal cord with both the cranial and spinal nerve roots are comparable to a uniform tissue tract which is rostrally firmly anchored at the mesencephalon and caudally by the attachment of the nerve roots. Due to this anchorage, the shape of the tract changes with each movement of the head or the spine.

As BREIG stated in 1960, the spinal cord adapts to shortening and lengthening during the flexion and extension of the spine. Many tissue structures are involved in this adaption process. Thus, apart from the compression and distorsion of the cord, axial and transverse tension forces are of major significance as a cause for spinal cord injury.

There is furthermore substantial evidence that not only mechanical but also circulatory factors play an important role in the pathogenesis of functional and anatomical lesions of the spinal cord as far as injuries or other affections of the spine are concerned.

From numerous experimental studies on spinal cord injuries, we know that damage to the spinal cord is caused by vascular breakdown with edema, by stasis in small vessels, by diapedetic hemorrhages, by petechiae, and by hemorrhagic necrosis.

These histological changes are initially to be found in the central grey matter where they are always more marked than in the white matter.

In their experimental compressive lesion to the spinal cord SCHRAMM et al. frequently found extensive hemorrhage or large hemorrhagic necrosis in the grey matter whereas the only findings in the white matter were edema and/or axonal swelling.

All of these observations and studies indicate that a spinal cord trauma caused by compression or strain through traction mainly causes damage to central areas if it does not lead to the rupture of the spinal cord matter. Possibly this can be ascribed to a greater vulnerability of the grey matter compared to the white matter. On the other hand, one has to take into consideration the disturbances in the arterial blood supply, such as inadequate circulation in the zone between the supply area of the A. spinalis anterior and the vascular network of the Aa. spinales posteriores (ZÜLCH, 1954; TURNBULL, 1971).

Conclusion

Central cervical spinal cord injuries obviously are far more frequent than has been realized. In our case histories their frequency was 28% of all cervical neurological impairments, caused by trauma. On the other hand only slight impairments can be clinically identified as such because serious impairments with hematomyelia lead to para/tetraplegia.

The diagnosis is made difficult by the fact that frequently head injuries are dominant and cover up the symptoms.

Prognosis seems to be good.

References

1. Breig, A.: Effect of histodynamic tension on the function of the central nervous system; with special reference to its analysis in spinal cord injury and skull traction. In: Preceedings of the German society for neurosurgery. Kuhlendahl, H., Hensell, V. (eds.), 3, pp. 36-54. Amsterdam: Excerpta Medica 1973
2. Brihaye, J., Flament-Durant, J., Retif, J.: Pathology of cervical spinal cord lesions without radiologically demonstrable injury of the cervical spine. In: Neurological surgery. Int. Congress Series 433. Carrea, R. (ed.), pp. 384-388. Amsterdam: Excerpta Medica 1978
3. Jellinger, K.: Pathomorphological aspects of the biomechanics of the CNS. In: Proceedings of the German society for neurosurgery 3. Kuhlendahl, H., Hensell, V. (eds.), pp. 27-35. Amsterdam: Excerpta Medica 1973
4. Karimi-Nejad, A.: Ergebnis der operativen Behandlung bei HWS-Verletzung. Hefte zur Unfallheilk. 132, 325-336 (1978)
5. Maynard, F.M., Reynolds, G.G., Fountain, St., Wilmot, C., Hamilton, R.: Neurological prognosis after traumatic quadriplegia. J. Neurosurg. 50, 611-616 (1979)
6. Schneider, R.C., Cherry, G., Pantek, H.: The syndrome of acute central cervical spinal cord injury. With special reference to the mechanisms involved in hyperextension injuries of cervical spine. J. Neurosurg. 11, 546-577 (1954)
7. Schneider, R.C.: The syndrome of acute anterior spinal cord injury. J. Neurosurg. 12, 95-122 (1955)
8. Schramm, J., Hashizume, K., Fukushima, T., Takahashi, H.: Experimental spinal cord injury produced by slow, graded compression. J. Neurosurg. 50, 48-57 (1979)

9. Turnbull, I.M.: Microvasculature of the human spinal cord. J. Neurosurg. 35, 141-147 (1971)

10. Zülch, K.J.: Mangeldurchblutung an der Grenzzone zweier Gefäßgebiete als Ursache bisher ungeklärter Rückenmarksschädigungen. Dtsch. Z. Nervenheilk. 172, 81-101 (1954)

Early and the Still Possible Late Surgical Treatment of Cervical Spine Injuries

A. KARIMI-NEJAD

Introduction

In recent years, early surgical treatment was performed in more than 100 patients with injuries to the cervical spine. The indication and the technique for the surgical measures could be worked out on the basis of the results, depending on the nature and level of the injury (KARIMI-NEJAD 1980, 1981). The results of the early surgical repositions are encouraging. With increasing experience, surgical treatment to eliminate the dislocations to a large extent has been successfully performed not only in the early phase after an injury, but even in further course up to seven years after trauma. In the following, in particular the surgical measures will be dealt with in relation to the nature and level of the injury as well as the time after the trauma.

Indication for Surgery/Injury Level

On the basis of the surgical consequences, but without taking into account the kind of injury and even the neurological deficits in the first instance, fundamental subdivision of the injuries in the upper cervical spine region will be undertaken solely on the basis of the anatomical situation and the pathomorphological alterations. The injuries must be subdivided into those above C3 and the injuries at and below C3. According to experience so far, we would regard the following injuries above C3 as requiring operation:

1. the *mobile* fractures or pseudarthrosis of the odontoid process,
2. the hangmans' fractures with additional damage to the axis body.

In typical hangmans' fractures without additional damage to the axis body, surgical repositioning should also be performed when an increasing dislocation occurs despite external fixation or when the external fixation hindering nursing attention to the injury cannot be optimally performed for other reasons.

Surgical Technique in Injuries of the Upper Cervical Spine

In injuries above C3, a dorsal stabilization (as shown schematically in Fig. 1) varied according to the time of injury is recommended. In the supine position and under general anesthesia, a CRUTCHFIELD forceps with an extension weight of about 1/10 of the body weight is applied primarily. Two bone grafts from the tibia of about three to six cm in length and 1 1/2 to 2 cm wide (corresponding to the intended fixation and the distances between C1 to C3 present) are taken from both legs roughly at the transition from the upper to middle third.

In extension in the supine position, the patient is repositioned into the abdominal position and the transverse arches from C1 to C2 (in fractures of odontoid process) or from C1 to C3 (in hangmans' fractures) were visualized on both sides by a midline exposure. With the aid of a Deschamps corresponding to the injury present and the fixation intended, wires with a diameter of roughly 0.5 to 0.7 mm are drawn through below the laminae C1 to C3 on both sides, if possible without injuring the musculature and ligaments. Having drilled the tibial grafts, previously removed (specified in Fig. 1), complete positioning is achieved first of all by traction on the dorsal arch of the atlas with simultaneous coordinated head positioning in retroflexion under X-ray control, and the anatomical position is restored again. In this position, firm internal fixation according to the specified scheme now follows.

In hangmans' fractures with additional injury to the axis body, a fixation of C1, C2 and C3 is performed (see Fig. 1a). In typical hangmans' fractures, the fixation of C1 and C3 (see Fig. 1b) is as a rule sufficient. The fractured bony parts of the dorsal arches of C2 are thereby pressed together by the tibial grafts.

On the other hand, in fresh "mobile" fractures and in pseudarthroses of odontoid process, a fixation of C1 and C2 is sufficient (see Fig. 1c).

If surgical repositioning is performed in the early phase of an injury, the tibial grafts should be applied with the cortical side to the laminae. In this way, a lasting spondylodesis is avoided as a rule since our own long-term observations show that these grafts situated in the soft tissue are fully resorbed in the due course. In this way, no additional limitation to movement in the injured or in the uninjured segment arises even after consolidation of the fracture. On the other hand, if the surgical repositioning is only performed more than six months after an injury because of increasing dislocation, a rapid consolidation of the fracture is not to be reckoned with. Here one is therefore dependent on a long-lasting or chronic dorsal fixation by osteosynthesis. In these cases and especially in pseudarthroses of odontoid process, the typical grafts are applied with the spongiosa side on to the lightly freshened up laminae and fixed.

Indication and Technique of Operation in Injuries of the Lower Cervical Spine

Of the injuries at and below C3, in our experience the following are to be regarded as requiring surgery:

1. axial deviation,
2. luxations,
3. luxation fractures,
4. compression fractures and
5. severe compression fractures.

Acute traumatic disc prolapses with neurological deficits *without* discernible radiological dislocation and/or bony injuries are rare according to our experience. On the other hand, isolated damage to an intervertebral disc which leads to a typical secondary radiological alteration (spondylosis deformans etc.) may occur due to trauma.

As stated in earlier communications (KARIMI-NEJAD 1980, 1981), the ventral access will have to be chosen on principle in injuries of the lower cervical spine region. In this narrow section of the spinal canal, damage to the affected intervertebral disc and the ligament apparatus with protrusion of soft tissue into the spinal canal are present in this region of the spinal canal in almost all injuries specified which require surgery. This protrusion of soft tissue leads to appreciable compression of the spinal cord. Furthermore, a repositioning into the normal anatomical position is frequently only possible intraoperatively.

In order to avoid any external fixation hindering nursing care and/or fresh dislocation or reluxation, on the basis of increasing experience we perform a stable internal fixation in addition to the blocking of the intervertebral space affected in injuries of the lower cervical spine requiring operation. If an elimination of the dislocation or a repositioning of the luxation has not occurred under preoperative extension, on the basis of our own experience we warn against any blind manual attempt at reposition. If it has not occurred spontaneously, the repositioning should always be performed intraoperatively. For this purpose, after typical ventral access the intervertebral space concerned is first of all exposed and cleared under supine extension traction of about 1/10 of the body weight. Under microscopic control, the epidural space is subsequently likewise freed of soft tissue. Only now is the dislocation or luxation which may still be present eliminated intraoperatively. As specified by SCHÜRMANN et al. (1978), the reposition is performed with a hook which is applied epidurally behind the dorsally luxated vertebral body. Here, the extension traction can be raised to 30 - 40 kg temporarily as required. Up to now we have always been able to perform the repositioning in this way even in locked luxations, even after passage of 6 to 12 months after the trauma.

Autogenic chips removed from the tibia are likewise used for fixation: the neighbouring luxated vertebral bodies are drilled through in the longitudinal direction (see Fig. 3) with a percussion drill specially constructed for this purpose (Fig. 2). A wire with a diameter of 0.5 to 0.6 mm is drawn through each of the prepared drill channels. The drilling is performed on the proximal vertebral body in the head-up and on the distal vertebral body in the head-down position.

The wire drawn through the distal vertebral body is at the same time drawn through the graft prepared to aid fusion. Afterwards, the vertebral bodies concerned are firmly anchored by means of the wires to a tibial graft used as a beam and apposed to the anterior edge of the vertebra with the cortical side ventral (see Fig. 3).

With increasing experience, we have been able to attain a complete fixation in the normal anatomical position in axial deviation luxations and luxation fracutres even months after the accident. An external immobilization was not necessary even in late operations. Thus for example in a 20 year old patient with sever luxation fracture and rupture of the joint surface of C5, an almost complete reposition with stable internal fixation could be performed even 8 months after the accident. Despite external fixation with a thorax cast the dislocation had increased. An increasing partial paraplegic syndrome was developing which completely regressed postoperatively.

In compression fractures and severe compression fractures, the compressed vertebral body is pulled back by means of the hook shown in Fig. 4, after prior clearance of the neighboring intervertebral spaces with freeing of the epidural space from soft tissue. After

Table 1. Level and nature of cervical spine injuries (93 patients)

Upper cervical spine C3 ↑	Fracture of the odontoid process e.i. pseudarthrosis					7
	Hangman's fracture without and with fracture of axis					9

Lower cervical spine C3 ↓	Level	Discs	Axial deviations	Dislocations	Fracture dislocations	Compression fractures	Total
	C3/4	2	1	1			4
	C4/5			6	3	3	12
	C5/6	4	1	9	7	9	30
	C6/7	1	1	14	10	1	27
	C7/Th1			3		1	4
	Total	7	3	33	20	14	93

the vertebral body has been restored to the normal position, two wires (likewise with a diameter of 0.5 to 0.6 mm) are drawn through epidurally by the hook behind the vertebral body. The hook developed for this purpose has a channel, so that the wire can be effortlessly drawn through behind the vertebral body and then finally through the proximal intravertebral space. Autogenous tibia grafts are also used in these cases for fusing the intervertebral spaces concerned on both sides. The wires are also drawn through the grafts so that they are fixed. Afterwards, the vertebral body which has been drawn forward is firmly fixed on a tibial graft which is likewise applied ventrally, and which is used as a beam.

With this technique, we have been able to attain an almost complete straightening of the cervical spine not only in the early phase, but also in the further course up to seven years after a compression fracture of a vertebra. The internal fixation in luxations, luxation fractures, compression fractures and severe compression fracture has been successfully performed in all segments of the cervical spine (see KARIMI-NEJAD 1981).

In a 32 year old patient, an extensive laminectomy was performed abroad primarily after a compression fracture of C5. Due to the surgical laminectomy, an increasing gibbus development occurred.

Seven years after the accident, a rapidly increasing incomplete paraplegia developed in consequence of the increasing gibbus development. Despite the lateness, we decided to perform a reposition of the compressed vertebral body with internal fixation. The compressed body was returned to its normal position and fixed in the typical way using the hook to pull forward of the compressed vertebral body (see Fig. 5). It was gratifying to observe that there was increasing regression of the incomplete paraplegia.

In Table 1, the nature and level of the cervical spine injuries in 93 patients with a follow-up of more than one to six years after the operation are listed. Presentation of the results of the neurological checkups has been dispensed with since these results have beeen presented in earlier communications (KARIMI-NEJAD 1980, 1981). Only in one case, in which we have attempted a blind reposition at the beginning of our practice, have the neurological findings deteriorated postoperatively.

References

1. Karimi-Nejad, A.: Indikation, Technik und Ergebnisse der operativen Behandlung von Halswirbelsäulen-(HWS)Verletzungen. Fortschr. Neurol. Psychiat. 48, 183-206 (1980)
2. Karimi-Nejad, A.: Internal fixation of cervical spine injuries. In Advances in neurosurgery, Vol. 9. Schiefer, W., Klinger, M., Brock, M. (eds.), pp. 479-489. Berlin, Heidelberg, New York: Springer 1981
3. Schürmann, K., Reulen, H.J., Busch, G.: Rekonstruktive und stabilisierende Maßnahmen bei Wirbelkörperverletzungen. Hefte Unfallheilk. 132, 336-342 (1978)

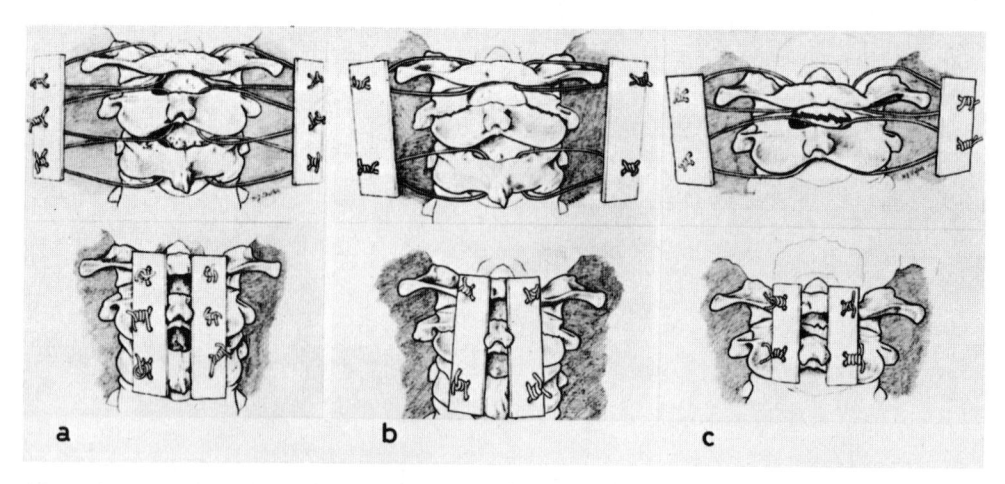

Fig. 1 a-c. Posterior fixation of upper cervical column: a For hangman's fracture accompanied by an additional fracture of the axis body; b for typical hangman's fracture; c for fracture of the odontoid process, i.e. pseudarthrosis of the odontoid process, see text

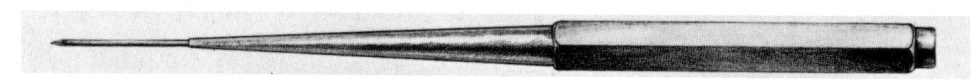

Fig. 2. Percussion drill for drilling the vertebral body for internal fixation in axial deviation, luxation and luxation fracture (length: 23.5 cm)

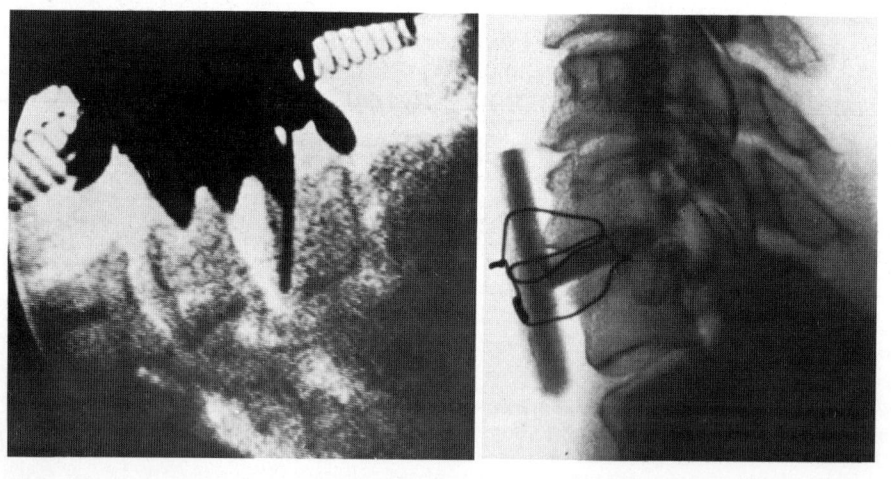

Fig. 3. Drilling of the vertebral body for internal fixation under X-ray control with subsequent internal fixation

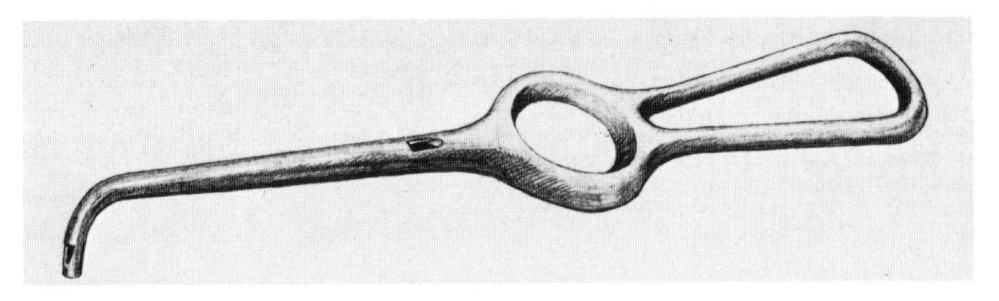

Fig. 4. Hook with a borehole for reposition of the vertebral body dislocated transversely into the spinal canal with internal fixation by epidurally located wires (length: 23.5 cm)

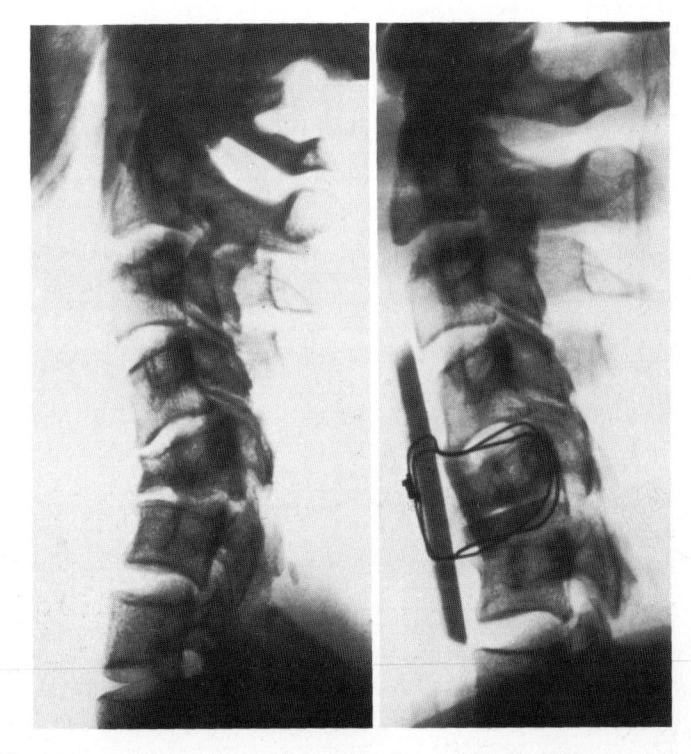

Fig. 5. Reposition and fixation of the compressed vertical body -C5- with primary surgical laminectomy *(left)*; reposition with internal fixation seven years after the accident *(right)*

Subluxations, Fracture Dislocations and Compression Fractures of Cervical Vertebral Column. Results of Surgical and Conservative Treatment

B. RAMA, H. KOCH, and O. SPOERRI

Introduction

Both, surgery and conservative therapy are practices in the treatment of lesions of cervical vertebral column (compared to decompressive surgery such as laminectomy). Both methods do not just stabilize the vertebral column but help to decompress the spinal cord and/or spinal nerve as well.

Regarding the results of both methods, we have to discuss the advantage of one of these methods compared with the other.

Material

56 patients were under treatment for a lesion in the segment C 2/3 and the caudal segments between 1970 and 1978. Time of follow-up is two to seven years. Four patients died because of this injury.

Conservative treatment comprised in 23 patients CRUTCHFIELD extension, followed by external stabilisation such as "diadem plaster" (craniocervico-thoracic plaster) in 19 cases. Four patients needed just external stabilisation. The indication for conservative treatment cannot be traced back in all cases. Serious injuries elsewhere determined conservative treatment in 14 patients.
29 patients *were treated surgically* because of lesions of the cervical vertebral column.
17 patients had CLOWARD ventral spondylosyndesis,
5 patients had VERBIEST vertebral fusion. Open dorsal exploration was necessary in 2 cases; it was done as well as CLOWARD's ventral spondylosyndesis in 5 patients.
Preoperative, 27 patients had CRUTCHFIELD, traction 22 patients were supplied with "diadem plaster" as postoperative treatment.

Brain injury II° was found as a complicating injury only in 2 surgically treated patients.

Surgery was indicated in 17 cases because of instability or unsatisfactory reduction by CRUTCHFIELD traction. One case needed dorsal decompression and dorsal repositioning because of incomplete paraplegia after turning in the paraplegia bed.
One case had a surgical complication: after CLOWARD's operation the bone dowel slid out and the patient had to be operated upon once again.

Results

Six conservatively treated patients showed a traumatic *radiculopathy* meaning sensory and motor paralysis, none of them became well. Even in one patient of the group of conservatively treated patients we later noticed a non-posttraumatic radiculopathy.

Considering a group of 17 surgically treated patients with radiculopathy, six of them became well, even in regard to "just" preoperative radicular pain (Table 1). Similar results can be found in regard to restitution of primary *incomplete paraplegia symptomatic* (Table 2). Whereas incomplete paraplegia regressed only uncompletely in 7 of our conservatively treated patients, restitutio ad integrum was noticed in 4 or 9 surgically treated patients. One patient shows discreet myelopathy that did not exist preoperatively; in the group of conservatively treated patients, however, discrete myelopathy had to be diagnosed metatraumatically in 2 cases.

Complete paraplegia did not show any improvement in 4 patients - as expected.

Table 1. Development of traumatic radiculopathy (No. of surgically treated patients in brackets)

	Luxation n = 2 (n = 9)	Dislocated fractures n = 3 (n = 7)	Compression fractures n = 1 (n = 1)
Not improved with complaints		(1)	
Improved with complaints	1 (5)	2 (3)	
Improved without complaints	1	(1)	1 (1)
Well (symptom free)	(4)	(2)	
Metatraumatic radiculopathy			1
No specification		1	

Table 2. Development of traumatic incomplete paraplegia syndrome (No. of surgically treated patients in parenthesis)

	Luxation n = 3 (n = 4)	Dislocated fractures n = 1 (n = 3)	Compression fractures n = 3 (n = 2)
Unchanged		(1)	(1)
Improved with rest symptoms	3 (1)	1 (1)	3 (1)
Well	(3)	(1)	
Metatraumatic myelopathy	1	(1)	1

Comparing the results of the different treatments, we also saw differences concerning X-ray pictures. Whereas kyphosis can be found in 1/4 of the cases in the group of conservatively treated patients as well as in the group of surgically treated patients, we did not find dorsal steps in surgically treated cases. (The other way, there are no additional damages to adjacent vertebral segments such as degenerative changes). Lordosis can be found in 11 of 29 surgically treated patients, but just in 5 of 23 conservatively treated patients (Table 3).

What about the patient's vocational capacity?

You may find remarkable differences at first sight. Whereas 25 of 29 surgically treated patients practised their original profession, only 13 of 23 conservatively treated patients did so. We have to point out, however, that 14 of these 23 conservatively treated patients suffered multiple and complicating injuries, which had an influence on vocational incapacity. So a comparison of vocational capacity between both groups is inapplicable.

Conclusion

We compared the results of 23 conservative with 29 surgical treatments of patients with subluxations, fracture dislocations and compression fractures of the segment C 2/3 and the caudal segments (C5, C6 and C4).

There was a better regression of radicular defects and incomplete paraplegia in the group of the surgically treated patients than in the group of conservatively treated ones. X-ray pictures show the same number of kyphosis in both groups, the position of the cervical vertebral column, however, is better in the group of surgically treated patients.

Nevertheless, this group shows more evident degenerative changes than the group of conservatively treated patients. Serious multiple injuries in the group of conservatively treated patients do not allow a comparison of both groups concerning vocational capacity.

Table 3. Radiological results (No. of surgically treated patients in parenthesis)

	Luxation n = 7 (n = 10)	Dislocated fractures n = 8 (n = 14)	Compression fractures n = 8 (n = 5)
Lordosis	1 (5)	2 (5)	2 (1)
Steep posture	2 (2)	(4)	1 (2)
Kyphosis	2 (3)	2 (2)	2 (2)
Dorsal steps	1	2	2
Additional lesions in adjacent segments	(4)	(1)	(2)
No information	1	2 (3)	1

Pathomorphological and Clinical Basis of the Prognosis in Cervical Injuries

V. REINHARDT, K. ROOSEN, H.-E. NAU, and L. GERHARD

Introduction

Occasionally a great discrepancy between clinically evaluated lesions and morphological findings seen in necropsy may occur (1, 2). This was the reason why we examined eleven patients out of 120 with cervical traumas who died and in whom necropsy was done.

Patients

The age of eleven patients with cervical traumas examined clinically and neuropathologically varied from 6 to 73 years. In 4 cases we found cervical trauma only, in 7 cases the additional skull brain injury grade 3 dominated the clinical picture. The survival time was 2 hours to 27 days.

In seven patients we found a complete transverse syndrome directly after the trauma, in one case a radicular lesion. In a further case the patient complained about pain only. In 2 cases the skull brain injury was so severe, that we had not thought of a cervical trauma immediately. An initial apnoe was diagnosed in 5 patients. In three we could not explain whether the breathing disturbance had to be due to the brain trauma or the cervical lesion. The diagnosis of spinal trauma could be confirmed by means of neuroradiology in 8 patients. In 2 cases the cervical lesion was suspected and discussed because of the clinical symptoms. In one case the cervical lesion was revealed at necropsy only. The diagnostic procedures showed bone lesions in 10 out of 11 patients, avulsions of the dens in 3, a dislocation fracture in 6 cases, and one compression fracture C3 to C5.

During the clinical stay those patients with initial radicular symptoms or isolated pain syndrome developed incomplete transverse lesions. Once apnoea appeared secondarily with a delay of 48 hours.

The reasons for the fatal outcome were medullary breathing disturbances in 6 cases, twice failures of central regulation. A 73 year old patient died because of pulmonary embolism on the 7th day, two patients because of bronchopneumonia due to central ventilation disturbances.

Case Reports

In these different clinical states it can be expected that the morphological sequelae, too, can differ enormously. Minimal morphological lesions were seen in a 73-year-old patient with a dislocation fracture C6/7 following a fall from a wall.

48 hours later the initial unsuspected neurological state turned to an incomplete transverse lesion. Five days later he died because of pulmonary embolism. In this case an oedema extending from the spinal medulla up to the medulla oblongata was found (Fig. 1). The development of the incomplete transverse lesion could be due to the secondary manifestation of oedema.

A more severe degree of tissue lesions with concomitant sequelae of the compression itself were seen in a 39 year old wife of a farmer who suffered a primarily complete transverse lesion distal to C5, when she was kicked by a cow during milking. She survived her fracture dislocation of C5/6 for 4 days. Histologically we found bleeding and necrosis. This could be recognized even macroscopically on the surface of the spinal cord (Fig. 2a, b). Hematomas of the wall of leptomeningeal and intraspinal vessels were a special microscopical finding in this case (Fig. 2c). Primary traumatic sequelae may immediately lead to a complete or nearly complete destruction of the medullary segments involved.

Of great interest were 2 patients with a complete transection of the medulla. The first case was a girl aged 6, who survived a car accident with dislocation of the dens for one day. The dislocation evoked a complete separation between cervical medulla and medulla oblongata with hemorrhagic necrosis of both ends.

An 11-year-old boy was comatose at first after a bicycle accident, regained consciousness in the following 6 days, remained however tetraplegic and showed apnoea during the whole clinical course. He died after another 8 days. In this case we found a complete separation again between the medulla oblongata and the cervical cord, but no bony lesion could be demonstrated even at necropsy. The hemorrhagic necrosis of the upper cervical medulla up to the inferior olive could also be recognized macroscopically (Fig. 3).

A 42-year-old man with a fracture dislocation C4/5 after diving into a swimming-pool and developed immediately a complete transverse lesion. After initial adequate diaphragmatic breathing he died in medullary failure. Histology revealed hemorrhagic necrosis and edema of the cervical medulla as well as edema of the medulla oblongata (Fig. 4).

Discussion

The morphological changes differ enormously. The mildest of them - possibly reversible - can be derived from the clinical course and symptoms only indirectly. As in cases of brain oedema (1, 2-4) within 48 to 60 hours too. This oedema can either evoke clinical symptoms or lead to the increase of already existing symptoms (3). Only the difference between initial neurological deficits and the later picture of morphological lesions allows of the possibility to assess the degree and extension of secondary alterations. An initially manifest post-traumatic apnoea with a primarily high transverse syndrome is of great importance, because in this case it is most probable that it is due to a primary, medullary lesion, irreversible, and prognostically infavourable (1). But also minor neurological deficits after high cervical medullary trauma have to be judged critically. In these cases it must be expected that the oedema extending mainly in a longitudinal direction through the spinal cord can reach the caudal medulla oblongata (3, 4). This causes a dysfunction of vital regulatory centres.

(The compensation of these disturbances even nowadays is still unsuccessful in contrast to the therapy of peripheral regulation disturbances).

These pathomorphological findings explain the clinical course of those patients who suddenly developed lethal breathing disturbances 2 or 3 days after the trauma.

References

1. Grote, W.: Fusionsbehandlung zervikaler Luxationsfrakturen. In: Die Wirbelsäule in Forschung und Praxis, Bd. 42. Junghanns, H. (ed.), pp. 104.109. Stuttgart: Hippokrates 1969
2. Jellinger, K.: Zur Morphologie und Pathogenese spinaler Läsionen bei Verletzungen der Halswirbelsäule. Acta Neuropath. $\underline{3}$, 451-468 (1964)
3. Lausberg, G.: Akutmaßnahmen bei Wirbelsäulenverletzungen mit und ohne Rückenmarksbeteiligung. Langenbecks Arch. klin. Chir. $\underline{327}$, 981-986 (1970)
4. Mayer, E.Th., Peters, G.: Pathologische Anatomie der Rückenmarksverletzungen. In: Neuro-Traumatologie, Bd. II. Kessel, F.K., Guttmann, L., Maurer, G. (eds.), pp. 39-61. München, Berlin, Wien: Urban & Schwarzenberg 1971

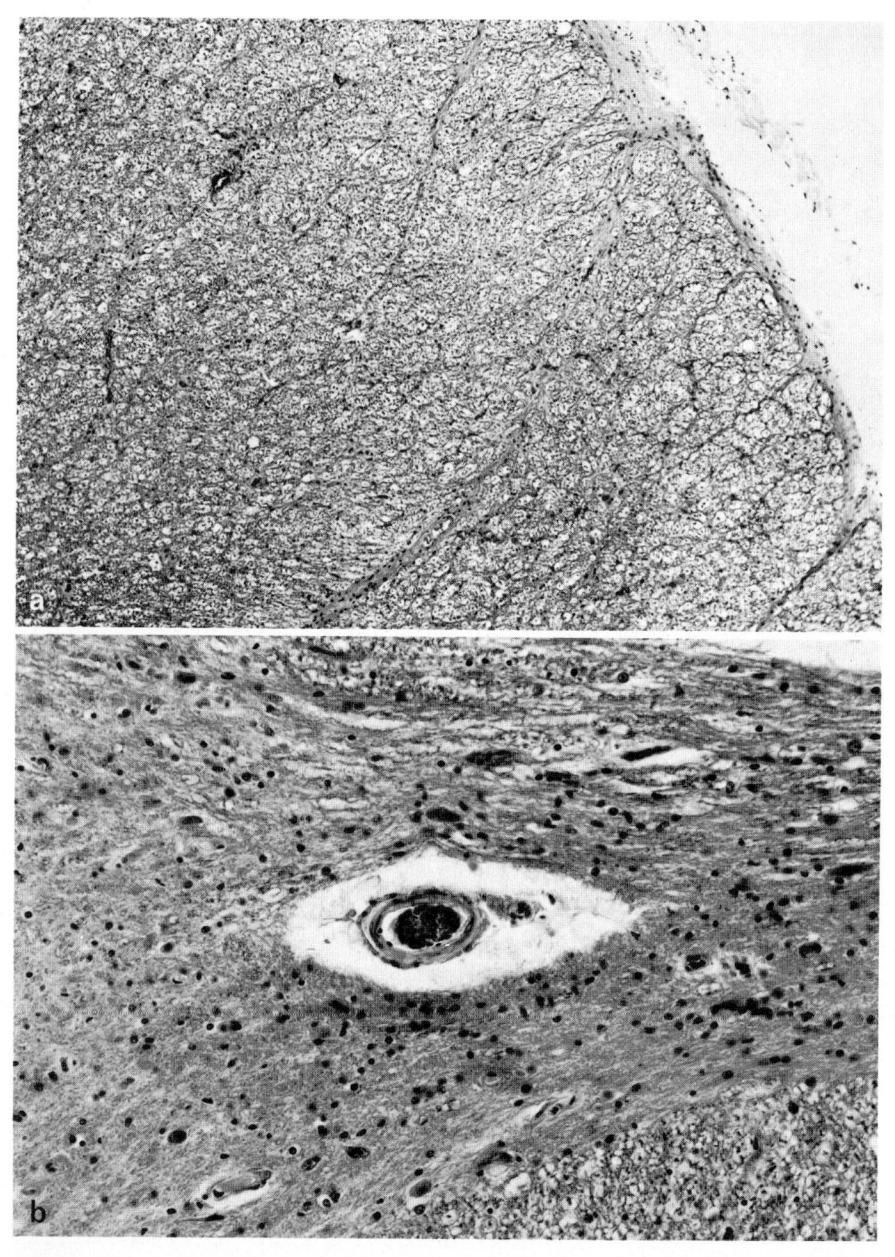

Fig. 1a, b. Cervical part of the medulla. a Minimal edema in the region of the lateral fascicle. HE; 150 x. b Perivascular edema in the grey commissure. HE; 430 x

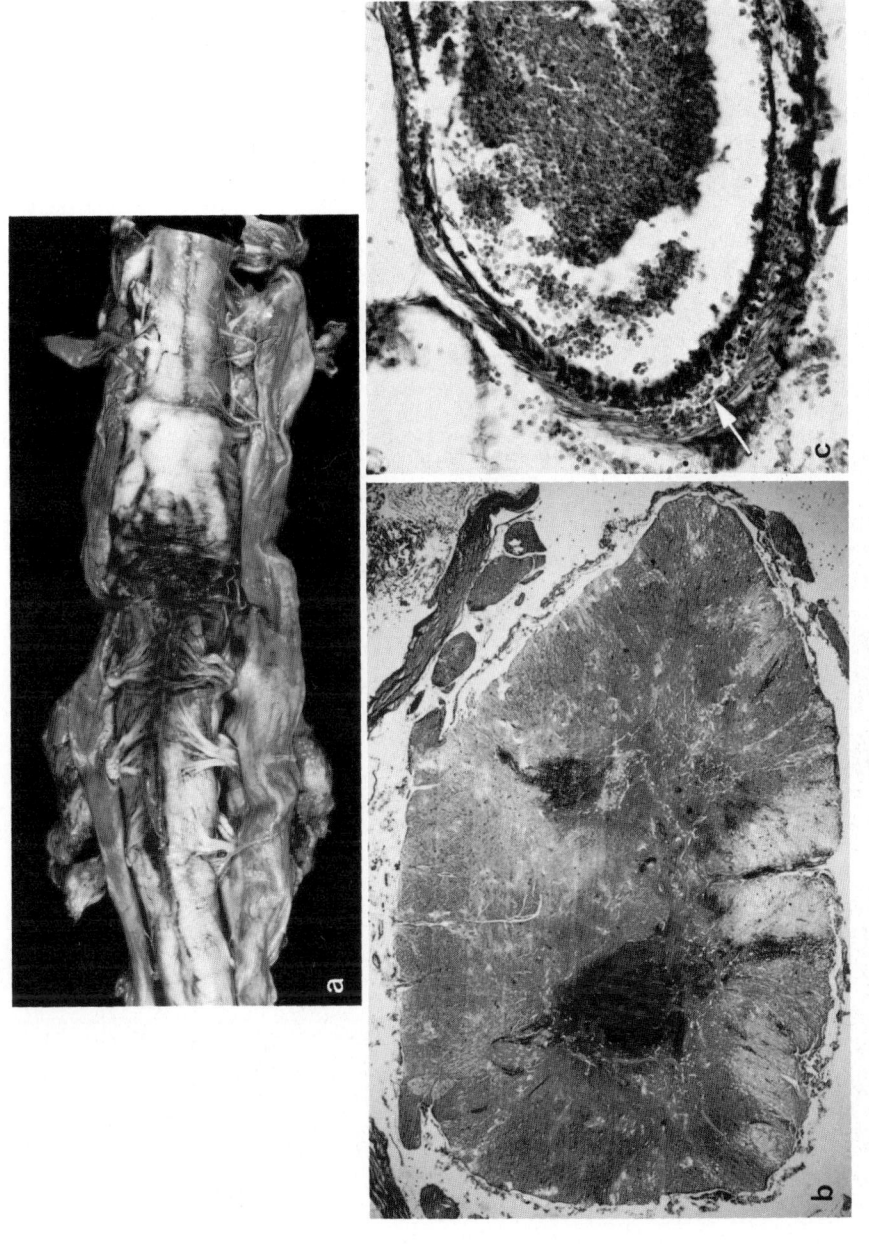

Fig. 2. a Macroscopic aspect of the injured cervical medulla. b Microphotograph of a cross section at the level of injury shows hemorrhages and necrosis mainly of the grey matter and edema. HE; 7x. c Hematoma (*arrow*) of the wall of an intraspinal artery between internal elastic and muscular layers. EvG; 430 x

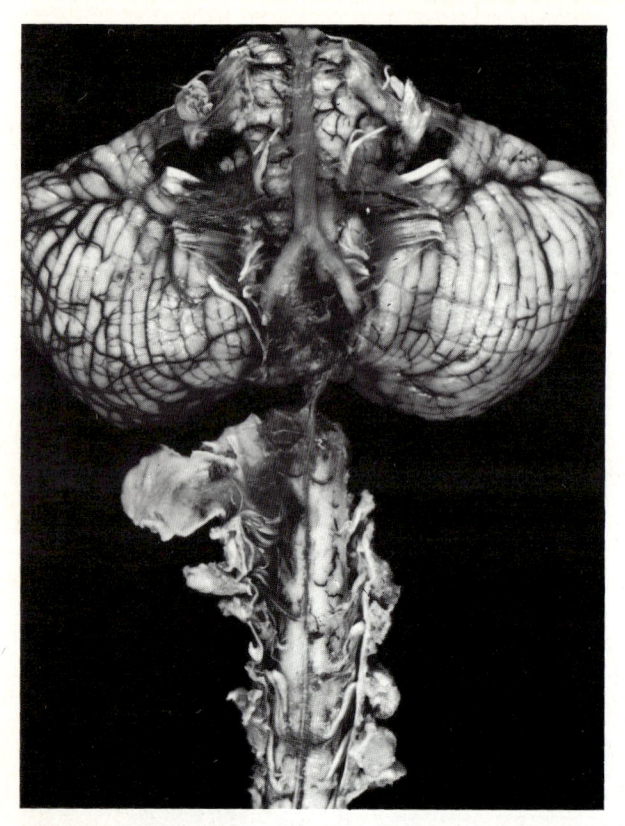

Fig. 3. Complete separation between medulla oblongata and cervical cord. Hemorrhagic necrosis of the upmost cervical medulla and inferior olive

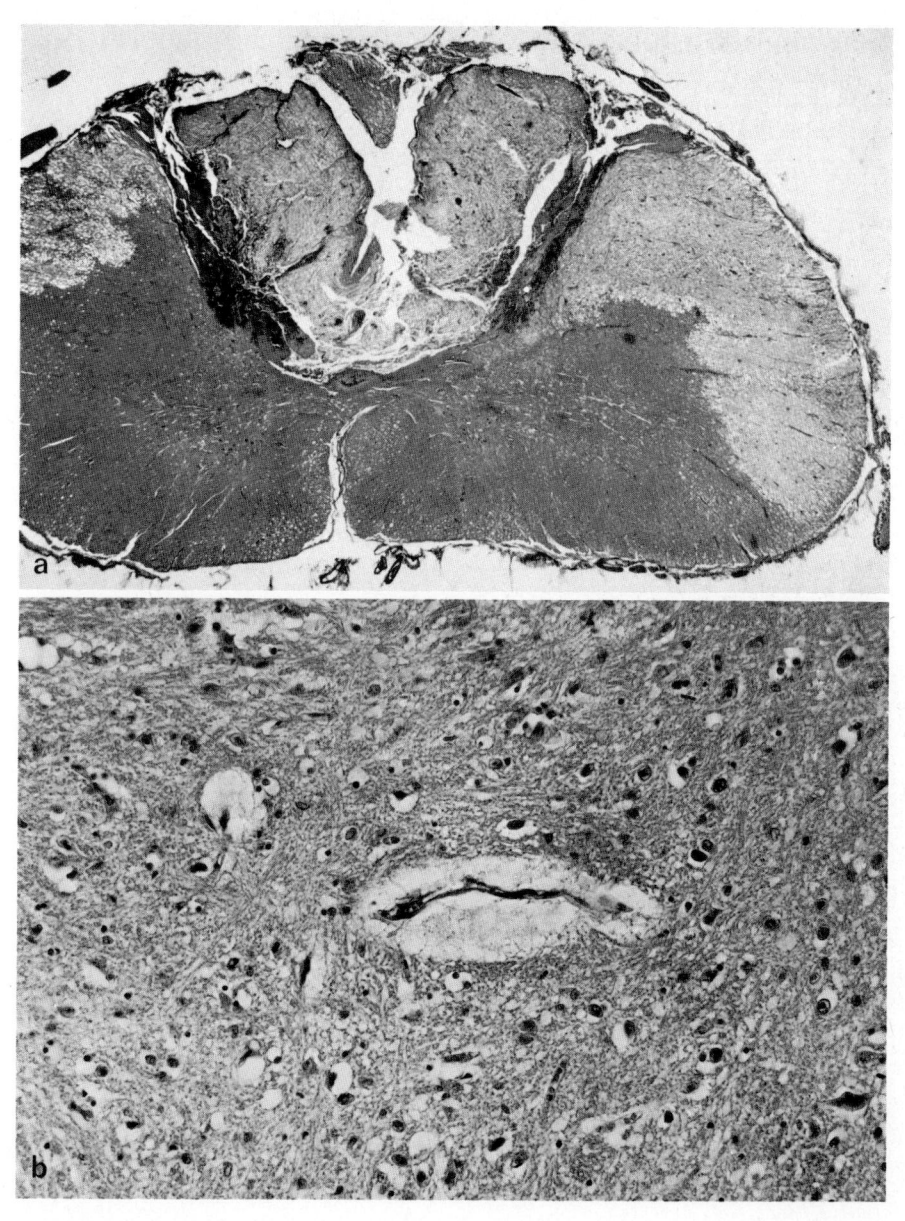

Fig. 4. a Hemorrhages and necrosis of posterior horns and posterior column. Severe edema. HE; 10 x. b Microphotograph of the medulla oblongata reveals a perivascular edema. EvG; 430 x

Surgical Treatment of Cervical Spine Injuries – Prognostic Aspects on Operative Procedure and Timing

K. ROOSEN and W. GROTE

The joint study of eight neurosurgical clinics regarding operative treatment of 283 cervical spine injuries which was reported at the 6th international neurosurgical congress in Sao-Paulo (10) shows that the prognosis of these cervical spine traumas in the first place depends upon the severity, the level of the lesion, and the duration of the accompanying spinal cord lesion. The type of bony injury and the kind of surgical approach had no significant influence on the late clinical results. In our opinion single factors like the period of recumbency, functional stability, complication rate will be different, yet this depends upon the specific clinical indications to operate and the operative technique (1-9, 12, 14-18, 20-23, 25-27).

Between 1969 and 1980 252 patients with cervical spine injuries were treated. The age curve and sex distribution correspond to the known statistical pattern of this disease group. For clinical evaluation the injuries are divided into 5 degrees depending upon the severity of the spinal cord lesion, - from normal neurological condition as degree I to complete cord transection syndrome, as degree V (13).

Grade	Neurological status
I	Normal
II	Radicular deficit
III	Incomplete transverse cord paralysis - able to walk
IV	Incomplete transverse cord lesion - incapable of walking
V	Complete transverse spinal cord lesion

The injuries of the cervical spine could be divided according to the plain diagnostic X-ray findings (Table 1). The X-ray pictures demonstrate depending upon the injured structure normal findings or axial deviations. The majority of patients operated upon had subluxations or fracture dislocations.

Table 1. X-ray findings of 132 patients surgically treated because of cervical spine injuries

Morphological damage	X-ray finding	Patients operated upon (n = 132)
Discogenic	Normal	22
Ligaments + disc	Axis deviation	5
	Dislocation (luxation)	38
Bony + ligamentous ± discogenic	Fracture dislocation	56
	Fragmented fracture	3
	Compression fracture	3

The rare surgical interventions in cases of vertebral body fractures verify that we presently give in these patients preference to conservative treatment.

Table 2. Surgical approaches to the cervical spine

Patients	132	
Operative method		
- Ventral		150
- Combined dorsal + ventral		8
Ventral fusion (v.F.) + 2/2 dorsal wire-(cerclage)	4	
Laminectomy + ventral fusion (v.F.)	4	
- Dorsal		3
Atlanto-axial fusion	1	
Laminectomy	2	

On 132 patients 150 segments were anteriorly fused; 142 times as the only measure (Table 2). In 4 cases decompressive laminectomy was performed, in 4 others additional dorsal fixation by means of circumferential wire was necessary. Three patients were operated upon using only the dorsal approach. We corrected an atlanto-axial subluxation in an 8 year old boy with autogenous bone graft, interposed in between the dorsal arches C1 and C2, which was additional secured by a circumferential wire (Fig. 1).

In most cases of 150 anterior cervical fusions on 129 patients alloplastic bone cement was used; a bone graft was implanted four times (Fig. 2).

Figure 2 shows the results 6 months to 8 years after the injury and surgery. The 100% increase to normal comes entirely from the group of patients, primarily classified as II because of radicular syndromes. Even though there were 9 improvements of conditions possible in degree III + IV, respectively 4 cases with normal findings, we saw no change however from degree V into degree I or II. The lethality rate of the total number of cases (Fig. 3) proves the prognostic importance of the early neurological findings. The probability of death through initial complete transverse cord lesion above C4 was approximately 94%.

In comparison with the results of the joint study (10), this shows no significant differences with regard to the prognosis. The analysis of our own therapeutic difficulties and complications as well as our discussion about the so far accepted contra-indications will make it perhaps possible to modify and improve the operative technique expecting thereby an improvement of clinical long-term results as well.

Complications	
Subluxation:	
Cement graft	9
Vertebral body	9
Rupture of the wire-(cerclage)	1
Death within 24 hours after operation	4

The ventral stabilization with bone cement has proved reliable as an alternative operative method in cases of traumatic disc lesions, axial angulations and subluxations (20) (Fig. 2).

Postoperative subluxation of bone cement - plombage out of the intravertebral space or dislocation of vertebral bodies (Fig. 3) as mechanical problems which we observed in 13.3% of cases occurred almost entirely after stabilization of fracture dislocations.

Vertebral body fractures and massive rupture of supportive ligaments and muscles aggravate the strain-stable anchorage of the PMMA-dowels. In these cases it should be primarily considered during the operation additional inner fixation on one side: i.e., ventral with AO-Plate or dorsal with wire-cerclage. In case of massive compression fracture the primary spondylectomy with autogenous bone replacement could be employed. The strain-dependent rupture of the wire-cerclage (Fig. 4) was only observed once among 4 patients. It could probably be prevented by reinforcement of wires with tibia bone grafts, bilaterally fixed to the dorsal arches; a procedure which has proved reliable in posterior blocking of atlanto-axial dislocations (13, 24).

For this kind of injuries there is available a dorsal fusion clip, developed by us as a team with Dr. TRAUSCHEL, head of the Central Technical Laboratory at the University Hospital Essen, which is simple to implant and because of its inner spring traction guarantees a long-lasting stability.

Four patients who died within 24 hours after the operation presented symptoms of degree V with segmental levels at C4/5. They could all be operated upon within 6 days after the symptoms of shock had subsided and the autonomic functions had stabilized. On the assumption that the indication to operate is thought of yet too early, we consider for that reason that in cases falling into degree V the suspension of operation has to be complied with for at least 7 days, which is not so in degrees I - IV. In these grades the timing of surgical fixation depends upon the ideal or at least sufficient repositioning of the cervical spinal column.

Operative treatment contra-indications	
Fixed luxation (locked subluxation)	8
Kind and extent of vertebral body injury (fragmented and compression fractures)	22
Level of complete transverse cord lesion + respiratory insufficiency	9
Severity of cerebral injury	6

Among the contra-indications "point 2" should be discussed with the question whether the early active stabilization by autogenous spinal body replacement with or without reliable osteosynthetic plate is advantageous even in those cases where no symptoms of myelopathy depending on mechanical compression are demonstrable. Extension for axial correction and external immobilization is so far preferred in cases of cervical fragmented and compression fractures without symptoms of cord compression, because of satisfactory conservative therapeutic results, despite its protracted clinical course.

References

1. Bürkle de la Camp, H.: Zur Behandlung der Halswirbelluxationen. Langenbecks Arch. Klin. Chir. 292, 514-522 (1959)

2. Cloward, R.B.: Treatment of acute fractures and fracture-dislocation of the cervical spina by vertebral-body fusion. J. Neurosurg. 18, 201-209 (1961)

3. Cloward, R.B.: Treatment of lesions of the cervical spine by the anterior surgical approach. In: The spinal cord, Austin, G. (ed.), pp. 389-440. Springfield: Thomas-Publication 1972

4. Grote, W., Wüllenweber, R., Bettag, W.: Behandlung cervikaler Luxationsfrakturen durch ventrale Fusion. Chirurg. 38, 138-140 (1967)

5. Grote, W.: Fusionsbehandlung zervikaler Luxationsfrakturen. In: Die Wirbelsäule in Forschung und Praxis, 42, pp. 104-109. Stuttgart: Hippokrates 1969

6. Grote, W., Roosen K.: Operative Behandlung der HWS-Verletzung. Monatsschr. Unfallheilk. 132, 318-325 (1978)

7. Hamel, E., Karimi-Nejad, A., Frowein, R.A., Kunst, H.: Results of conservative and surgical early treatment of cervical spine injuries. Adv. Neurosurg. 4, 185-190 (1977)

8. Junghanns, H.: Verblockungsoperationen bei Frakturen der Halswirbelkörper. Wschr. Unfallheilk. 73, 443-452 (1970)

9. Junghanns, H.: Operative Behandlungen für die Schleuder- und Abknickverletzungen der Halswirbelsäule. Wschr. Unfallheilkd. 74, 485-494 (1971)

10. Karimi-Nejad, A.: Ergebnis der operativen Behandlung bei HWS-Verletzung. Monatsschr. Unfallheilk. 132, 325-335 (1978)

11. Karimi-Nejad, A., Frowein, R.A., Roosen, K., Grote, W., Schumacher, W., Lausberg, G., Pia, H.W., Lorenz, R., Busch, G., Schürmann, K., Hübner, B., Hermann, H.D., Loew, F., Wüllenweber, R., Menzel, J., Penzholz, H.: The treatment of fracture dislocations of the cervical spine. In: Neurological surgery. Carrea, R. (ed.), pp. 347-354. Amsterdam-Oxford: Excerpta Medica 1978

12. Karimi-Nejad, A.: Indikation, Technik und Ergebnisse der operativen Behandlung von Halswirbelsäulen-(HWS)-Verletzungen. Fortschr. Neurol. Psychiat. 48, 183-206 (1980)

13. Karimi-Nejad, A.: Internal fixation of cervical spine injuries. In: Advances in neurosurgery, Vol. 9. Schiefer, W., Klinger, M., Brock, M. (eds.), pp. 479-489. Berlin, Heidelberg, New York: Springer 1981

14. Kuhlendahl, H.: Schleudertrauma der HWS. Neurochirurgische Probleme. Langenbecks Arch. klin. Chir. 316, 470-475 (1966)

15. Lausberg, G.: Akutmaßnahmen bei Wirbelsäulenverletzungen mit und ohne Rückenmarksbeteiligung. Langenbecks Arch. klin. Chir. 327, 981-986 (1970)

16. Lausberg, G.: Die operative Therapie bei Verletzungen der Halswirbelsäule. Z. Orthop. 112, 899-903 (1974)

17. Pia, H.W.: Halswirbelsäulenschäden und ihre operative Behandlung. Wien. Med. Wschr. 123, 597-600 (1973)

18. Raynor, R.B.: Severe injuries of the cervical spine treated by early anterior interbody fusion and ambulation. J. Neurosurg. 28, 311-316 (1968)
19. Robinson, R.A., Walker, A.E., Ferlic, D.C., Wiecking, D.K.: The results of anterior interbody fusion of the cervical spine. J. Bone Jt. Surg. 44-A, 1569-1587 (1962)
20. Roosen, K.: Experimentelle, klinische und radiologische Langzeituntersuchungen zum Ersatz zervikaler Bandscheiben durch Knochenzement (Polymethylmethacrylat). Habil.-Schrift, Essen 1979
21. Schlegel, K.F.: Die akuten Schleuderverletzungen der Halswirbelsäule und ihre Behandlung. Beitr. Z. Orthop. 104, 293-303 (1968)
22. Schürmann, K., Busch, G.: Die Behandlung der zervikalen Luxationsfrakturen durch die ventrale Fusion. Chirurg. 41, 225-228 (1970)
23. Schürmann, K., Reulen, H.J., Busch, G.: Rekonstruktive und stabilisierende Maßnahmen bei Wirbelkörperverletzungen. Hefte Unfallheilkd. 132, 336-342 (1978)
24. Schürmann, K.: Atlanto-axiale dislocation in rheumatoid arthritis with cervical cord compression (myelopathy). In: Advances in neurosurgery, Vol. VII. Marguth, F., Brock, M., Kazner, E., Klinger, M., Schmiedek, P. (eds.), pp. 151-154. Berlin, Heidelberg, New York: Springer 1979
25. Verbiest, H.: Anterolateral operations for fractures and dislocations in the middle and lower parts of the cervical spine. J. Bone Jt. Surg. 51-A, 1489-1530 (1969)
26. Verbiest, H.: Antero-lateral operations for fractures or dislocations of the cervical spine due to injuries or previous surgical interventions. Clin. Neurosurg. 20, 334-336 (1973)
27. Wiesner, H., Mumenthaler, M.: Schleuderverletzungen der Halswirbelsäule. Eine katamnestische Studie. Arch. orthop. Unfall-Chir. 81, 13-36 (1975)

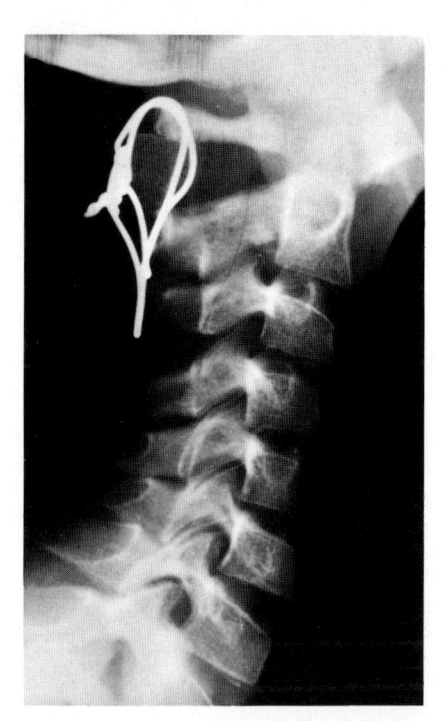

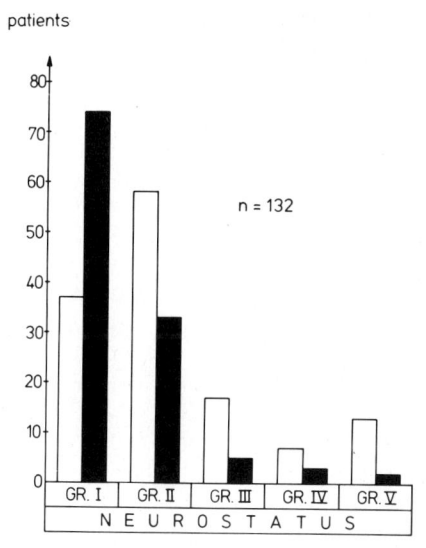

Fig. 1. Dorsal stabilization of a traumatic atlanto-axial deviation using an autogenous bone-graft and wire (cerclage) (Arcodesis C 1/2)

Fig. 2. Anterior cervical spine fusions in 129 patients. Neurological status; □ = admission (n = 132); ■ = follow-up (n = 117)

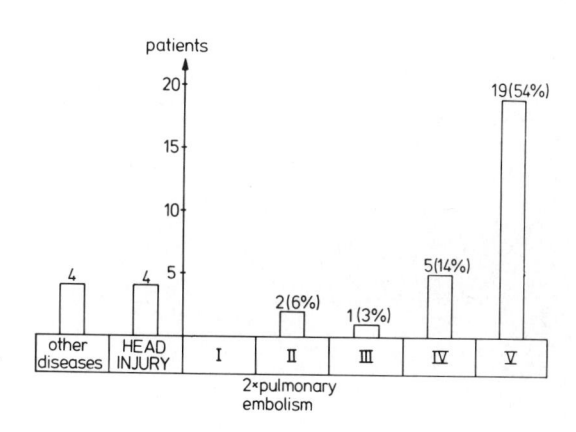

Fig. 3. Lethality (n = 35 ≙ 14%)

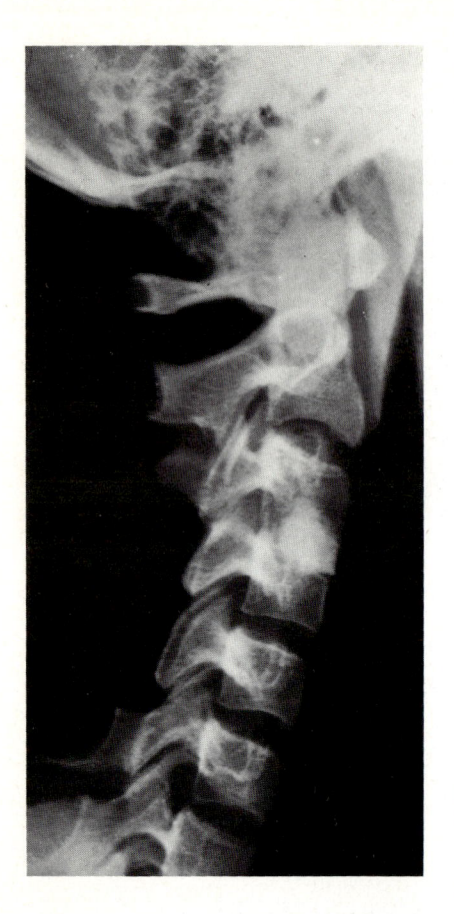

Fig. 4. Ideal bony integration of an alloplastic implant (PMMA). Subluxation fracture C 3/4; lateral X-ray view 18 months after operation

Fig. 5. Lateral xerotomogram. Partial reluxation of vertebral body and PMMA-dowel after anterior fusion because of dislocations fracture c 6/7

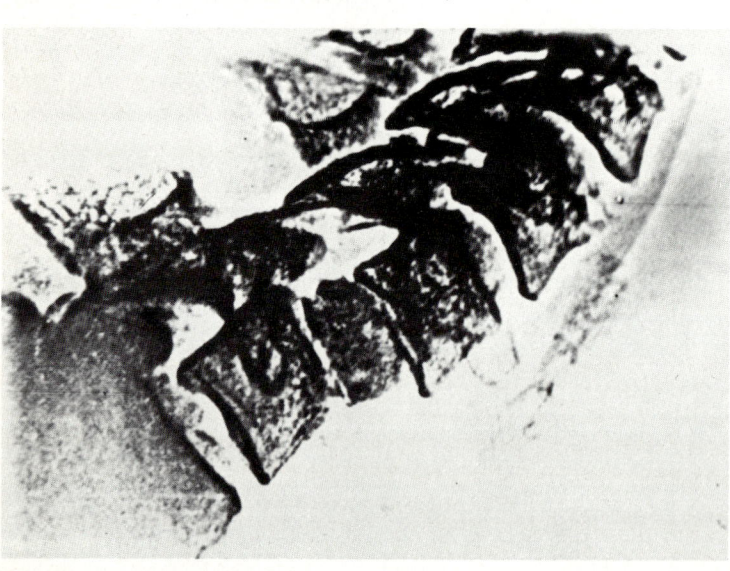

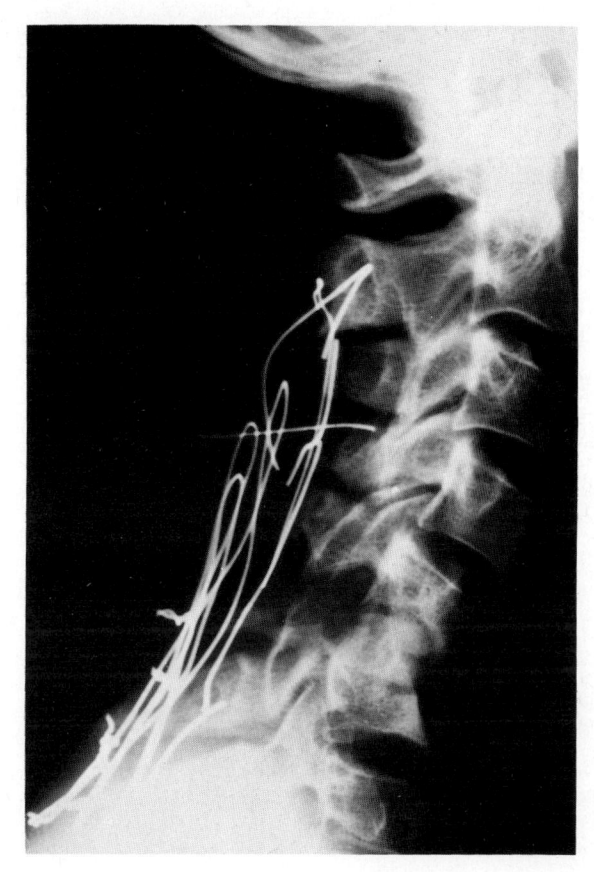

Fig. 6. Rupture of the wire-cerclage 6 months after surgery

Free Topics

Regional Cerebral Blood Flow and Extra-Intracranial Bypass Surgery

J. BOCKHORN, A. BRAWANSKI, and M. R. GAAB

The extra-intracranial arterial bypass surgery as a method for treating disturbances of the cerebral perfusion has a certain place in the repertoire of neurosurgical operations for improving the cerebral blood flow.

Nevertheless there are again and again questions as to whether extensive and sweeping diagnostic methods like cerebral angiography have to be undertaken in patients suffering from cerebral ischemia. Those questions are certainly pertinent for cerebral angiography with a considerable complication rate followed by worsening of the neurological status. The frequency of those complications is given in the literature ranging from 0.2 to 4.5% (4, 6). In these figures complications caused by allergies to the contrast media are not taken into account. There are no large differences in the complication rate for the different routes of angiography by catheter from the femoral artery, by direct carotid puncture or by the retrograde brachial artery angiography (6, 8). Patients after a stroke seem especially endangered by angiographic study for in those patients the cerebral perfusion is already diminished. The hypotensive situations caused by the application of the contrast medium during the angiography or by medication for performing the angiography, or even by direct reaction of the cerebral vascular system to the contrast medium may precipitate further strokes. The data of the literature are obtained from the primary diagnostic procedures prior to an appropriate medical or surgical treatment. Certainly those figures are also valid after performing surgery especially after an extra-intracranial bypass.

The angiography is of course unavoidable for the detailed presentation of the anatomic lesions which led to the cerebral ischemia. It is defintely not sufficient to trust alone the non-invasive methods: the auscultation and the ultrasound-Doppler-sonography.

But there are patients in whom the considerable deficit of cerebral function makes surgical intervention questionable. In these situations the regional cerebral blood flow measurement helps in deciding in which patients a surgical measure is useful before employing angiography. In certain cases the risk of angiography can be avoided. The regional cerebral blood flow measurement in its non-invasive fashion by the inhalation method gives sufficiently detailed informations. By decreases of the regional cerebral blood flow values below about 25 ml/ 100 g tissue/min in the calculation of the Initial Slope Index (ISI) of RISBERG (9) - this value can be termed "stroke threshold" - one can assume that sufficient perfusion of the region of the brain involved which allows a certain basic metabolism of the nervous cells to take place no longer exist (Fig. 1) (2).

At the Neurosurgical University Hospital Würzburg the regional cerebral blood flow measurement is performed with 133-Xenon using the inhalation technique[1]. The calculations are done using the FOURIER transformation program of the RISBERG group (3, 10). In addition we have combined the 32 single detectors to certain detector groups corrosponding to the anatomical and functional brain regions and to the different vascular areas to make the measurement with 32 detectors more easily understandable and more useful for the clinician (1).

As well as preoperative diagnostic measurement the non-invasive blood flow measurement is useful in the postoperative follow-up of patients after extra-intracranial bypass surgery as a method which does not burden or endanger the patient (5, 7). Additionally follow-up examinations are possible in short or long-term intervals (Fig. 2). Other non-invasive diagnostic procedures like the ultrasound-Dopplersonography of the vessel used for the anastomosis do not give sufficient accuracy in their statements. The diameter of the superficial temporal artery increases and so changes of the flow velocity do not represent the actual anastomotic function.

Angiography is risky as mentioned above. Besides that angiography does not give the proper clue of the actual haemodynamic function of the anastomosis. Using high pressure while injecting the contrast medium in the course of direct carotid angiography an overflow of the contrast to the intracranial vascular bed can occur owing to the unphysiological pressure situation during the injection. In contrast to this the Xenon method has the advantage of giving statements on the haemodynamic efficiency of the anastomosis.

About 30 patients in whom extra-intracranial bypass surgery had been performed were examined pre- and postoperatively with rCBF-measurement. The first postoperative measurement was done about one week following the surgery, usually one or two days after the regularly performed treatment with dextrane for increasing the microcirculation was finished. In most of the cases an increase of the perfusion values was found compared to the preoperative study (Fig. 3). But even when the first postoperative measurement during the first week after surgery does not show an increase of the cerebral perfusion this is not equivalent to failure of the operative procedure. About this, only a later measurement some 8 to 10 weeks after surgery can give information.

With a functioning anastomosis a distinct increase is found on the operated side as well as on the opposite side (Fig. 4). The increase of the contralateral perfusion values can be seen as an expression for undoing a preoperative existing intracerebral and interhemispheric steal effect, that now, with a sufficiently functioning anastomosis is no longer present, and that in this way the "healthy" hemisphere is getting its total perfusion.

We have nearly given up postoperative angiography following a surgically created extra-intracranial arterial bypass. Only in cases with combined vascular lesions which made a vascular surgical intervention necessary to the internal carotid artery of the one side after an extra-intracranial arterial bypass on the opposite side did we carry out angiography.

---

[1] Supported by the "Stiftung Volkswagenwerk"

Conclusion

The rCBF measurement is very useful in the follow-up after extra-intracranial bypass surgery. Blood flow measurement shows the hemodynamic efficiency of the bypass in contrast to angiography which reveals the patency of the anastomosis. The exact intracranial vascular pattern of perfusion seen on angiography does not show the extent of useful perfusion as the rCBF measurement does.

In addition the blood flow measurement as a non-invasive technique using inhalation of 133-Xe can be repeated in the sense of a follow-up study without endangering the patient. That is not possible to the same extent with angiography. There is a certain risk of deterioration in the neurological condition of the patient when using angiography.

References

1. Brawanski, A., Gaab, M., Bockhorn, J.: Nichtinvasive Messung der regionalen cerebralen Durchblutung. Acta medicotechnica (in press)
2. Deshmukh, V.D., Meyer, J.S.: Noninvasive measurement of regional cerebral blood flow in man. New York, London: Spectrum Publications 1978
3. Jablonski, T., Prohovnik, I., Risberg, J., Stahl, K.-E., Maximilian, V.A., von Sabsay, E.: Fourier analysis of 133-Xe inhalation curves: accuracy and sensitivity. Acta Neurol. Scand. 60, 216 (1979)
4. Kohlmeyer, K.: Invasive Neuroradiologie: Risiken und Aufklärung des Patienten. Neurol. Psychiat. 6, 61-62 (1980)
5. Little, J.R., Yamamoto, Y.L., Feindel, W., Meyer, E., Hodge, C.P.: Cerebral blood flow in superficial temporal artery to middle cerebral artery anastomosis. In: Microsurgery for cerebral ischemia. Peerless, J.S., McCormick, C.W. (eds.), pp. 59-66. New York, Heidelberg, Berlin: Springer 1980
6. Maurer, H.-J.: Risiken bei Kontrastmitteluntersuchungen. Dtsch. Ärztebl. 77, 1555-1564 (1980)
7. Meinig, G., Fenske, A., Schürmann, K.: The value of noninvasive regional CBF measurement in diagnostic and follow-up studies in cerebral vascular disease with special regard to EIAB. In: Microsurgery for cerebral ischemia. Peerless, J.S., McCormick, C.W. (eds.), pp. 80-86. New York, Heidelberg, Berlin: Springer 1980
8. Reisner, H., Samec, P., Zeiler, K.: On the complication rate of cerebral angiography. Neurosurg. Rev. 3, 23-29 (1980)
9. Risberg, J., Ali, Z., Wilson, E.M., Wills, E.L., Halsey, J.H.: Regional cerebral blood flow by 133-Xenon inhalation. Stroke 6, 142-148 (1975)
10. Risberg, J.: Regional cerebral blood flow measurements by 133-Xe inhalation: Methodology and applications in neuropsychology and psychiatry. Brain and Language 9, 9-34 (1980)

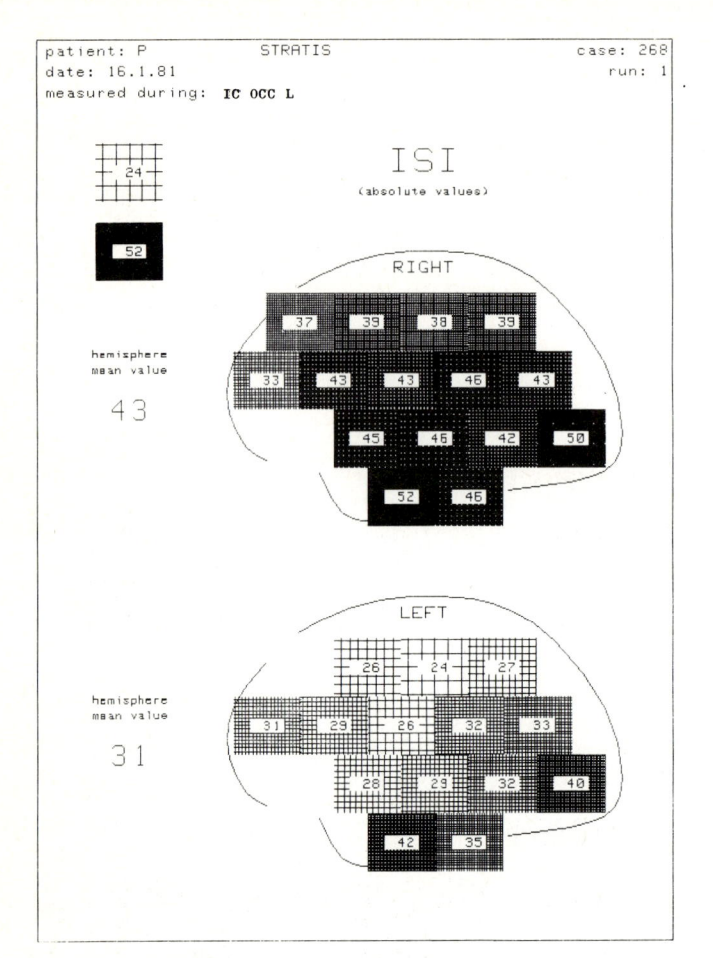

Fig. 1. rCBF measurement in a case with completed stroke on the left side. Severe depression of rCBF values to about 25 ml/100 g tissue/min

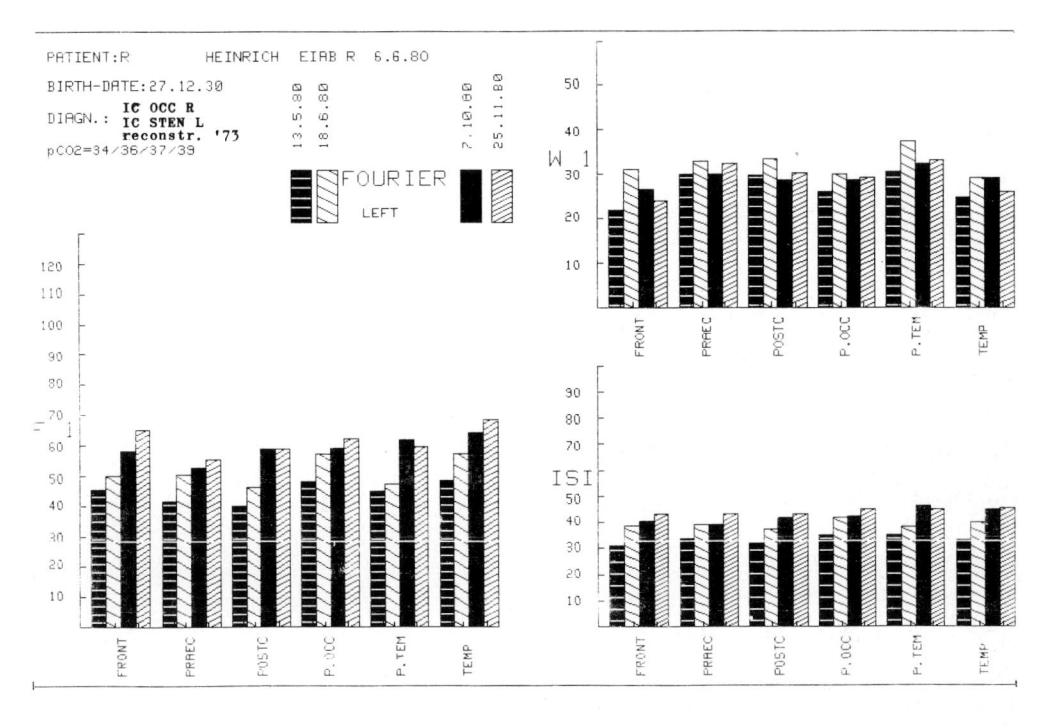

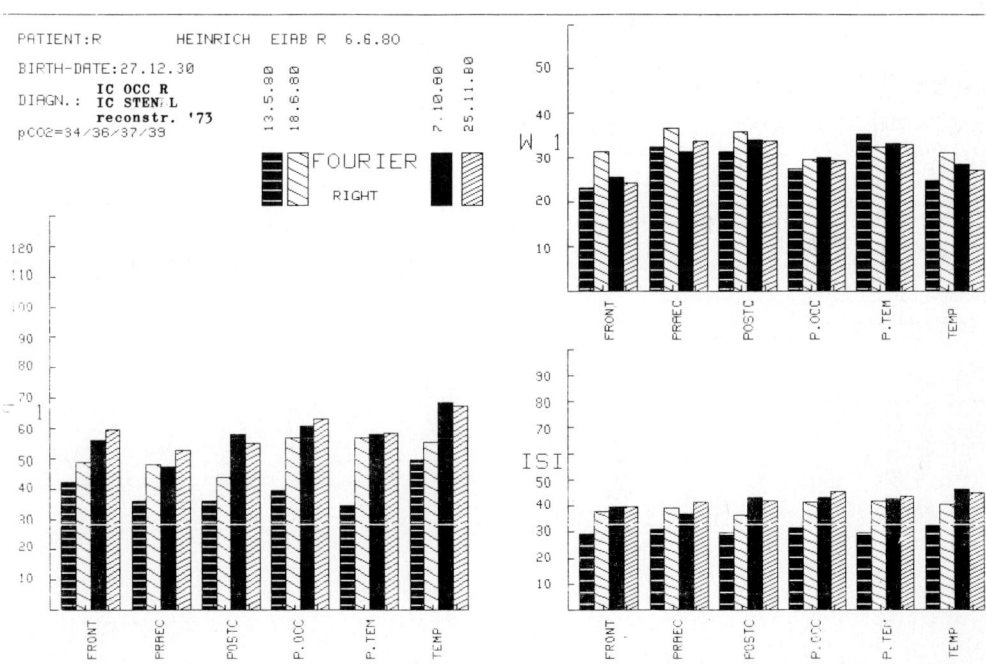

Fig. 2. Follow-up by rCBF measurements on a course of 6 months with continuous increasing of rCBF values

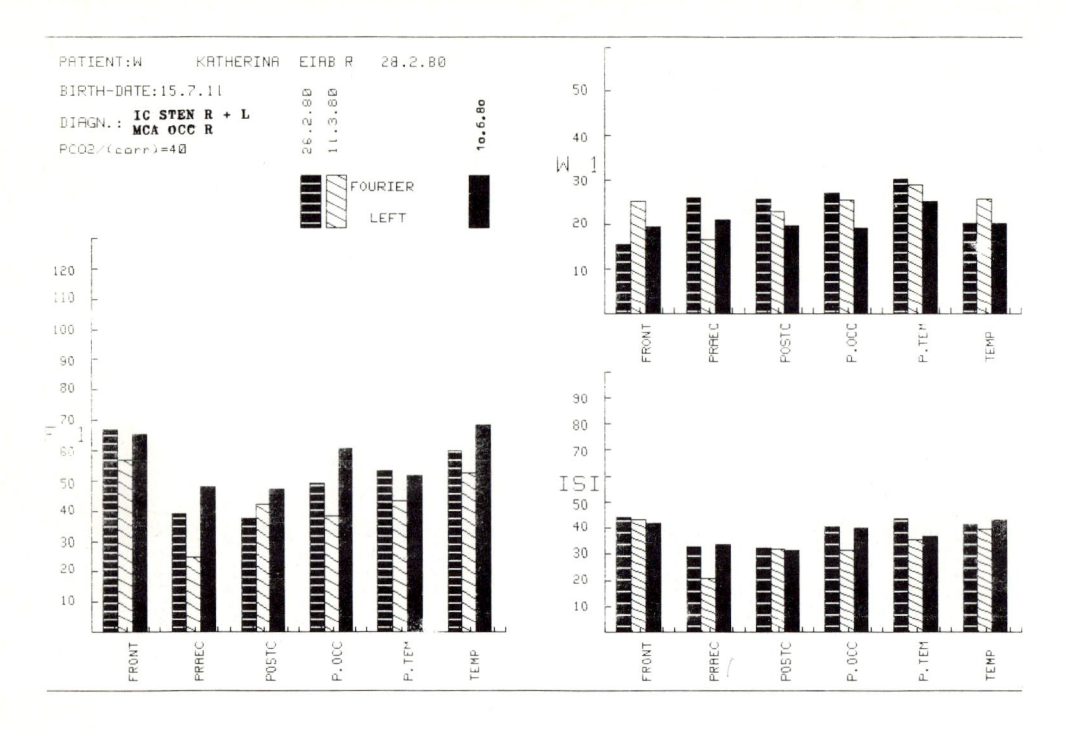

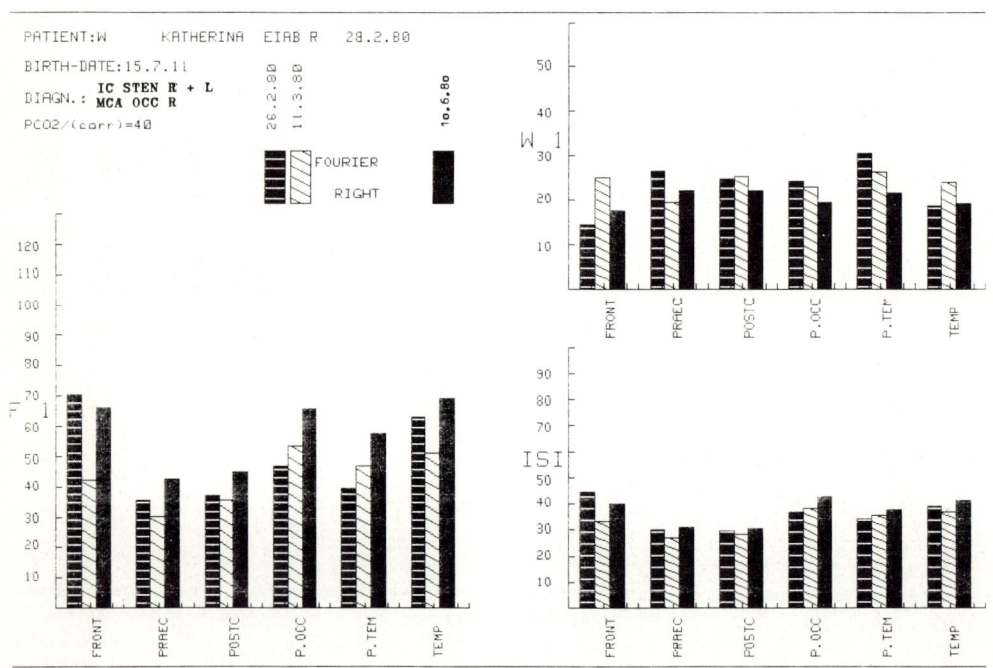

Fig. 3. Decrease of rCBF values immediately after right sided bypass with increased values three months later

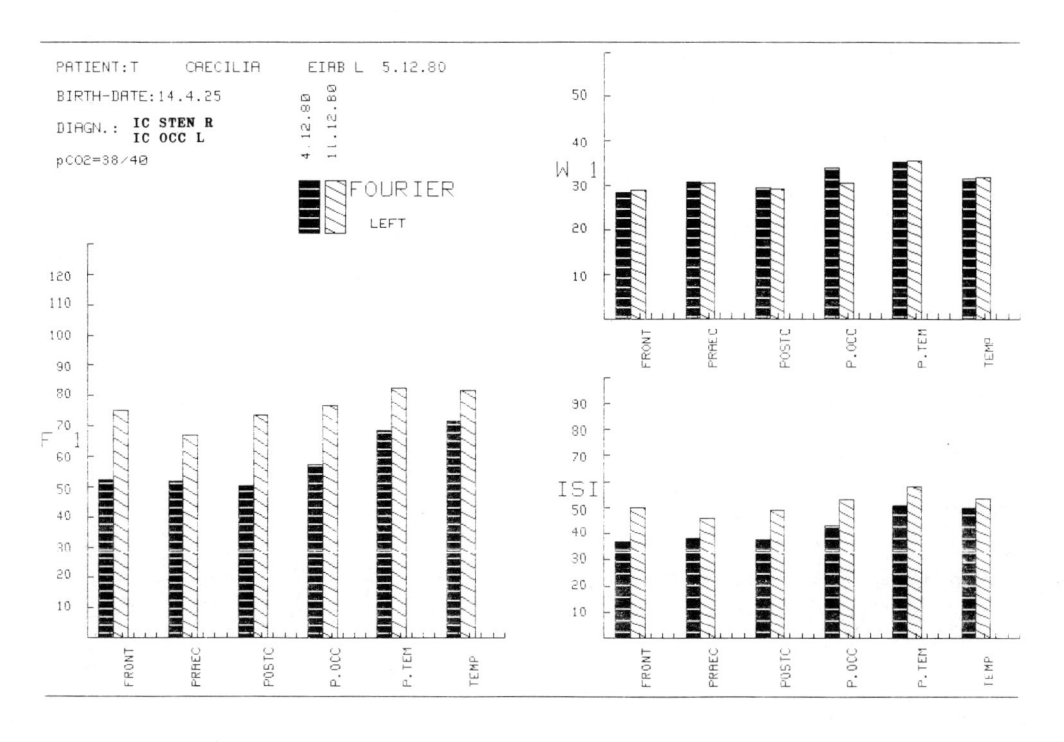

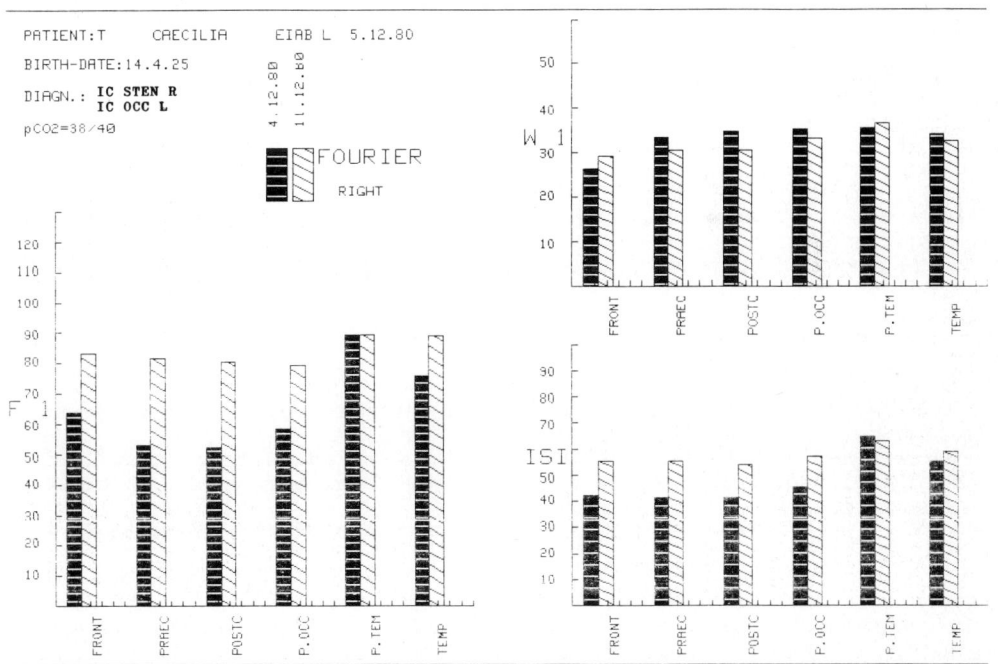

Fig. 4. Increase of rCBF values bilaterally; sign of diminishing intracerebral steal phenomenon after establishing an extra-intracranial bypass

Early Morphological Changes in Microvascular Anastomoses

H. Wismann and R. Meyermann

The extra-intracranial arterial bypass (EIAB) is a shunt, which detours a stenosed or occluded brain-supplying artery. If, in the end, there is still an occlusion at the bypass, then its therapeutic value is worthless.

A few long-term studies and autopsies enable us to see that at the end 0-22% of the EIAB's had been clotted (2, 6, 10, 13, 17, 20, 23). Unfortunately there is no clear information about this process and its causes, even when one studies the few pathological examinations so far known (5, 11). There is no other way to attain new information about the underlying causes without looking at previous studies, involving vessels in other parts of the body (1, 3, 4, 14, 16, 21, 25, 26). In conclusion, nearly all occlusions in the first 2 postoperative weeks are caused by thrombosis, and technical reasons (especially the mobilization of the vessel stumps) have been isolated as the main cause. On the other hand atherosclerosis is blaimed for the occurrence of late occlusions, but there is less knowledge of the aetiology of the latter.

We studied the question of atherosclerotic wall changes at microarterial anastomoses, which are similar to the EIAB. So we anastomosed the arteria carotis communis, which we previously ligated at the bulbus and put it under the clavicula, with the arteria subclavia in 5 rats, which we anaethetized with ether. Each anastomosis was shown with 10/0 ethicon suture material. In order to differentiate as to whether the expected lesions are caused by the special haemodynamic condition of an end-to-side anastomosis, or whether they are caused by the mobilization of the vessel stump, we performed 5 similar end-to-end anastomoses between the carotis and the sublcavia. In the third case we performed 5 end-to-end anastomoses at the immobilizated carotis (Fig. 1).

The rats were killed 2 weeks after the operation by an intracardial perfusion of glutaraldehyde the vessel specimens were fixed with osmiumtetroxyd and contrasted with uranylacetat and were embedded in araldid blocks. For the "light-microscope"-examination the thick sections were studied with hematoxylin eosin and toluidin blue. The thin sections were studied under the transmission electron microscope ZEISS EM 9.

The results are as follows: All anastomoses were patent. There were no stenoses or dilatations evident. There was no sign of intraluminal thrombosis, but eventually there were adhesions of thrombocytes, which occasionally ejected their granules.

To make it possible to describe atherosclerotic wall lesions in vessels, which were only 2 weeks old (postoperatively!), we had to follow

HAUST's definition of the atherosclerotic early lesion (15). In his words the early lesion consists of either a microthrombus or an edema of the intima (especially the proliferation of neo-intimal cells), or a third possibility, it consists of a fatty streak. Microthrombi or fatty streaks were not evident. But the intimal edema occurred regurarly in the anastomotic region. The endothelial layer wasn't smooth and closed, the adjacent endothelial cells overlapped inadequately. The subendothelial space was enormously wide, profusely filled with extracellular material and neo-intimal cells. Endothelial cells and neo-intimal cells showed many vesicles and occasionally swollen mitochondria. The lamina elastica interna showed extraneous cavaties. Occasionally one could observe a collection of mediamyocytes adjacent to these cavaties. In other regions of the operated vessels we found a normal morphology like in control vessels. Regularly we established a topographical pattern of the intimal edema, i.e. it was very tiny in the immediate anastomotic region, adjacent there was a large area of intimal edema with an extreme proliferation of neo-intimal cells, and then there was a normal morphology again. We observed this topographical pattern in all three types of anastomoses, especially prevalent in the end-to-side anastomosis.

Other authors previously described degenerative changes of the vessel wall, when they examined anastomoses performed on other parts of the body; from our experiment we came to a similar conclusion. This observation was possible, because we used young animals in our experiment, that means we were able to deal with a fresh vasculature. In older individuals a similar topographical pattern was observed in non-operated vessels, i.g. there were intimal cushions at the apex of bifurcations and circularly situated around ostia of small branches (8). Simply the exogenous trauma is not singularly important for the development of such intimal cushions, but endogenous factors, like a specifically hemodynamical situation, have the same effect. We, too, found in our experiment subtle indications that hemodynamical forces are involved in the development of degenerative vessel wall changes (7, 9, 12, 18, 19, 22, 24). Namely there was a difference in respect to the intima proliferation between the end-to-side anastomosis on the one hand and the end-to-end anastomosis on the other. But there was no difference between the end-to-end anastomoses, which were performed on the mobilized or the immobilized carotid artery (Fig. 2).

On the whole, the atherosclerotic early lesions were not so impressive in our experiments since the changes had no immediate effect. But what will happen with the patency of an anastomosis, which had been performed on a preoperatively degenerative vessel system, which had been damaged by the above mentioned factors, is questionable. It would not be surprising, if these arteries - through further atherosclerotic stages - occluded.

References

1. Acland, R.D., Trachtenberg, L.: The histopathology of small arteries following experimental mocrovascular anastomosis. Plast. Reconstr. Surg. 60, 868-875 (1977)
2. Auer, L.: Surgical treatment of cerebrovascular insufficiency - a follow-up sutdy. Acta Neurochir. 46, 85-92 (1979)

3. Baxter, Th.J. et al.: The histopathology of small vessels following microvascular repair. Brit. J. Surg. 54, 617-622 (1972)
4. Björkerud, S., Bonders, G.: Arterial repair and atherosclerosis after mechanical injury. Atheroscl. 13, 355-363 (1971)
5. Bodosi, M., Merie, F.T.: Development of histological structure of microanastomoses. 5th Intern. Symp. on Microvasc. Anast. for Cerebr. Ischemia (1980)
6. Chater, N. et al.: Microvascular bypass for cerebral ischemia - an overview, 1966-1976. In: Microsurgery for stroke. Schmiedek, P., Gratzl, O., Spetzler, R. (eds.), pp. 79-88. Berlin, Heidelberg, New York: Springer 1977
7. Collatz Christensen, B., et al.: Repair in arterial tissue. Acta Path. Microbiol. Scand. Sect. A 87, 265-273 (1979)
8. Cornhill, J.F. et al.: Localization of atherosclerotic lesions in the human basilar artery. Atheroscl. 35, 77-86 (1980)
9. Dahm, H.H. et al.: Das Endothel der A. carotis communis im Bereich experimenteller Stenosen - Rasterelektronenmikroskopische Untersuchungen. Verh. Dtsch. Ges. Kreislaufforschg. 40, 222-224 (1974)
10. Deruty, R.: La revascularisation cérébral par anastomose artérielle extra-intra-crânienne. Acta Chir. Belg. 2, 85-93 (1979)
11. Deruty, R., Pialat, J.: Histological study of EIAB in man (2 cases). 5th Intern. Symp. on Microvasc. Anast. for Cerebr. Ischemia (1980)
12. Fox, J.A., Jugh, A.E.: LOcalization of atheroma: a theory based on boundary layer separation. Brit. Hea-t J. 28, 388-399 (1966)
13. Gratzl, O. et al.: Clinical experience with extra-intracranial arterial anastomosis in 65 cases. J. Neurosurg. 44, 313-324 (1976)
14. Grondin, C.M. et al.: Atherosclerotic changes in coronary vein grafts six years after operation. J. Thorac. Cardiovasc. Surg. 77, 24-31 (1979)
15. Haust, M.D.: Zur Morphologie der Arteriosklerose. Internist 11, 621-626 (1978)
16. Kern, W.H. et. al.: The intimal proliferation in aortic-coronary saphenous vein grafts. Am. Heart. H. 84, 771-777 (1973)
17. Lee, M.C. et al.: Superficial temporal to middle cerebral artery anastomosis. Arch. Neurol. 36, 1-4 (1979)
18. Moore, S.: Endothelial Injury and atherosclerosis. Exp. Molec. Pathol. 31, 182-190 (1979)
19. Mustard, J.F., Packham, M.A.: The role of blood and platelets in atherosclerosis and the complications of atherosclerosis. Thromb. Diathes. Haemorrh. 33, 444-456 (1975)
20. Redondo, A. et al.: Ischémie cérébrlae: traitment par microanastomoses vasculaires extra-intra-crâniennes. Nouv. Presse Méd. 7, 1625-1630 (1978)
21. Rosenbaum, Th.J., Sundt, Th.M.: Thrombus formation and endothelial alterations in microarterial anastomoses. J. Neurosurg. 47, 430--41 (1977)
22. Sandmann, W. et al.: Arteriosklerose durch Strömung? Vasa 6, 321-327 (1977)

23. Spetzler, R.: Extra-intracranial arterial anastomosis for cerebrovascular disease. Surg. Neurol. 11, 157-161 (1979)
24. Staubesand, J.: Intra- und extrazelluläre Lysosomen bei myozytären Reaktionen der Arterienwand. Med. Welt 28, 1470-1474 (1977)
25. Stolte, M.: Morphologische Analyse der Koronarchirurgie. Baden-Baden: Witzstrock 1975
26. Tritthart, H., Auer, L.: Entwicklung histologischer Veränderungen nach mikrochirurgischer Gefäßnaht. Acta Chir. Austr. 3, 64-66 (1978)

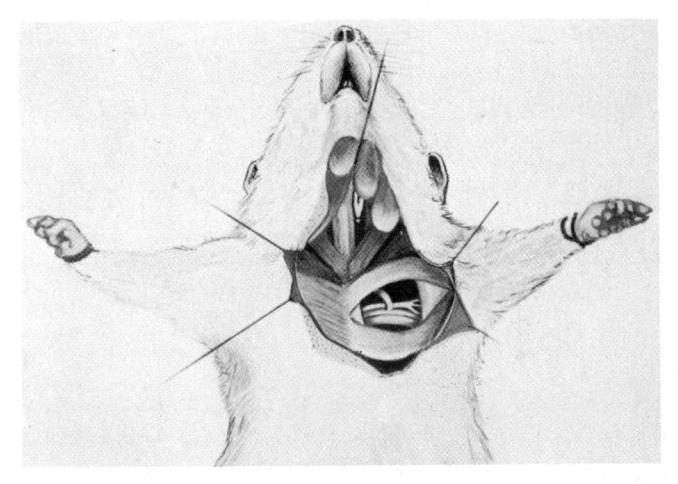

Fig. 1. Retroclavicular end-to-side anastomosis between Art. carotis communis (∅ 1.2 mm) and ARt. sublcavia (∅ 0.8 mm)

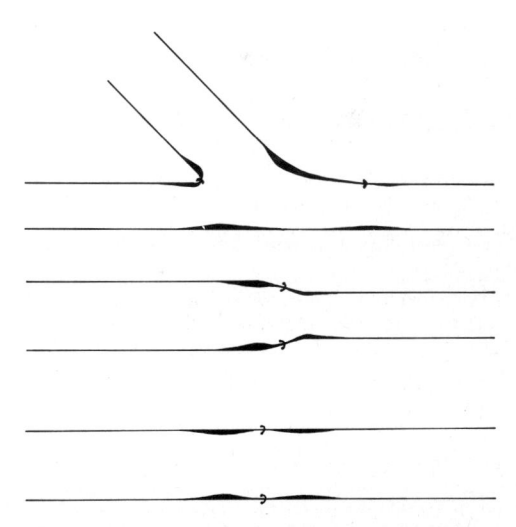

Fig. 2. End-to-side and end-to-end anastomosis between Art. carotis communis and Art. subclavia. Note prevalent areas of intimal edema (especially intima proliferation)

Diaphanoscopy of Blood Vessels, Visualization of Emboli Originating from Blood Clots Formed Close to Suture Lines

E. WINTERMANTEL

Introduction

Different methods of analyzing the quality of microsurgical anastomoses are known: angiography and microradiography as invasive methods, electromagnetic flow measurements and microvascular auscultation with a diplo-microphone (1) as non-invasive methods. An additional method which can be harmful to the endothelium is the radical pressure test performed with forceps. These methods can be called *indirect methods* as injections of contrast medium or use of an apparatus or instuments are necessary to get data such as angiograms or auscultation curves. Errors in measurement and analysis of the data may occur. In order to avoid these errors a method for *direct observation* of the blood stream in vivo was developed.

Materials and Approach

In order to obtain a transillumination of the blood flow a micro-bulb (2) was fixed in a small transparent plastic tube isolated from any liquid (Fig. 1). Dimensions of the micro-bulb are 2 mm in width and 5.7 mm in length. Candle power is indicated with 0.1 MSCP (= 0.1 cd). Micro-bulb is put behind the vascular segment of interest and the blood stream is observed through the operating microscope (x 40 magnification adjustment). The blood stream in 20 end-to-end anastomoses performed on carotid arteries of Wistar rats have been observed.

Results

Some of the following results have been recorded cinematographically. Photos (Figs. 3, 4) are taken from this movie film.

In all anastomoses thrombus formation was observed. Immediately after performing the anastomosis a ring thrombus close to the suture line and along the entire inner anastomotic line is formed. Within seconds later various shapes of blood clots are formed distal to the suture line and originating from this ring thrombus. Coming up to a certain size their resistance against the blood flow seems to be sufficient to be broken into parts which are swept along with the blood stream as emboli. Two main types of break-off of an intravascular originating from the suture line can be differentiated:

1. *Top Break-Off*. Immediately after suturing the top of a blood clot is broken off and swept along with the blood stream leaving a thrombus-base on the inner vascular surface. A new top is formed on this base and again broken off.

2. *Longitudinal Axial Break-Off*. Later on also the part of the thrombus closest to the vascular wall, the thrombus base, is broken axially leaving a canal between the two parts of the original thrombus. Formation of new thrombus shapes with top break-offs and longitudinal axial break-offs can now be observed.

The postoperative observation time was 30 min. Thrombus formation always occurred at the same areas on the inner vessel surface during this period. Initially free areas distal to the suture line stayed free from blood clots even 30 min p.o.

Discussion

ACLAND (3) and STEPHENS (4) mention a side lightening method for observation of blood clots in small vessels. STEPHENS describes symmetrical formation of blood clots proximal and distal to the suture which are swept away. This vessel was cleared after 5 min of flow. However no photographic documents of the phenomena could be presented.

This result does not completely correspond to the findings in this study as even at the end of the observation period of 30 min thrombus formation was seen independent of the extent of the blood clot and of the quality of the suture. No symmetrical thrombus formation proximally and distally of the suture line could be seen in this study.

In one artery a total occlusion could be observed. In this case the original distally formed thrombus "grew backwards" across the suture line and against the blood flow thus occluding the artery.

The swept out emboli may cause regional hypoxic tissue damage through occlusion of smaller arteries.

References

1. Wintermantel, E.: Microvascular auscultation. A new technique, using a diplo-microphone, for analysis of blood flow at suture lines in small arteries. Acta Neurochir. 53, 25-37 (1980)
2. Miniature bulb manufactured by MGG Micro-Glühlampengesellschaft, P.O. Box 80 07 60, D-2050 Hamburg 80, Federal Republic of Germany
3. Ackland, R.: The use of side lightening in observing blood flow in small vessels. (Personal communication to H.W. Stephens Jr., June 1973). In: Microvascular anastomoses for cerebral ischemia. Fein, J.M., Reichman, O.H. (eds.), p. 185. Berlin, Heidelberg, New York: Springer 1978
4. Stephens, H.W.: Electromagnetic blood flowmetry in microvascular anastomosis. In: Microvascular anastomoses for cerebral ischemia. Fein, J.M., Reichman, O.H. (eds.), pp. 181-194. Berlin, Heidelberg, New York: Springer 1978

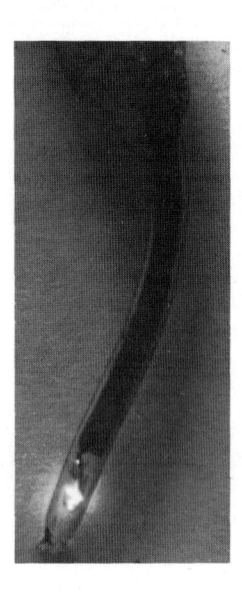

Fig. 1. Miniature electric bulb within a small transparent plastic tube isolatred from liquids. The diameter of the bulb is 2 mm, the candle power is 0.1 MSCP (= 0.1 cd)

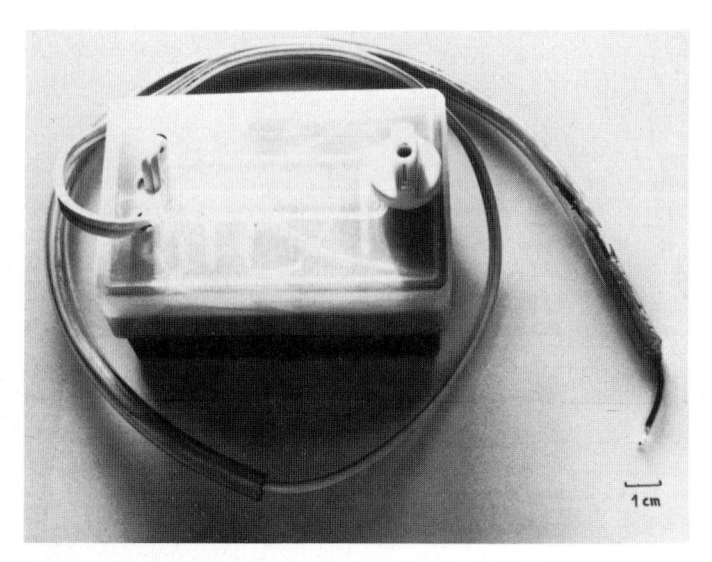

Fig. 2. Miniature electric bulb and power source assembled as a unit. Fixation of the small plastic tube containing the bulb within a larger one allows one to clamp the light source onto a laboratory stand for permanent fixation during filming through the operating microscope with high magnification (x 40)

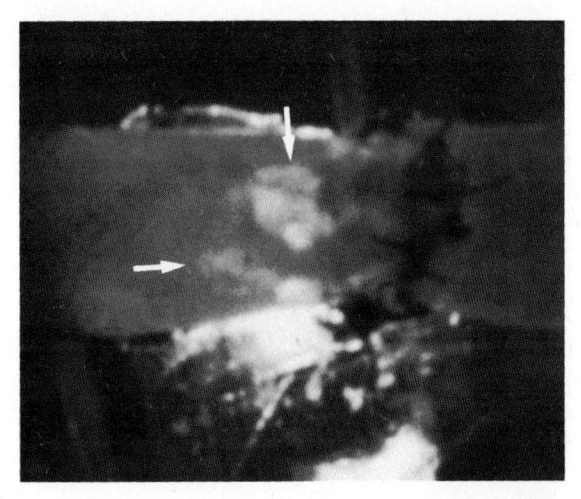

Fig. 3. Diaphanoscopy of a rats carotid artery distal to a microsurgical end-to-end anastomosis. Blood flow is from the right to the left. A big blood clot has been broken into two parts indicated by *arrows* leaving a canal in between. Small canals are formed within the bigger part *(upper arrow)*. Later on this blood clot was broken into numerous fragments along these small canals. The bigger the blood clots are, the brighter they appear, as the dark blood stream between the top of the thrombus and the opposite vascular wall is a thin layer thus absorbing less light. Reproduction from a 16 mm Ektachrome Video News Film

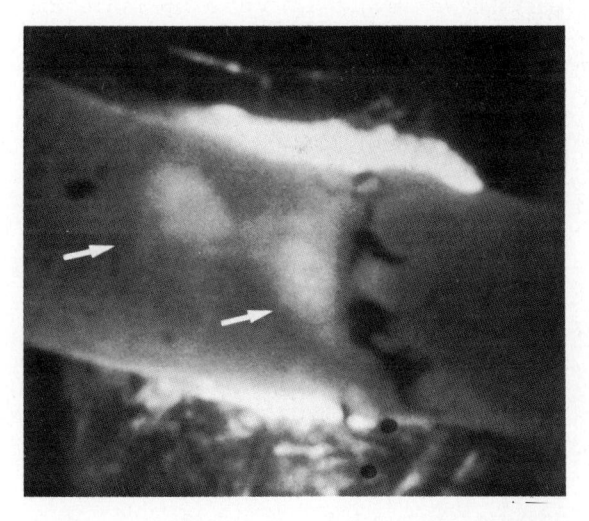

Fig. 4. Another specimen. Blood flow is from the right to the left. The more distal part of the blood clot is floating within the blood stream before being washed away. Reproduction from a 16 mm Ektachrome movie film

Shunt Therapy in Medulloblastoma?

D. VOTH, M. SCHWARZ, N. HÜWEL, and E. MAHLMANN

Introduction

Palliative treatment of hydrocephalus internus occlusus in space-occupying processes of the posterior cranial fossa before operation has proved of value in treatment of cerebellopontine tumors in adults. It was accordingly also recommended in tumors of the posterior fossa in childhood. Whereas such a procedure still appears to be justifiable in benign processes, we have rejected the application of a ventriculoatrial or ventriculoperitoneal drainage in medulloblastoma. Apart from the familiar high susceptibility to disturbances and high complication rate of such shunt systems (3-5, 9-12, 14, 20, 22, 23, 26), there is a danger of generalized tumor metastasis (19). We had to observe this ourselves in one case.

For this reason, we have looked for a drainage system for this group of patients which is not susceptible to disturbances and which does not induce the danger of generalized metastasis. The interventriculostomy (15) described by LEKSELL (1949) meets these requirements (1, 2, 17). We report on our experience and the technical procedure and comment on the indications.

Materials and Results

We performed ventriculocisternostomy in 21 patients. Details are to be seen in Table 1. The treatment of a hydrocephalus internus occlusus which may be present was always performed via a preliminary ventricular drainage with the MEDITEK system (24). After opening the posterior fossa and exposing the tumor with very extensive or total exstirpation of the process, a lamellar catheter according to PORTNOY (19) or a modification suggested by ourselves (CODMAN) is introduced through the (almost always dilated) aqueduct, the third ventricle and through the foramen of MONRO into the posterior horn of the ventricular system. The distal end is placed into the cervical CSF space at the level of the 2nd or 3rd vertebral body. The wound is afterwards closed. Measured of intracranial pressure according to the LUNDBERG method (16, 25) is continued up to normalization of the pressure conditions.

In all cases, there was a free passage through the drainage and pressure normalization. The drainage functioned without disturbances during the period of observation. An additional shunt therapy or a local revision did not prove to be necessary in any case. This also applies to the cases in which a tumor recurrence in the region of the rhombencephalon later blocked the 4th ventricle again. The tumor grew around the catheter in the floor of the rhomboid fossa, but the patency remained unimpaired.

Table 1. Survey of the patients with a ventriculocisternostomy

Number	Patient	Male (m) female (f)	Age (years)	Observation (year, month)	State	Recurrence
Medulloblastoma						
1.	D. M.	m	6	1 4	Good	–
2.	W. Th.	m	13	10	Good	–
3.	S. B.	m	3	6	Good	–
4.	P. B.	f	10	8	Good	–
5.	E. M.	m	7	2	Poor	–
6.	F. H.	m	11	1 3	Good	–
7.	V. V.	f	13	8	Poor	–
8.	W. S.	f	14	5	Good	–
9.	Sch. S.	f	13	1	Good	–
10.	W. Ch.	m	5	5	Died	+
11.	B. O.	m	15	1	Died	+
Pilocytic astrocytoma						
12.	R. A.	m	9	1 2	Good	–
13.	H. H.	m	19	6	Satisfactory	–
14.	E. S.	f	6	3 5	Satisfactory	–
15.	W. M.	m	8	2 6	Good	–
Ependymoma						
16.	D. A.	m	13	2 3	Died	+
17.	M. G.	f	23	1 1	Good	Subtotal resect.
18.	B. A.	f	3	10	Good	–
Other indications						
19.	E. M. Mesencephalic cyst	m	12	4	Good	–
20.	K. K. IVth ventricle arachnoid cyst	f	9	3 9	Good	–
21.	L. H. Membranous aqueduct occlusion	f	21	1	Good	–

A LEKSELL drainage with correct position according to our method is shown in Fig. 1. In the lateral projection, the total course of the catheter can be seen well. In the anteroposterior projection, the proximal end deviates with the lamellae from the midline. Sliding back of the catheter is revealed by a median position of the proximal end and in the lateral picture by the position of the lamellar portion in the third ventricle or at the entrance to the aqueduct (Fig. 2).

The exact course of the LEKSELL drainage is also well documented in the computer tomogram (Fig. 3). We have only observed a sliding back of the end of the catheter up to the entrance of the aqueduct in one case. Here there was likewise no functional disorder. Finally, it is mentioned that the introduction of the catheter into the aqueduct did not lead in any case to any undesired reactions.

Discussion

For several reasons, space-occupying processes of the posterior cranial fossa may require shunt therapy, thus for example when the aqueduct is blocked by edema or a reactive gliosis, or when a subtotally resected malignant tumor (e.g. medulloblastoma) gives rise to the expectation of a recurrence with new blockage of the CSF drainage pathways. The ventriculoatrial and ventriculoperitoneal systems which are frequently chosen have the disadvantage that their revision rate is very high, and that there is also danger of generalized tumor metastasis. For this reason, besides the indication worked out by LEKSELL, e.g. in aqueduct stenosis or in a membranous occlusion, we have emphasized above *two further indications*:

1. the possibility of a late recurrence with fresh blocking of the aqueduct and of the 4th ventricle, e.g. in medulloblastomas and ependymomas; in this case, the intraoperatively inserted LEKSELL drainage renders a latershunt application superfluous.

2. There may be a renewed blockage or a stenosis of the aqueduct due to edema development and later due to a reactive gliosis also after resection of a benign process, e.g. of a pilocytic astrocytoma in the immediate vicinity of the aqueduct exit. In these cases, prophylactic application of the LEKSELL drainage is indicated.

In our patients, this procedure has proved itself both in adults and above all in children (6-8, 18) with tumors of the posterior cranial fossa (Fig. 4). (We should like to have the method discussed once more in the indications specified).

Formulated exactly, our modification of the LEKSELL drainage is a ventriculocisternostomy, whereas the original technique is appropriately designated as interventriculostomy. In the procedure we describe, an additional fixation of the catheter is superfluous; with exact placing of the distal end into an anterior horn, we have not observed any sliding away in anyone case.

Conclusions

The interventriculostomy described by LEKSELL was applied in a modification of our own as ventriculocisternostomy in 21 patients with a tumor in the region of the posterior cranial fossa. We give this method definite preference over the usual shunt systems (27). As new indications, we should like to mention the probability of a tumor recurrence, e.g. in medulloblastomas or ependymomas, and furthermore the possibility of a postoperative occlusion of the aqueduct exit by edema or gliosis even in benign tumors reaching up to the rostral end of the 4th ventricle. The drainage functioned without disturbances in all cases. Their application did not lead to any undesired reactions.

References

1. Dandy, W.E.: The diagnosis and treatment of hydrocephalus resulting from structures of the aqueduct of sylvius. Surg. Gynec. Obstet. 31, 701-704 (1969)
2. Elvidge, A.R.: Treatment of obstructive lesions of the aqueduct of sylvius by interventriculostomy. J. Neurosurg. 24, 11-23 (1966)
3. Foltz, E.L., Shurtleff, D.B.: Conversion of communicating hydrocephalus to stenosis or occlusion of the aqueduct during ventricular shunt. J. Neurosurg. 24, 520-529 (1966)
4. Forrest, D.M., Cooper, D.G.W.: Complications of a ventriculoatrial shunt: A review of 455 cases. J. Neurosurg. 29, 506-512 (1968)
5. Gardner, P., Schoenbaum, S.D., Shillito, J.: Infections of cerebrospinal fluid shunts: epidemiology, clinical manifestations, and therapy. J. Infectious Dis. 131, 543-552 (1975)
6. Gutjahr, P., Voth, D., Neidhardt, M.: Ergebnisse der kombinierten Behandlung (Operation, Radio- und Chemotherapie) bei 132 Kindern mit primären ZNS-Tumoren. Therapiewoche 28, 4346-4352 (1978)
7. Gutjahr, P., Voth, D.: Erfolgreiche Medulloblastom-Therapie - und danach? Adv. Neurosurg. 5, 257-258 (1978)
8. Gutjahr, P., Voth, D.: Treatment and prognosis of childhood brain tumors: Experience with 140 cases. Verhdlg. Dtsch. Krebsges. 2, 434-435 (1979)
9. Hakim, S., de la Roche, F.D., Burton, J.D.: A critical analysis of valve shunts used in the treatment of hydrocephalus. Dev. Med. Child Neurol. 15, 230-255 (1973)
10. Hemmer, R.: Complications of atrial-ventricular shunts and their prevention. Kinderchirurgie 5, 10-24 (1967)
11. Ignelzi, R.J., Kirsch, W.M.: Follow-up analysis of ventriculoperitoneal and ventriculo-atrial shunts for hydrocephalus. J. Neurosurg. 42, 679-682 (1975)
12. Illingworth, R.D.: Subdural hematoma after the treatment of chronic hydrocephalus by ventriculocaval shunts. J. Neurol. Neurosurg. Psychiat. 33, 95-99 (1970)
13. Kessler, L.A., Dugan, P., Concannon, J.P.: Systemic metastases of medulloblastoma promoted by shunting. Surg. Neurol. 3, 147-152 (1975)
14. Leem, W., Miltz, H.: Complications following ventriculo-atrial shunts in hydrocephalus. Adv. Neurosurg. 6, 1-5 (1978)
15. Leksell, L.: A surgical procedure for atresia of the aqueduct of sylvius. Acta Psychiatr. (Kobenh.) 24, 559-568 (1949)
16. Lundberg, N.: Continuous recording and control of ventricular fluid pressure in neurosurgical practice. Acta psychiat. Scand. (Suppl. 149) 36, 1-193 (1960)

17. Norlen, G.: Contribution to the surgical treatment of inoperable tumors, causing obstruction of the sylvian aqueduct. Acta psychiatr. (Kobenh.) 24, 629-637 (1949)
18. Otte, J., Emmrich, P., Schwarz, M., Voth, D., Gutjahr, P.: Zur postoperativen Behandlung von Kindern mit Tumoren des ZNS. In "Pädiatrische Intensivmedizin" 8, Georg Thieme Verlag, Stuttgart. Im Druck
19. Portnoy, H.D.: New ventricular catheter for hydrocephalic shunts. J. Neurosurg. 34, 702-703 (1971)
20. Samuelson, S., Long, D.M., Chou, S.N.: Subdural hematoma as a complication of shunting procedures for normal pressure hydrocephalus. J. Neurosurg. 37, 548-551 (1972)
21. Steinbock, P., Thomson, G.B.: Complications of ventriculo-vascular shunts: Computer analysis of etiological factors. Surg. Neurol. 5, 31-35 (1976)
22. Strahl, E.W., Liesegang, J., Roosen, K.: Complications following ventriculo-peritoneal shunts. Adv. Neurosurg. 8, 6-9 (1978)
23. Voth, D.: Nuklearmedizinische Funktionsprüfung ventrikulo-atrialter und ventrikulo-peritonealer Anastomosen. Klinische Wertung. Pädiatr. Nuklearmed. 1, 40-45 (1979)
24. Voth, D., Nakayama, N.: Ein neues ventilgesteuertes System für die präliminare Ventrikeldrainage (Technische Beschreibung und klinische Erfahrungen). Neurochirurgia 19, 196-201 (1976)
25. Voth, D., Hey, O., Nakayama, N., Emmrich, P.: Die kontinuierliche Registrierung des intrakraniellen Druckes (Intraventrikuläre Messung) im Rahmen der pädiatrischen Intensivmedizin. Pädiatr. Intensivmed. ___, 104-109 (1977)
26. Voth, D.: Über die körperliche Belastbarkeit von Kindern mit einem Shuntsystem zur Behandlung des Hydrocephalus internus. Sozialpädiatrie (1981) (in press)
27. Voth, D., Schwarz, M.: New aspects concerning the technique and indication for ventriculo-cisternal drainage according to Leksell (Interventriculostomy). Neurosurg. Rev. (1981) (in press)

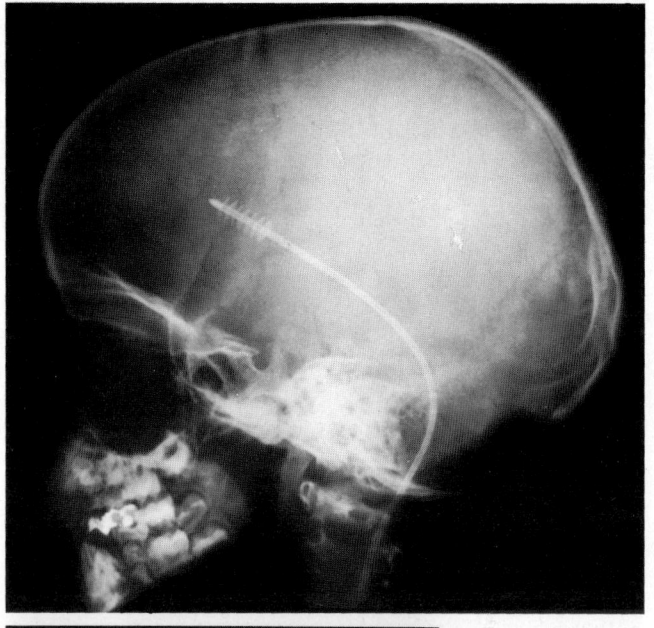

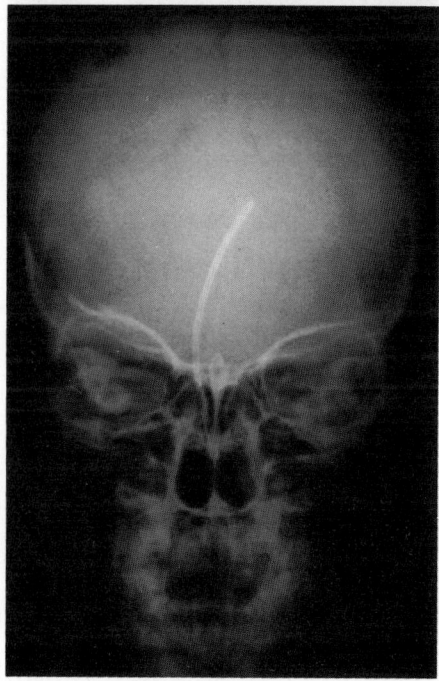

Fig. 1. *Above:* In the lateral projection, the course of the catheter becomes clear from the anterior horn up to the cervical CSF space. *Below:* In the ap projection, the distal end of the catheter with lamellae deviates from the midline when it was correctly placed in one of the two anterior horns

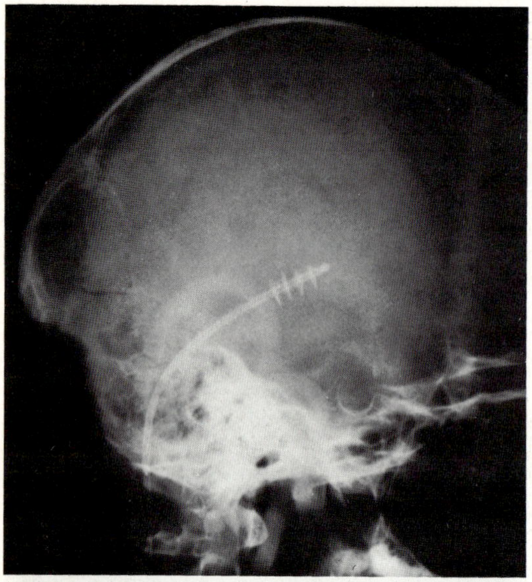

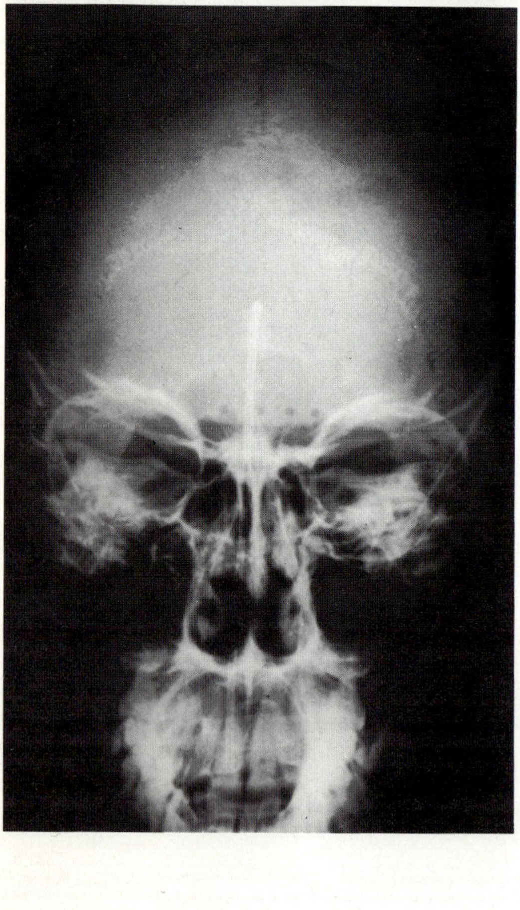

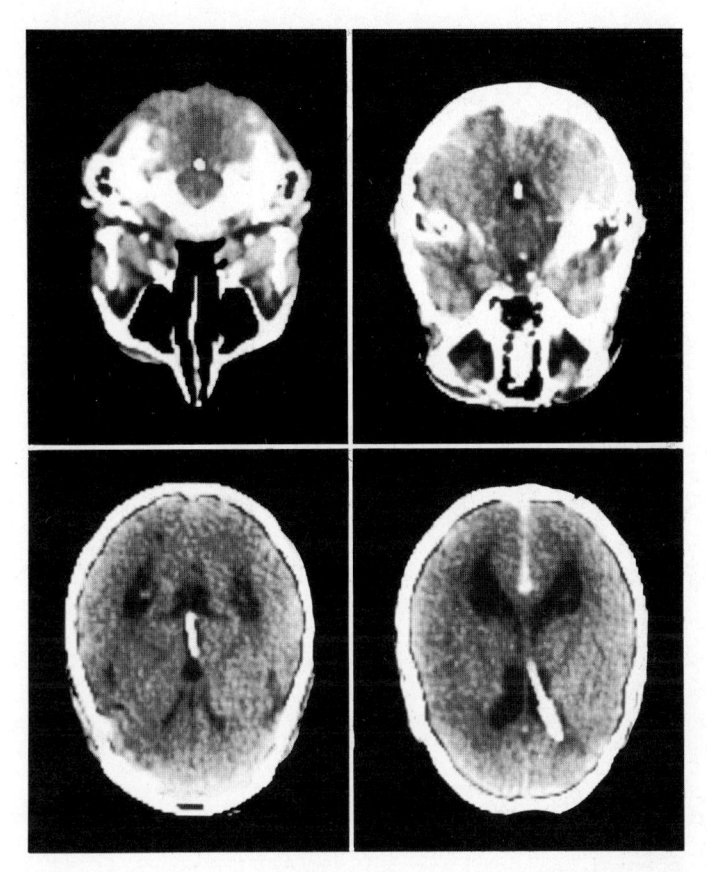

Fig. 3. The pictures show the correct course of the catheter from the left anterial horn up to the transition into the foramen occipitale magnum in the computer tomogram

Fig. 2. *Above:* Despite perfect function of the drainage, this localization is not desired; the lamellar portion is situated in the aqueduct entrance. *Below:* In the ap projection, this position is revealed by a median location of the catheter. In this case, the catheter had not been pushed forward far enough into one of the anterior horns

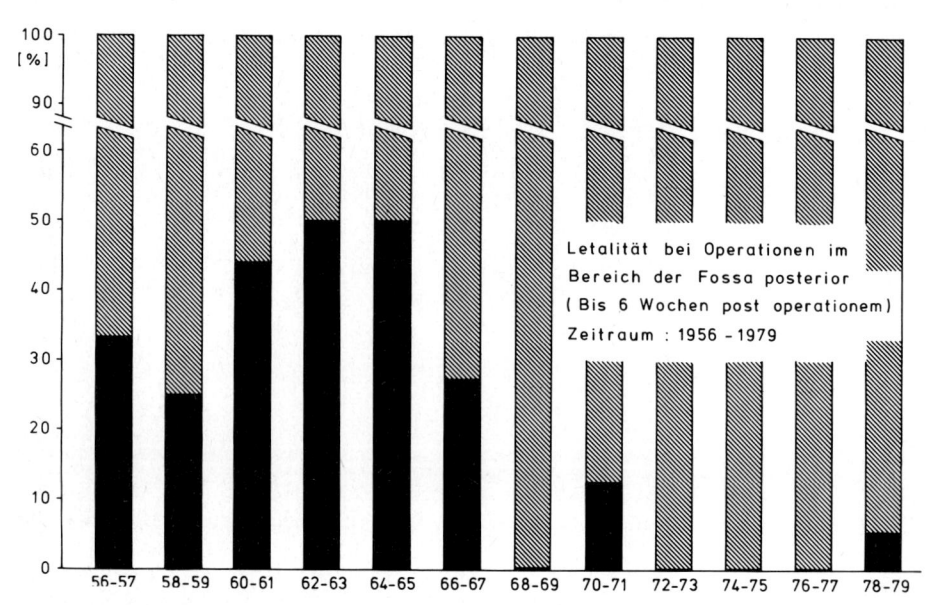

Letalität bei Operationen im Bereich der Fossa posterior
(Bis 6 Wochen post operationem)
Zeitraum : 1956 - 1979

Fig. 4. The mortality within the first six weeks in patients with brain tumors (ependymomas, medulloblastomas, astrocytomas, angioblastomas etc.) in the region of the posterior fossa. The compilation reveals that the mortality (which was very high in the 1960's) has fallen in the mean time to values between zero and 5%. A large number of reasons is responsible for this, e.g. the improvement of the intensive care, a consistent edema therapy, application of intracranial pressure measurement, refinement of the surgical techniques, additional measures (including the procedure described here) as well as a clearer demarcation between maximum and total extirpation

Effect of 6-Methylprednisolone on the Brain Function in Patients with Solitary Circumscribed Supratentorial Tumors

K. VON WILD, L. GLUSA, A. SEPEHRNIA, and M. SAMII

Introduction

The use of corticosteroids has been accepted a beneficial adjunct for the management of brain tumors since their introduction in clinical practice by KOFMAN et al. (1957), GALICICH et al. (1961), and RASMUSSEN et al. (1962). Methylprednisolone (MP) has been noted to have different effects pharmacologically when compared to dexamethasone (DM), for instance no sodium retention or edema at pharmacological doses, short adrenal suppressive activity, and higher inhibition of glial tumors (6, 8, 10, 19). Although there seems to be some good qualities of MP most of the clinical studies report on the effects of DM during the last years (4, 11, 15). Our study is based on the experience of LIEBERMAN et al. (1977) with high dose MP in patients with inoperable brain tumors on the one hand and on the EEG findings under steroids in experimental brain edema of PAPPIUS (1972) and JAMES (1978) on the other. Clinical observations and experimental studies suggest that the effects of steroids seen clinically in brain tumors can not be explained by their effect on cerebral edema alone but on central pharmacological effects. The latter mechanism remains unclear. As the functional state of the brain can be estimated by EEG recordings (3, 5, 7, 12, 16) central pharmacological effects can be demonstrated by common and computerized EEG analysis (2, 13). In order to prove the response of patients with brain tumors to high dose MP treatment during the preoperative course in respect to reduce postoperative morbidity and mortality we performed a polygraphic study. This paper describes some data of EEG changes under MP medication estimating its central pharmacological effect on brain function in supratentorial tumors.

Patients and Methods

The effects of MP were studied in 5 male and 5 female patients with solitary circumscribed supratentorial tumors, who were admitted for brain surgery. According to CT findings 4 tumors were of the right and 4 of the left hemisphere, 1 glioma of the right frontal lobe extented slightly into the left frontal lobe, and 1 meningioma was located in the middle of the frontal skull base. They were histologically 5 meningiomas and 5 gliomas[1]. The age of our patients ranged from 21 to 67 years with an average age of 40.9 years, which was higher in the meningiomas (51.8 years) than in the gliomas (30 years).

---

[1]We thank Prof. LÖBLICH, Chairman of "Pathologisches Institut der Landeshauptstadt Hannover", for the macro- and histopathological findings

A Statham SP 50 transducer for epidural ICP measurement was implanted over the contralateral hemisphere one day before the EEG examination started. Pressure values ranged below 10 mm Hg in 3 gliomas and 1 meningioma, between 10 and 20 mm Hg in 1 glioma and 4 meningiomas, and between 20 and 30 mm Hg in 1 glioma. Our technique has been described before (18).

Clinical examinations showed signs and symptoms of brain tomours in all patients: 6 suffering from headaches, 2 with an impairment of visual function, 3 with vertigo, 2 with hemiparesis, and 5 patients with a psychosyndrome.

The schedule of 6a-methylprednisolone (URBASON, HOECHST) medication was as follows: 1000 mg at 10 p.m. on the first day and from the 2nd to 5th day 40 mg at 6 a.m., 2 and 10 p.m. Drug administration i.v. in bolus technique.

EEG records were performed at 6 - 8 p.m. on the 1st - 7th day under steady state conditions, so we had one record before and two examinations after medication. EEG was recorded bipolar fronto-temporal, fronto-parietal, and cetro-auricular over both hemispheres according to the 10 - 20 system (Figs. 1, 2) on a Hellige Neuroscript 1010. Channels 7, 8 and 10 served for polygraphic recording of ECG, ventilation and epidural pressure. The paper speed used was 30 mm/sec, filter 70 Hz, and time constant 0.3 sec for the EEG. Polygraphic records were stored on a magnetic tape for off-line computer analysis. Visual and computer-based EEG analysis was done on 10 min epochs. General slowing was classified as slight, moderate or severe abnormalities and a focus of continuous polymorphic delta activity, as first described by WALTER, was differentiated from focal theta activity (3, 5, 7, 12).

Focal signs were present in 9 of 10 patients. Besides that 4 patients showed slight, 2 moderate, and another 2 patients severe abnormalities.

Power spectral analysis, using Fast Fourier Transformation (FFT), was done on a BIO 16 computer with aid of program ESAP (AEG-Telefunken). Sampling rate of artefactfree EEG recording was 180 sec total analysis time. The power contained in the frequency bands, delta (0.5 - 3.5 Hz), theta (3.5 - 7.5 Hz), alpha (7.5 - 12.5 Hz) and beta (12.5 - 32 Hz) was calculated every 4 sec with a resolution of 0.25 Hz. Power spectra were plotted (Fig. 3). Data of calculated EEG intensity were proven statistically[2] to evaluate EEG changes under MP treatment on both hemispheres (17).

CT examination was performed from the first to the seventh day after EEG recording. These results will be reported elsewhere in detail (Part 2: CT Analysis). Before the study 5 patients showed a slight peritumoral edema that was found to be moderate in 2 and severe in another 2 patients.

Results

All patients put on MP medication showed an improvement in their general condition and neurological deficits. No worsening or unwanted side-effects were observed.

---

[2] We thank Dr. C. G. BÜCHEL, Hoechst AG, Frankfurt am Main

EEG studies demonstrated an improvement of abnormalities to next better group or normal findings, especially in the slow theta and delta frequency bands with an icrease of faster frequencies (alpha band), with a maximum at the fourth day of MP treatment. This effect seemed to be more pronounced over the tumor involved hemisphere, however it was even marked over the contralateral side. EEG changes were mostly independent of both the size of the tumor and the perifocal edema. These changes in electrical activity occurred at the first day of medication, whereas two days after withdrawl of MP we could observe the same pattern of abnormalities as before. Focal slow wave pattern showed a similar behaviour under MP treatment (Figs. 1, 2). Computerized EEG analysis showed a significant improvement of the abnormalities over the two hemispheres. There was a marked decrease of the delta portion and slow theta activity with a significant increase in the faster frequencies (theta and alpha portions). These changes are proven statistically to be dose and so time dependent (Table 1). Calculating the ratio of delta/theta intensity (B1/B2) a significant decrease of the ratio could be evaluated in all patients over both hemispheres (Table 2). These findings are prominent when the calculated EEG intensity in frequency band is plotted (Fig.3). Power spectra demonstrate decrease in amplitude and increase in frequency with a tendency to normalization under MP medication as well as the relaps after MP withdrawl.

In gliomas (percentage of power in frequency band demonstrated) a decrease of 30% of delta intensity was demonstrated with an increase of 6% in the theta and 100% in the alpha intensity under medication, whereas in meningiomas decrease in delta intensity was 10% with an increase in theta of 3% and alpha intensity of 10%. These findings were found over the tumor involved hemisphere, however similar effects, even not so prominent, were revealed over the contralateral hemisphere as well (Fig. 4). Withdrawl of MP led to an increase in slow wave intensity as seen before.

Contrary to our EEG findings the evaluation of epidural pressure measurements did not reveal a statistically significant trend under medication. However there was a tendency to lower values obvious under medication. No patient showed an increase in ICP during MP treatment.

Discussion

EEG abnormalities and focal continuous polymorphic delta activity are common pattern in brain tumors and are related to disturbed brain function (3, 5, 7, 12, 16). It has been well known that severe EEG abnormalities in patients with brain tumors correlate with a hazardous postoperative course and high mortality (3, 12). Based on EEG and CT findings of 127 supratentorial tumors GASTAUT et al. (1979) have proven that there is no correlation obvious between the degree and the extent of slow wave activity and the severity and size of the peritumoral edema. Therefore the neurosurgeon has to improve the patient's brain functions in order to put him in an optimal general condition for brain surgery. RASMUSSEN and GULATI were the first who reported beneficial effects of steroids on the postoperative course in brain surgery. Potent corticosteroids with minimal side effects have been proven experimentally and clinically during the last two decades. DM and MP are documented to be effective on brain edema, to alleviate signs and symptoms of increased intracranial pressure, to improve neurological deficits, and to reduce postoperative morbidity (15). Besides that especially MP is reported to in-

Table 1. Statistical remarkable and significant temporal trend

Tumor	Channel 1 or 2 with	Channel 1 or 2 without	Channel 3 or 4 with	Channel 3 or 4 without	Channel 5 or 6 with	Channel 5 or 6 without
δ	Significant decrease					
ϑ	Significant increase	Significant increase	Remark increase	Significant increase		Remark increase
α	Significant increase		Significant increase			
β	Significant increase	Significant increase	Significant increase		Remark increase	Significant increase
ϑ/α		Significant increase				
P total	Significant decrease	Significant decrease				

Table 2. Ratio of delta/theta intensity. Test for temporal trend. Rank correlation according to SPEARMAN

Channel	Tumor	r_s	$p<$	
1 or 2	Without	-0.4143	0.01	Significant decrease
	With	-0.4964	0.001	Significant decrease
3 or 4	Without	-0.3946	0.01	Significant decrease
	With	-0.4143	0.01	Significant decrease
5 or 6	Without	-0.2071	Not s.	No trend
	With	-0.3196	0.05	Stat. remark decrease

hibit growth of gliomas and to reduce their size in high dose steroid treatment (6, 9, 19). As MP has an excellent antiinflammatory effect and its antiedematous effect seemed to be superior to DM in cerebral cytotoxic edema in the experimental studies of JAMES (1978) one may conclude different pharmacological mechanisms of both steroids in cerebral edema and brain function. JAMES has shown that under medication the behavioural and EEG changes were far less in the DM group when compared with the MP group, even though MP was the only one to reduce the water content in the grey matter in his experimental setup. On the other hand PAPPIUS in 1972 reported on the studies of G.J. BALL and H.P. TUTT who have proven that DM improved EEG abnormalities in freezing brain lesion, independent from the effect on cerebral edema.

Our results confirm the hypothesis of a central pharmacological effect of MP, may be on brain metabolism, which leads to changes in the brain's functional state. As the EEG represents the brain function and EEG abnormalities are signs of disturbed brain function one may conclude that a decrease of slow wave activity under MP medication can be interpreted as a tendency to normalization. A decrease in EEG abnormalities with an increase in faster frequency intensity, as it can be shown in computerized EEG power spectra analysis, express an increase in vigilance. So we may conclude from our studies in patients with supratentorial brain tumors, who showed more or less EEG signs of impaired brain function, that high dose URBASON medication (MP) has proven statistically to increase the vigilance due to a central effect of the drug. As EEG abnormalities are related to thalamic and brain stem structures (3, 7) one may speculate that these regions respond to MP in case of impaired brain function. This can be underlined by our EEG findings which gave significant effects over the tumor involved as well as over the contralateral hemisphere even in patients with small tumors and mild peritumoral edema.

Besides these results we want to emphasize the value of EEG examination as a helpful adjunct in the preoperative and postoperative course to estimale the patients brain function and general condition even though EEG might be neglected now that CT is available.

References

1. Allegre, G.: Utilisation du Methyl-6-Prednisolone Hemissucinate de Sodium (Solumedrol) dans le traitement de l'hypertension intracranienne et de differents etats neurologiques graves. Lyon Med. 225, 6, 553-558 (1971)

2. Dolce, G., Künkel, H.: Computerized EEG analysis. Stuttgart: Fischer 1975

3. Duensing, F.: Das Elektrencephalogramm bei Störungen der Bewußtseinslage. Arch. Psychiat. u. Z. Neur. 183, 71-105 (1949)

4. Galicich, J.H., French, L.A.: Use of dexamethasone in the treatment of cerebral edema resulting from brain tumors and brain surgery. Amer. Pract. 12, 169-174 (1961)

5. Gastaut, J.L. et al.: Electroencephalography in brain edema. Electroenceph. Clin. Neurophysiol. 46, 239-255 (1979)

6. James, H.E.: Effects of steroids on behaviour, electrophysiology, water content and intracranial pressure in cerebral cytotoxic edema. Pharm. Biochem. Behavior 9, 653-657 (1978)

7. Jung, R.: Neurophysiologische Untersuchungsmethoden. II. Das Elektroencephalogramm (EEG). In: Handbuch der inneren Medizin, Vol. V/1, pp. 1216-1325. Berlin: Springer 1953
8. Kleeman, C.R., Koplowitz, J. et al.: Metabolic effects of two newer adrenal analogs, 6-methylprednisolone (medrol) and 6-methyl-9α-fluoro-21-desoxyprednisolone (9α-fluoro-21-desoxy-medrol). Metabolism 7, 425-440 (1958)
9. Kofman, S., Garvin, J.S. et al.: Treatment of cerebral metastases from breast carcinoma with prednisolone. J.A.M.A. 163, 1473-1476 (1957)
10. Lieberman, A., Le Brun, Y. et al.: Use of high dose corticosteroids in patients with inoperable brain tumors. Journal of Neurol., Neurosurg, Psych. 40, 678-682 (1977)
11. Meinig, G.: Beurteilung der antiödematösen Therapie bei Hirntumorpatienten. Neurochirurgie 23, 212-218 (1980)
12. Niebeling, H.-G.: Einführung in die Elektroenzephalographie. Leipzig: Johann Ambrosius Barth 1968
13. Pappius, H.M.: Effects of steroids on cold injury edema. In: Steroids and brain edema. Reulen, H.J., Schürmann, K. (eds.), pp. 57-63. Berlin, Heidelberg, New York: Springer 1972
14. Rasmussen, T., Gulati, D.R.: Cortisone in the treatment of postoperative cerebral edema. J. of Neurosurg. 19, 535-544 (1962)
15. Reulen, H.J., Schürmann, K.: Steroids and brain edema. Berlin, Heidelberg, New York: Springer 1972
16. Ruf, H.: Das Elektrencephalogramm beim Hirntumor. Dtsche. Z. Nervenheilk. 162, 60 (1950)
17. Sachs, L.: Statistische Auswertungsmethoden. Berlin, Heidelberg, New York: Springer 1971
18. von Wild, K., Samii, M. et al.: Zur Indication, Technik und praktischen Bedeutung des Monitoring bei Patienten mit Schädelhirntraumen. In: Neurotraumatologie. Wieck, H.H. (ed.), pp. 193-196. Stuttgart, New York: Georg Thieme 1980
19. Wilson, C.B., Barker, M. et al.: Steroid-induced inhibition of growth in glial tumors: a kinetic analysis. In: Steroids in brain edema. Reulen, H.J., Schürmann, K. (eds.), pp. 95-100. Berlin, Heidelberg, New York: Springer 1972

Fig. 1. Patient D., 25-year-old man, left frontal astrocytoma. Polygraphically registration of EEG (channel 1-6), ECG (channel 7), respiration (channel 8), and ICP (channel 10). Sections of 20 sec of the 1st day (before methylprednisolone medication), 4th day (under mp medication), and 7th day (40 h after withdrawl of mp). The EEG shows a reduction of delta- and theta-waves as well as a decrease of delta foci and an increase of alpha- and betawaves under mp-treatment. The ICP of 10 - 15 mm Hg on the 1st day was reduced to 4 - 9 mm Hg on the 4th day and 3 - 8 mm Hg on the 7th day. There were no changes in ECG- and respiration-values

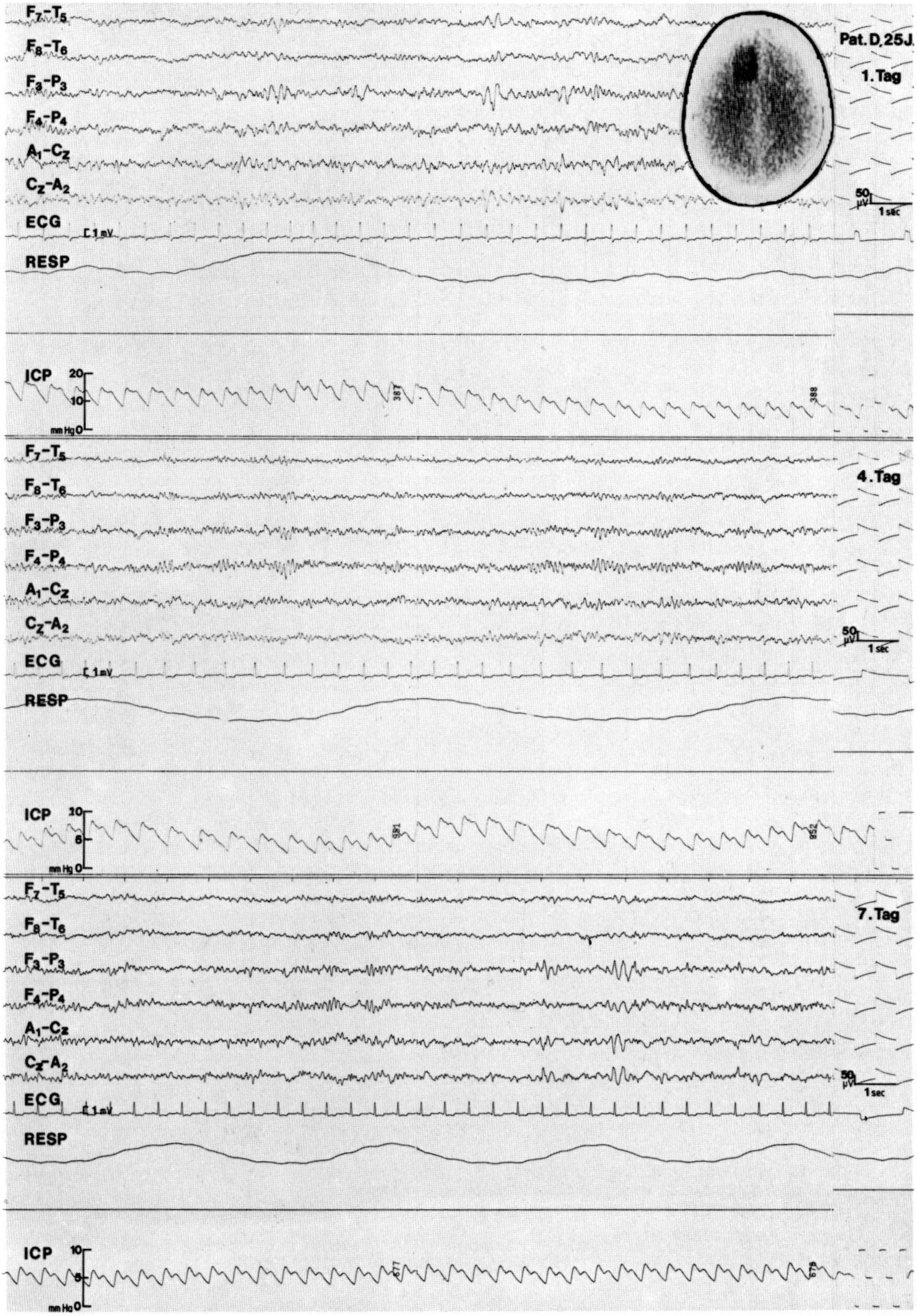
Pat. D, 25 J.
1. Tag
4. Tag
7. Tag
F7-T5
F8-T6
F3-P3
F4-P4
A1-Cz
Cz-A2
ECG
1 mV
RESP
ICP
mm Hg
50 µV
1 sec

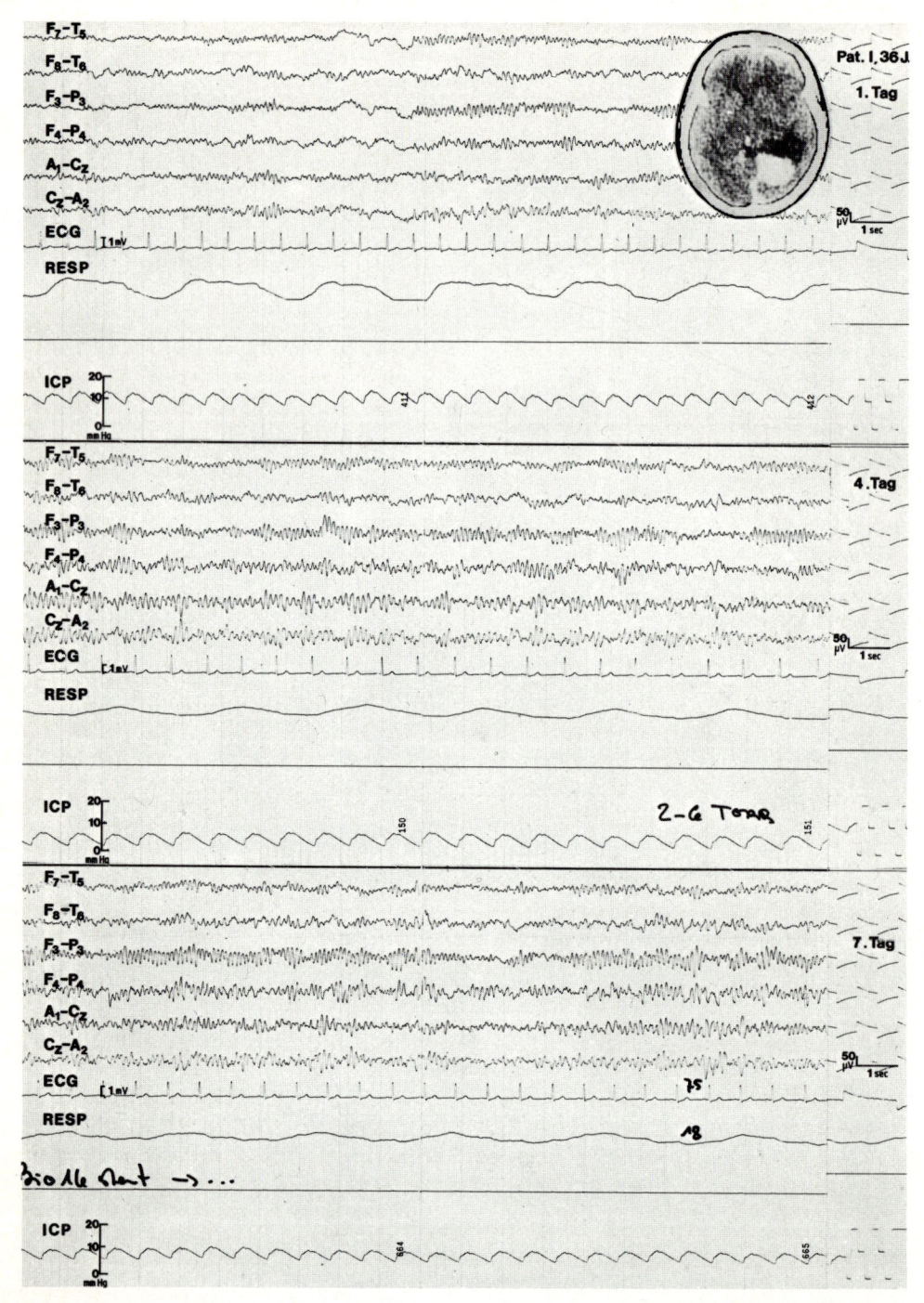

Fig. 2. Patient I., 36-year-old woman, tentorium meningioma right occipital. (Registration see Fig. 1). Under mp-treatment the delta-portion as well as the slow theta-waves decreased. We noticed an increase in the faster frequencies especially in the alpha-band

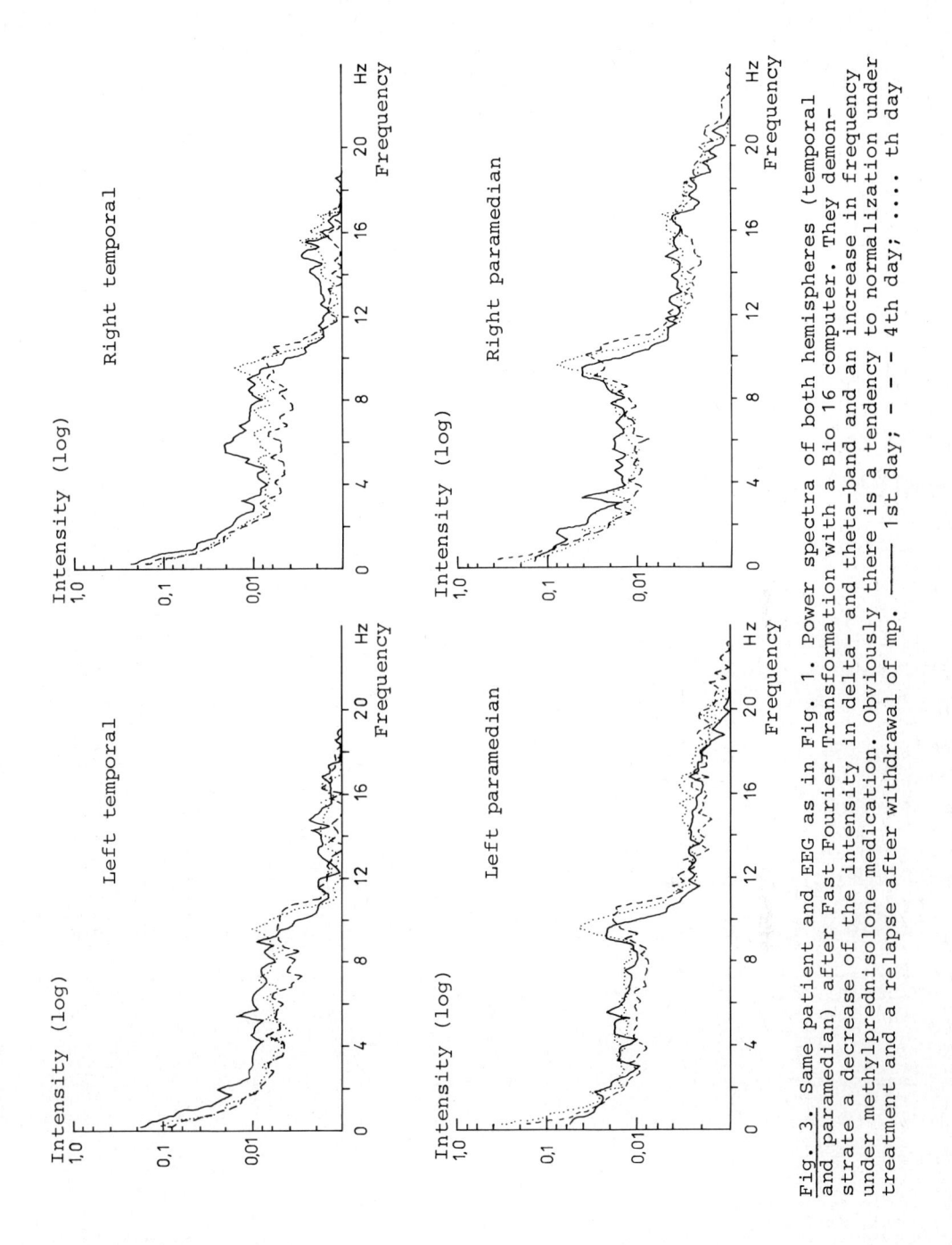

Fig. 3. Same patient and EEG as in Fig. 1. Power spectra of both hemispheres (temporal and paramedian) after Fast Fourier Transformation with a Bio 16 computer. They demonstrate a decrease of the intensity in delta- and theta-band and an increase in frequency under methylprednisolone medication. Obviously there is a tendency to normalization under treatment and a relapse after withdrawal of mp. —— 1st day; - - - 4th day; ·········· th day

◁ Fig. 2 (continued). These findings were more prominent over the contralateral hemisphere. The ICP of 8-15 mm Hg on the 1st day was reduced to 2-6 mmHg on the 4th day and 5-10 mm Hg on the 7th day. There are no significant changes in ECG- and respiration-values

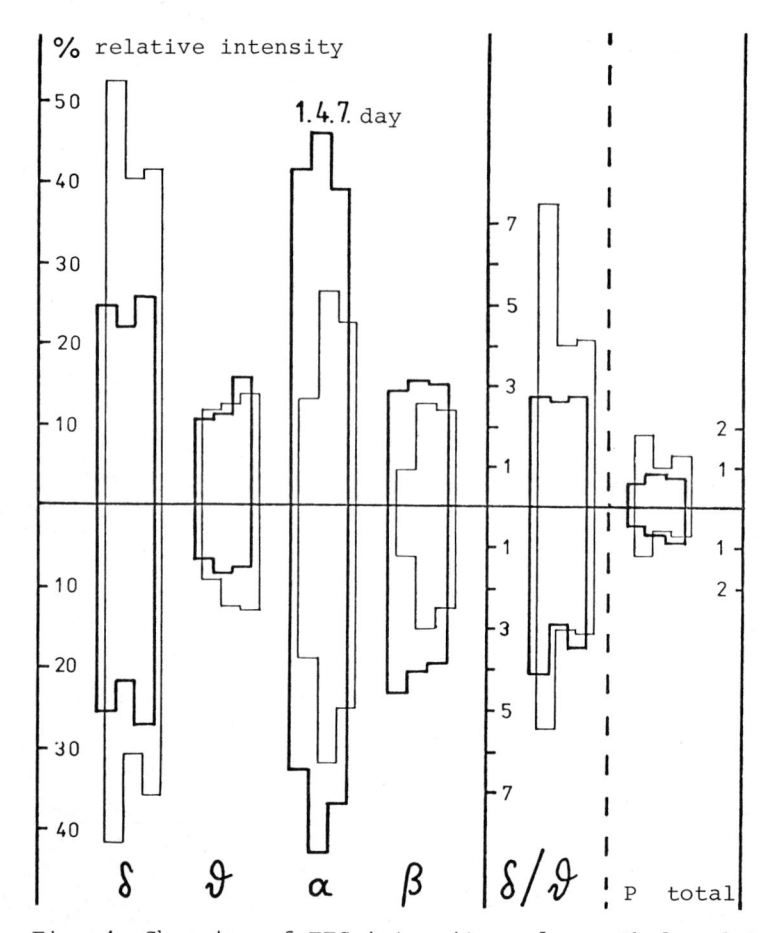

Fig. 4. Changing of EEG intensity under methylprednisolone medication (4th day) and after withdrawl (7th day) on 5 meningiomas (───) and 5 gliomas (───). The upper part of the figure shows the relative intensity of the δ-band (0.5 - 3.5 Hz), ϑ-band (3.5 - 7.5 Hz), α-band (7.5 - 12.5 Hz), and β-band (12.5 - 32 Hz), the δ/ϑ-quotient and the total power of the 4 bands on the tomour-side, the lower part of the contralateral side. We chose the EEG-channel that located the tumour and the contralateral one. In gliomas (percentage of power in frequency band demonstrated) a decrease of 30% of delta intensity with an increase of 6% in the theta and 100% in the alpha intensity under medication was demonstrated, whereas in meningiomas decrease in delta intensity was 10% with an increase in theta of 3% and alpha intensity of 10%. These findings were more prominent over the tumour involved hemisphere

Pressure/Volume (P/V)-Test and Pulse Wave (PA)-Analysis of ICP[*]

M. R. Gaab, I. Haubitz, A. Brawanski, J. Faulstich, and H. E. Heissler[**]

Introduction

The clinical value of continuous intracranial pressure (ICP) registration is widely accepted, especially in intensive monitoring of cerebral diseases and in neurological evaluation. The recording of mean ICP alone, however, is often *insufficient* due to the *exponential relationship* between intracranial volume increase and ICP (9, 11, 14): in cerebral monitoring, the onset of a progressive space consuming complication may be compensated in the mean ICP for a long time and therefore initially remains undetected (2, 5). The continuous decrease in intracranial compliance often leads to sudden and critical rises in ICP following further growth of the lesion. During diagnosis, the reduced intracranial compliance e.g. in low pressure hydrocephalus (LPH), is also often masked by a "normal" mean ICP, even though the disease is progressive and requires operative therapy (5, 8, 16).

An objective evaluation of the actual intracranial *compliance* is therefore of clinical importance. Direct measurement is performed by constructing a *pressure-volume* (P/V)-*diagram* following artificial intra-arachnoidal fluid injection (2, 4, 5, 12). One disadvantage of this procedure is that it is invasive. It distresses the patient, may initiate high secondary pressure waves or induce infection, and cannot be repeated frequently (2, 5). In addition, the mathematical method of MARMAROU (4, 5), using a mono-exponential regression, has limited accuracy (5).

We therefore tried to improve the technique and evaluation of the invasive pressure-volume-test. In order to obtain a non-invasive compliance parameter, the *waveforms* of ICP were analysed following previous experimental investigations (2, 3, 13, 17).

The Pressure-Volume (P/V)-Test

In 54 patients with chronic intracranial disease (hydrocephalus, subdural effusion or chronic subdural hematoma, Fig. 1) the pressure-volume-relationship of ICP was tested by lumbar *bolus injection* (a rapid injection of the volume is necessary for compliance evaluation, 4, 11). Rapidly growing intracranial processes and high intracranial hypertension were excluded by CAT scan and ICP monitoring over several

---

[*]Supported by grants from Deutsche Forschungsgemeinschaft (DFG, Ga 273/1) and from the Federal Ministry for Research and Technology (BMFT, project MMT 19)
[**]We gratefully acknowledge the competent technical assistance of Miss Doris Kern and Miss Marianne Barbian

days using miniaturized epidural pressure transducers (5, 6, 7). In a lateral recumbent position, a lumbar puncture was performed using 20 G-needles, usually at 2 levels (technique comp. 5). With continuous and *simultaneous lumbar-spinal* and *cranial-epidural* pressure recordings (Fig. 1), mock CSF (5) was injected or withdrawn within a few seconds as a "bolus". The volume was increased geometrically (+/-1,2,4,8 ml) following an initial estimate of the max. tolerable injection volume (increase in ICP not above 40 mm Hg (5)) based on the first 1-ml-injection and the formulas shown in Table 1 (5). The P/V-diagram was computed according to the accpeted method of MARMAROU with exponential curve fitting and following our own *new* (5) *technique* using *Newton's approximation* (Table 1). With both methods the complete P/V-diagram, PVI, compliance and elasticity (Table 1) are calculated using the basic ICP level (P_0) and the peak ICP (P_p) following a volume injection ΔV; thus, P_0, V, and P_p are the test data.

MARMAROU's method using exponential regression assumes a zero-assymptotic ICP course with negative ΔV values in every P/V-diagram. This simplifying assumption of exponential regression is generally *not* accepted in the demonstration of correlations between biological parameters (15); a zero-asymptotic curve fitting results in considerable inaccuracy (Fig. 1b). The advantage of this mathematically simple method, however, is the easy and rapid evaluation. We therefore use MARMAROU's technique for an immediate bedside estimate of the compliance. An HP 9845 calculator lists the values together with additional liquordynamic parameters (method 4, 5) in a clear synopsis of cranial and spinal measurement (Table 2).

The P/V-diagram is not computed by curve fitting, but by calculating a mean PVI from the different sets of P_0, V and P_p data (Table 2). This mean PVI is transformed into the exponential slope k of the P/V-curve (Table 1), which defines the complete diagram together with the know initial ICP (before artificial volume change). With this technique, a pressure drop to the level before bolus injection must not be waited for, and the entire investigation is performed *within a few minutes*.

A more precise P/V-diagram (Fig. 1a, b) is achieved by NEWTONIAN approximation (Table 1) using a TR 440 computer with the programme SAUSGL from AEG-Telefunken. With this mathematical procedure (details see (5)), two parameters (P_{eq} and k) are derived from the independent data P_0, V and P_p; this results in an *individual asymptomatic baseline* (= P_{eq}), which is approached with negative ΔV values (Fig. 2a). The (inter)individual differences, and the influences of the various hydrostatic levels of the ICP recording points are taken into consideration. The *improved accuracy* of our method can also be demonstrated quantitatively (5).

An attempt to determine a P/V-curve with two inflection points as proposed by (4, 10), corresponding to a hyperbolic function (P_p = P_{eq} + sin h ($\overline{k.V+b}$), without plateau, or accuracy.

Pp = (A-B·V) + sin h (k.V+b), with a plateau in the pressure compensation range), always resulted in greater curve deviations (5).

The main advantage of our P/V-diagram with Newton's approximation is the clear distinction between cranial and spinal pressure responses following lumbar volume load (Fig. 1a). The different slopes of cranial and spinal curves allow a differentiation between communicating hydrocephalus and *disturbances of CSF circulation* (Figs. 1c, d). With this investigation, 20% of 48 patients with suspected communi-

Table 1. Parameters and formulas of intracranial compliance: calculation of the P/V-diagram according MARMAROU or with NEWTON's approximation (own method)

Parameters	Marmarou's method (Exponential regression)	Own technique (Newton's approximation)
Basic formula	$ICP = b \cdot e^{k \cdot V}$	$ICP = P_{eq} + b \cdot e^{k \cdot V}$
P/V-diagram calculation	$P_p = P_o \cdot e^{k \cdot \Delta V}$	$P_p = P_{eq} + (P_o - P_{eq}) \cdot e^{k \cdot \Delta V}$
PVI (press. vol. ind.)	$PVI = \dfrac{\Delta V}{\lg(P_p/P_o)} = \dfrac{\ln 10}{k}$	$PVI = \ln 10 \cdot \dfrac{P_o - P_{eq}}{P_o - P_{eq}} \cdot k^{-1} \approx \dfrac{\Delta V}{\lg\dfrac{(P_p - P_{eq})}{(P_o - P_{eq})}}$
k – slope of P/V c.	$k = \ln\dfrac{P_p}{P_o} \cdot \Delta V^{-1} = \dfrac{\ln 10}{PVI}$	$k = \ln\dfrac{P_p - P_{eq}}{P_o - P_{eq}} \cdot \Delta V^{-1}$
E ("elastance")[a]	$E = k \cdot P_m = \dfrac{P_m}{0.4343 \cdot PVI} = \dfrac{1}{C}$	
C ("compliance")[a]	$C = \dfrac{1}{k \cdot P_m} = \dfrac{0.4343 \cdot PVI}{P_m} = \dfrac{1}{E}$	

[a] Value varies with different P_m, therefore limited clinical significance

Table 2. Bedside evaluation of bolus injection- and constant-speed-infusion test: clear survey on cranial as well as spinal PVI, k-slope, pulse amplitude behaviour and CSF outflow resistance (R_O) or conductance (C_O) using a HP 9845 computer

```
              * * *   BOLUSINJECTION-TEST   * * *
PAT. NAME:B.R.     BD :55 y.           INVEST. DATE:      20.04.80
CRANIAL RECORD: Pp = 11.0000 *EXP( .0792 *V )   TRANSDUCER GAELTEC#

BOLUS(ml) P0    Pp     PVI    Pa1    Pa2    Pa1/P0  Pa2/Pp   Aa1    Aa2
-----------------------------------------------------------------------
  -1.0    11.0  10.0   24.2   1.8    1.3     .2      .1      0.0    0.0
   1.0    11.5  13.0   18.8   1.8    2.5     .2      .2      0.0    0.0
  -1.0    11.5  11.0   51.8   1.8    1.6     .2      .1      0.0    0.0
   1.0    11.0  12.0   26.5   1.7    2.3     .2      .2      0.0    0.0
  -2.0    11.5  10.5   50.6   1.9    1.5     .2      .1      0.0    0.0
   2.0    12.5  14.5   31.0   2.2    2.8     .2      .2      0.0    0.0
  -2.0    14.0  12.0   29.9   2.7    1.7     .2      .1      0.0    0.0
   2.0    12.0  16.0   16.0   1.7    3.1     .1      .2      0.0    0.0
  -4.0    13.0  10.0   35.1   2.2    1.7     .2      .2      0.0    0.0
   2.0    13.0  15.0   32.2   1.8    2.8     .1      .2      0.0    0.0
   4.0    15.0  22.5   22.7   2.8    5.0     .2      .2      0.0    0.0
   4.0    16.0  25.0   20.6   3.0    5.7     .2      .2      0.0    0.0
   8.0    18.5  50.0   18.5   3.3   10.7     .2      .2      0.0    0.0


PVI MEAN =  29.1  ml    [+/-(25-30 ml)]
K=  .079210


SPINAL RECORD : Pp = 15.5000 *EXP( .0673 *V )     LP,NEEDLE 2xG 20

BOLUS(ml) P0    Pp     PVI    Pa1    Pa2    Pa1/P0  Pa2/Pp   Aa1    Aa2
-----------------------------------------------------------------------
  -1.0    15.5  14.0   22.6   1.3    1.0     .1      .1      0.0    0.0
   1.0    16.0  18.0   19.5   1.7    2.5     .1      .1      0.0    0.0
  -1.0    17.0  16.0   38.0   2.0    1.4     .1      .1      0.0    0.0
   1.0    16.0  17.0   38.0   1.6    2.4     .1      .1      0.0    0.0
  -2.0    17.0  15.5   49.9   1.8    1.3     .1      .1      0.0    0.0
   2.0    17.5  19.5   42.6   2.0    2.9     .1      .1      0.0    0.0
  -2.0    17.5  16.0   51.4   2.0    1.6     .1      .1      0.0    0.0
   2.0    16.0  20.0   20.6   1.6    3.4     .1      .2      0.0    0.0
  -4.0    17.0  13.5   40.0   1.8    1.3     .1      .1      0.0    0.0
   2.0    15.5  17.0   49.9   1.7    2.0     .1      .1      0.0    0.0
   4.0    16.5  22.5   29.7   2.0    4.3     .1      .2      0.0    0.0
   4.0    17.0  25.0   23.9   3.3    5.5     .2      .2      0.0    0.0
   8.0    19.0  50.0   19.0   4.0   11.0     .2      .2      0.0    0.0


PVI MEAN =  34.2  ml    [+/-(25-30 ml)]
K=  .067267

RESISTANCE/CONDUCTANCE            P0=  11.00      PA=   0.00

In(ml/min)  PA(c)  Pst(c)   PA(s)  Pst(s)   Ro(c)  Co(c)   Ro(s)  Co(s)
-----------------------------------------------------------------------
  1.50      0.00   50.00    0.00   47.00    26.00   .04    20.67   .05


Ro mean(cr)= 26.00    [3-10 mmHg*ml/min]    Co mean(cr)= .04   [0.1-0.35]
Ro mean(sp)= 20.67                          Co mean(sp)= .05
```

cation LPH showed clear signs of "compartment-block" (1, 5). A definite cranio-spinal dissociation is also often demonstrated in *Syringomyelia* (5). This is of pathophysiological and therapeutic value.

Analysis of the ICP Pulse Wave (PA)

The intracranial pressure *pulse amplitude* (PA) is generated mainly by the arterial cerebral *pulse volume* ("endogenous bolus test" by the volume amplitude VA) (2, 3, 5). With decreasing intracranial compliance, the ICP pulse amplitude therefore increases as long as the arterial inflow is not reduced by an extreme ICP elevation (above 50 mm Hg, 3, 17). PA thus is a function of VA and the man ICP (P_m); it is defined as (see our formula for the P/V-diagram):

$$PA = 2(P_m - P_{eq}) \frac{e^{k \cdot VA} - 1}{e^{k \cdot VA} + 1} = 2(P_m - P_{eq}) \cdot \text{arc tgh}\left(\frac{k}{2} \cdot VA\right).$$

With a continuously constant VA, the PA would be linearly dependent on P_m,

$$PA = c_1 \cdot P_m + c_2 \qquad (c_1, c_2 = \text{const.}),$$

and the P/V-diagram could be derived continuously from the PA/P_m-relationship without any invasive procedure according to:

PVI = VA · ln 10/ ln (c_1 + 1).

In our 54 patients, we registered the ICP pulse amplitude PA during the bolus injection test and the mean ICP P_m simultaneously (Fig. 2). Following computation of the P/V-diagram, the generating pulse volume VA for each PA can be calculated from the P/V-curve (Fig. 2b, e'). Unfortunately, this evaluation shows, that the VA does *not* remain constant, even at lower ICP values up to 50 mm Hg: VA generally *rises* with increasing P_m (Fig. 2b) (5), but may also decrease at higher P_m without any predictable regularity (5). A direct and quantitative calculation of the actual intracranial compliance is therefore *impossible* without a known VA. However, despite a variable VA, the pulse amplitude PA was *linearly correlated* with the mean ICP (P_m, Fig. 2c,f) in almost every patient (5, 17). This concurs with previous experimental investigations (3, 13). A comparison of the slope c of this Pa/P_m-regression with the exponential slope k from the corresponding P/V-diagram (Fig. 3) shows an approximate, but nevertheless significant correlation between pulse amplitude analysis and compliance!

We therefore routinely (5, 7) use an ICP wave form analysis (Intertechnique IN 110 computer) as an *indirect* and *continuous compliance parameter*, especially in intensive monitoring, where invasive P/V-studies cannot be performed. The PA/P_m relationship, computed as a regression line (Fig. 4), often indicates expanding intracranial lesions much earlier than the course of the mean ICP (5) with an increasing slope. The renormalization of this PA/P_m-slope is also often correlated with clinical improvement (Fig. 4). In addition to a PA/P_m-regression, the change in ICP waveform with variations of intracranial compliance and clinical course can also be demonstrated by a *Fourier analysis* of ICP fluctuations (Fig. 4). An increase in pulse amplitude is associated with a decrease in ICP breathing amplitude (AA).

---

[1] Mathematical derivation see (5)

Discussion

Evaluation of intracranial compliance supplements the mere ICP recording and has clinical significance. The lumbar bolus injection test is suitable for a quantitative calculation of the P/V-diagram. It is therefore helpful in diagnosis, especially in determining the activity and indication for surgery in LPH or cystic intracranial processes (4, 5, 7, 8, 16). Simultaneously, parameters of CSF dynamics such as resistance/conductance can easily be measured (Table 2; 4, 5, 11). The MARMAROU' method only allows an approximate bedside compliance testing, our mathematical model with Newton' approximation is more accurate. However, the latter method requires a considerable computer capacity, and some variations from "normal values" as reported in the literature must be considered (e.g. the lower PVI limit, 5). Continued intracranial ICP recording prior to and during the P/V test is low in risk and easily performed using miniaturized epidural transducers (5, 6, 7). It not only excludes acute elevations in ICP as a *contraindication* for the bolus test, but also allows a simultaneous demonstration of the spinocranial *pressure transmission* during lumbar bolus injection. This evaluation of spino-cranial communication disturbances is of clinical value in hydrocephalus and syringomyelia (5).

A non invasive and continuous estimate of intracranial compliance variations, particularly in intensive care monitoring with rapidly fluctuating intracranial volumes, is possible by an ICP pulse waveform analysis. In addition to the intracranial compliance, *cerebral vasoregulation* also influences the intracranial pulse amplitude, and therefore provides further information about vasoparalysis or cerebral vasospasm (2, 5). Because of its complexity, the ICP amplitude is only of relative prognostic value, which may perhaps be increased and differentiated by simultaneous investigation of arterial pulsation and arterial-intracranial transfer function (coherence analysis, 2).

Conclusions

The actual intracranial compliance cannot be derived from the registration of mean ICP. The calculation of a P/V-diagram and other compliance parameters is possible using the lumbar bolus injection test. Using our mathematical method with Newton's approximation, a more precise P/V-curve is computed; the simultaneous spinal and cranial pressure recording thereby allows the demonstration of CSF circulation disturbances, e.g. in hydrocephalus and syringomyelia. A continuous, non invasive estimate of intracranial compliance is achieved by an ICP waveform analysis using pulse amplitude/mean ICP regression and Fourier transformation. The regression slope is correlated with the P/V-course and also provides information about cerebral vasoregulation.

References

1. Brawanski, A., Gaab, M.: Intracranial pressure gradients in the presence of various intracranial space-occupying lesions. In: Advances in neurosurgery, Vol. 9. Schiefer, W., Klinger, M., Brock, M. (eds.), pp. 355-362. Berlin, Heidelberg, New York: Springer 1981

2. Chopp, M., Portnoy, H.D.: Analysis of intracranial pressure waveforms, comparison to the volume pressure test. Biomed. Sci. Instrum. 16, 149-158 (1980)

3. Eijndhoven, J.H.M., Avezaat, C.J.J.: The analogy between CSF pulse pressure and volume-pressure response. In: Intracranial pressure IV. Shulman, K., Marmarou, A., Miller, J.D., Becker, D.P., Hochwald, G.M., Brock, M. (eds.), pp. 173-176. Berlin, Heidelberg, New York: Springer 1980

4. Ekstedt, J.: CSF hydrodynamic studies in man. 2. Normal hydrodynamic variables related to CSF pressure and flow. J. Neurol. Neurosurg. Psychiat. 41, 345-353 (1978)

5. Gaab, M.R.: Die Registrierung des intrakraniellen Druckes. Grundlagen, Techniken, Ergebnisse und Möglichkeiten. Habilitationsschrift, Würzburg: Fachbereich Medizin 1980

6. Gaab, M.R., Knoblich, O.E., Dietrich, K.: Miniaturisierte Methoden zur Überwachung des intrakraniellen Druckes. Techniken und klinische Ergebnisse. Langenbecks Arch. Chir. 350, 13-31 (1979)

7. Gaab, M.R., Sörensen, N.: Extradurale Langzeit-Messung des intrakraniellen Druckes in der Pädiatrie. Methodik und klinische Anwendung. Kinderarzt 11, 11-20 (1980)

8. Gruss, P., Gaab, M., Sörensen, N., Wodarz, R.: Zum Begriff des "arrested hydrocephalus". Neurochirurgia 22, 85-95 (1979)

9. Langfitt, T.W., Weinstein, J.D., Kassell, N.F.: Cerebral vasomotor paralysis produced by intracranial hypertension. Neurology 15, 622-641 (1965)

10. Löfgren, J., Essen, C.v., Zwetnow, N.N.: The pressure-volume curve of the cerebrospinal fluid space in dogs. Acta Neurol. Scand. 49, 557-574 (1973)

11. Marmarou, A.: A theoretical and experimental evaluation of the cerebrospinal fluid system. Ph. D. Thesis: Drexel University 1976

12. Marmarou, A., La Morgese, J.: Compartmental analysis of compliance and outflow resistance of the cerebrospinal fluid system. J. Neurosurg. 43, 523-534 (1975)

13. Nones, H., Aaslice, R., Lindegoard, K.: Intracranial pulse pressure dynamics in patients with intracranial hypertension. Acta neurochir. 38, 177-180 (1977)

14. Shulman, K.: Pressure/volume relationships in intracranial disease. Z. Kinderchir. 25, 289-303 (1978)

15. Sprent, P.: Models in regression and related topics. London: Methuen 1969

16. Symon, L., Hinzpeter, Th.: The enigma of normal pressure hydrocephalus: Tests to select patients for surgery and to predict shunt function. Clin. Neurosurg. 24, 285-315 (1977)

17. Szewszykowski, J., Sliwka, S., Kunicki, A., Dytko, P., Korsak-Sliwka, J.: A fast method of estimating the elastance of the intracranial system. J. Neurosurg. 47, 19-26 (1977)

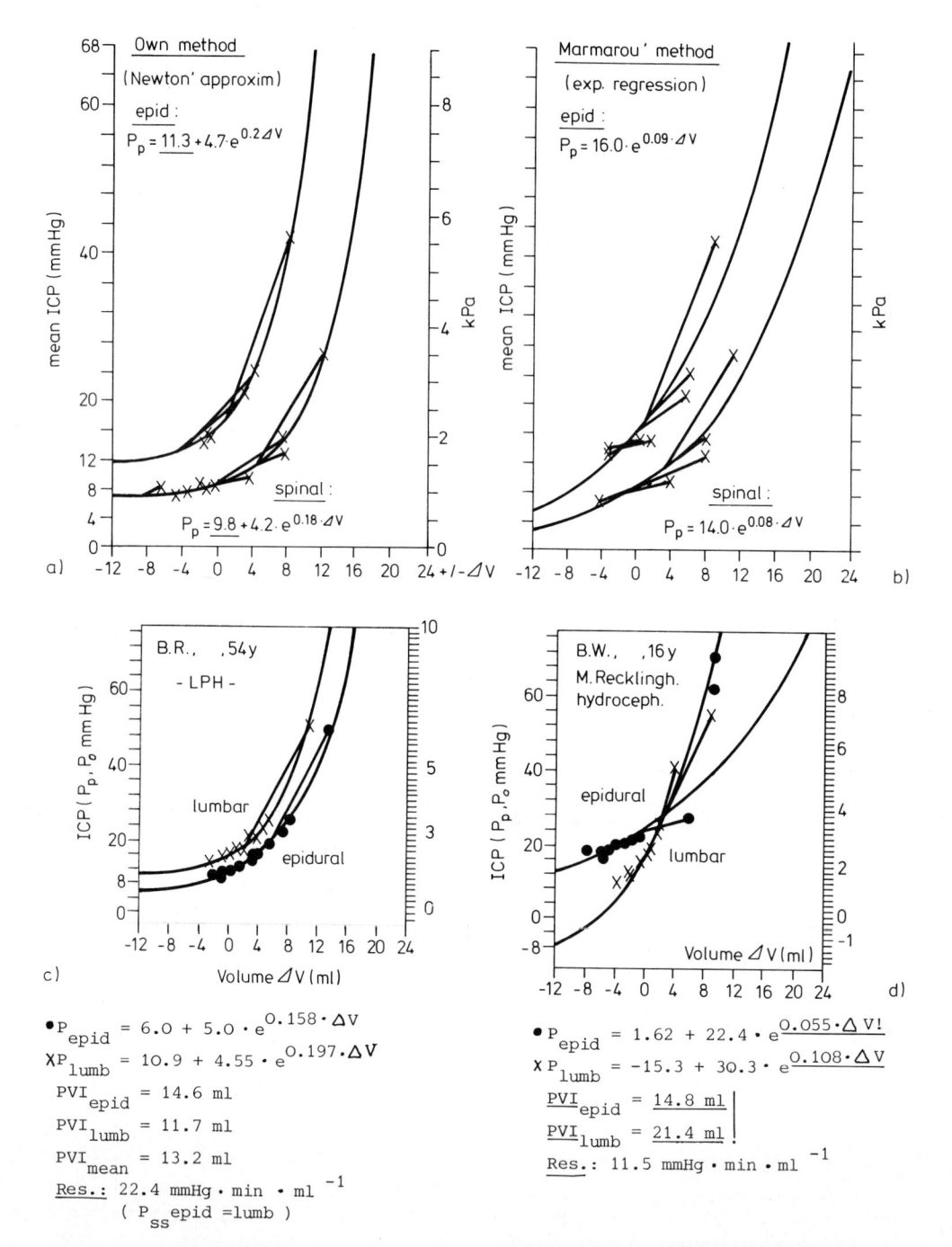

a) Own method (Newton' approxim)
epid: $P_p = 11.3 + 4.7 \cdot e^{0.2 \Delta V}$
spinal: $P_p = 9.8 + 4.2 \cdot e^{0.18 \cdot \Delta V}$

b) Marmarou' method (exp. regression)
epid: $P_p = 16.0 \cdot e^{0.09 \cdot \Delta V}$
spinal: $P_p = 14.0 \cdot e^{0.08 \cdot \Delta V}$

c) B.R., 54y – LPH –

• $P_{epid} = 6.0 + 5.0 \cdot e^{0.158 \cdot \Delta V}$
x $P_{lumb} = 10.9 + 4.55 \cdot e^{0.197 \cdot \Delta V}$
$PVI_{epid} = 14.6$ ml
$PVI_{lumb} = 11.7$ ml
$PVI_{mean} = 13.2$ ml
Res.: 22.4 mmHg · min · ml^{-1}
(P_{ss} epid =lumb)

d) B.W., 16y M.Recklingh. hydroceph.

• $P_{epid} = 1.62 + 22.4 \cdot e^{0.055 \cdot \Delta V !}$
x $P_{lumb} = -15.3 + 30.3 \cdot e^{0.108 \cdot \Delta V}$
$PVI_{epid} = 14.8$ ml
$PVI_{lumb} = 21.4$ ml !
Res.: 11.5 mmHg · min · ml^{-1}

Fig. 1a-d. Simultaneous spinal and cranial P/V-diagram following bolus injection. The low accuracy of MARMAROU's method of exponential regression b is significantly improved by our method with Newton' approximation a. The clear separation of spinal and cranial P/V-reaction by this method allows a demonstration of spino-cranial communication disturbances (c, d; same patient as Table 2)

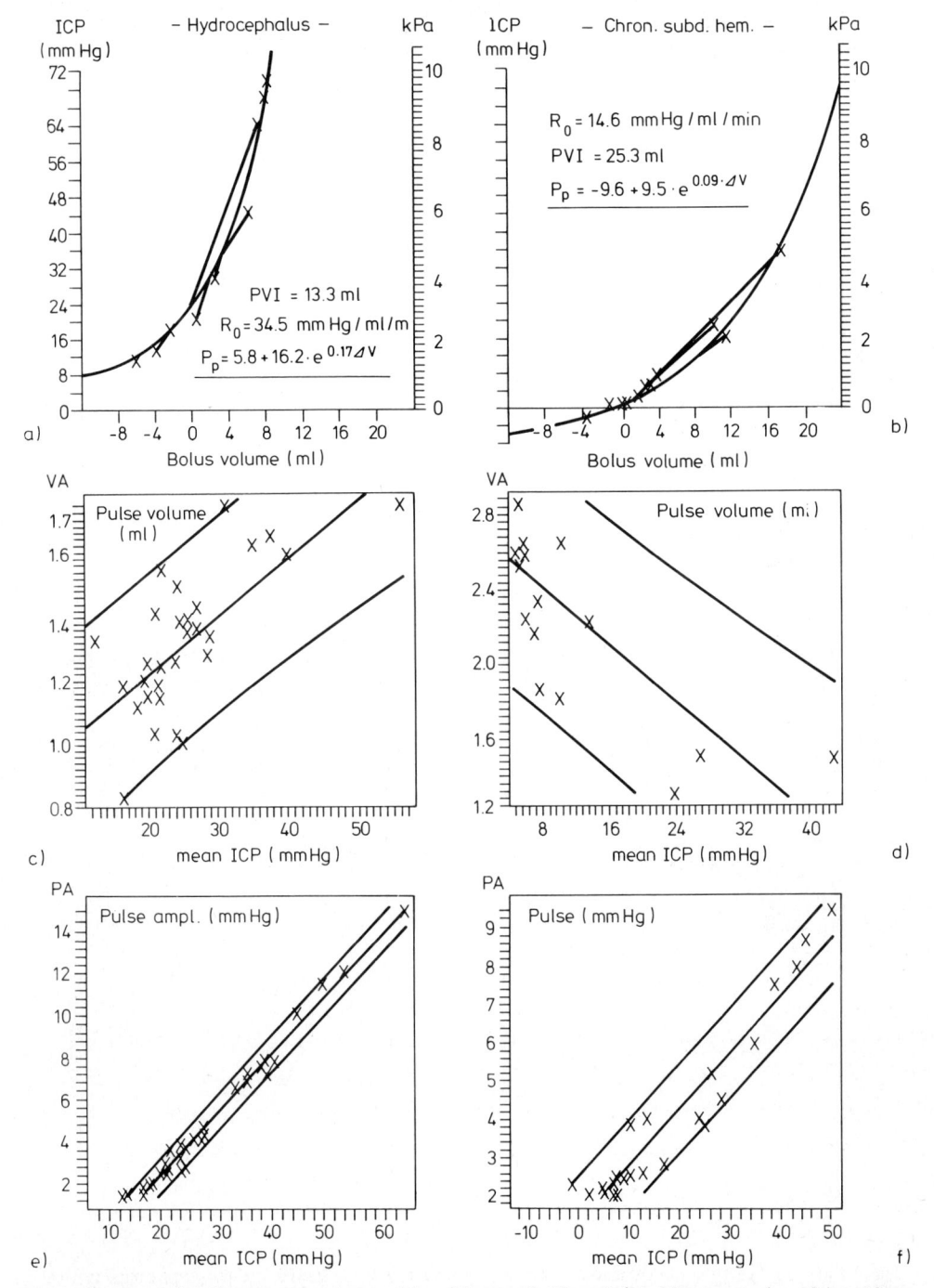

Fig. 2a-f. Simultaneous investigation of the P/V-diagram (a, b), the intracranial pulse volume VA (c, d) and the pulse amplitude-mean ICP ($\overline{PA}/\overline{P}_m$) relationship (e, f) during lumbar bolus injection. In spite of inconstant VA, the $\overline{PA}/\overline{P}_m$ regression gives a significantly linear correlation

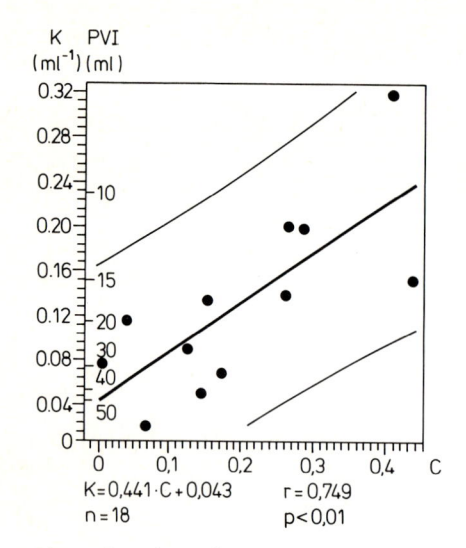

Fig. 3. The slopes of the P/V-diagram (k) and of the PA/P_m-regression show a significant, but approximate correlation

Fig. 4a-f. Clinical significance of ICP pulse wave. The slope of the pulse amplitude/mean ICP (PA/P_m)-regression varies with intracranial edema formation (steep slope = low compliance) and is more correlated with clinical symptoms (a-e) than the mean ICP (P_m, a-d). With Fourier analysis (f), the increase of the pulse amplitude (PA) concurs with a decreasing breathing amplitude (AA)

Pat. A.K. Head injury, hematoma, edema

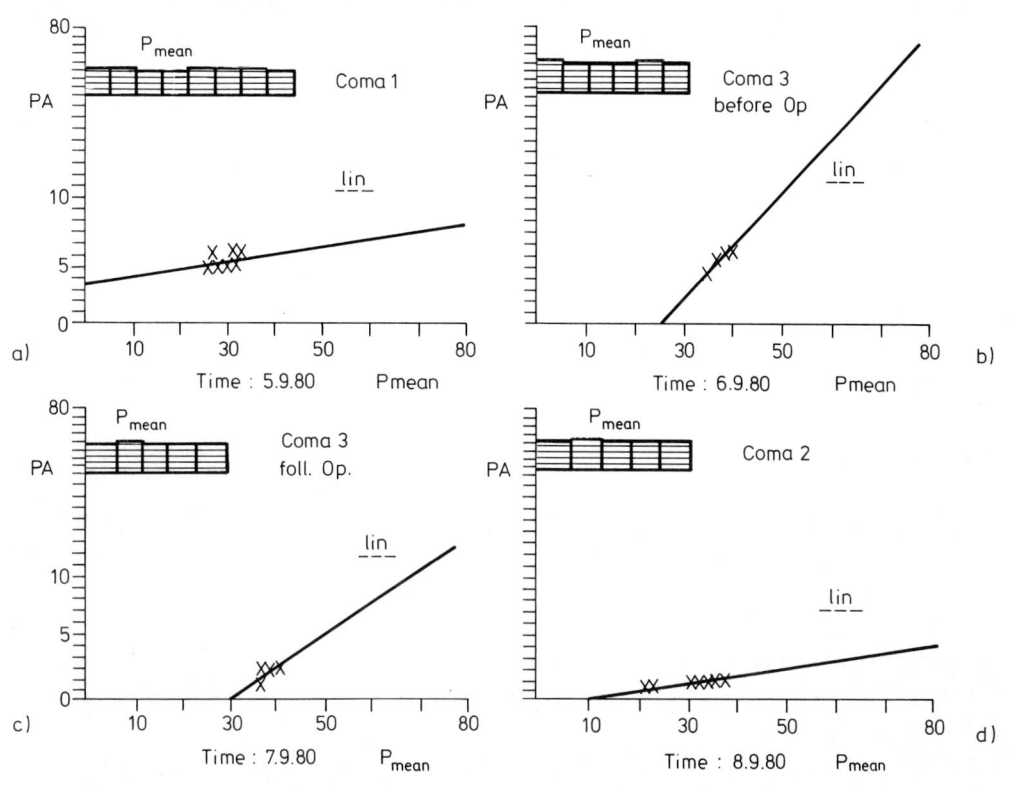

Pat. M.S., ♀, 51 y., after op. olf. meningeoma-edema

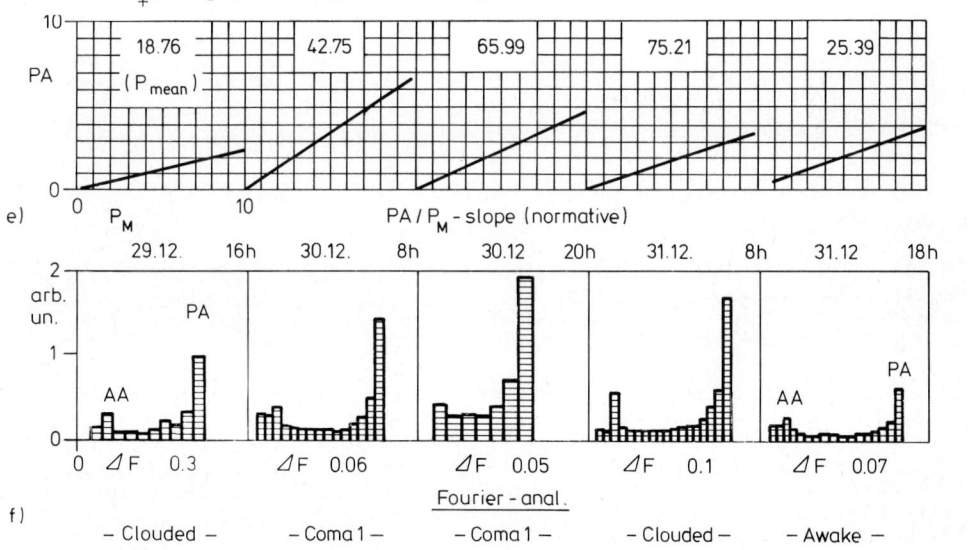

Clinical Application of Computer Assisted Continuous Monitoring of Intracranial Pressure

F. MÜNCH, K. VAN DEYK, D. RINKER, E. EPPLE, and H. JUNGER

Introduction

The importance of continuous recording of the intracranial pressure (ICP) in the intensive care of patients with severe head injury is generally accepted. Influences of head position, mechanical ventilation and hemodynamic alterations on the ICP become more evident. To emphasize the advantage of simultaneous recording of the ICP with other vital parameters, two examples are demonstrated in this study.

Material and Methods

In two patients with severe head injury, 19 and 16 years old, ICP was recorded continuously from the epidural space. Following parameters were simultaneously measured: heart rate (HR), blood pressure (BP), pulmonary arterial pressure (PAP) and central venous pressure (CVP). All measured parameters were registered by the Hewlett-Packard 5600 Intensive Care System with a sampling rate of two values per minute. The data were printed out in a computer generated patient chart developed by the Institut für Biomedizinische Technik Stuttgart and the Department of Paediatric Cardiology of the University of Tübingen. Cardiac output (CO) was determined by thermodilution with the Edwards Cardiac Output Computer 9520; additional measurements were performed when sudden alterations of the ICP had occurred. Arterial and mixed-venous blood gas samples were analyzed. Alveolar-arterial O_2 difference ($AaDO_2$), arterio-venous O_2 content difference ($avDO_2$), oxygen consumption (VO_2), pulmonary shunt (Qs/Qt), cardiac index (CI) and left ventricular stroke work index (LVSWI) were calculated.

Results

Figure 1 shows part of the computer chart of the 19-years old patient. The left half seems to exhibit an accumulation of artefacts. When extended on the time axis, however (Fig. 2), it reveals a specific relationship of the elevation of ICP to the peaks of HR.

Figure 3 displays part of the computer chart of the second patient. It demonstrates the dependence of ICP on the character of artificial ventilation used. The arrows point out the moments when the single-ventilation has been prolonged by increase of tidal volume and decrease of peak flow, keeping in this manner the minute ventilation constant. The result is a marked elevation of the ICP.

Figure 4 shows an other part of the computer chart of the same patient. The increase of HR at about 9.10 a.m. is followed by a decrease of BP and an elevation of ICP and PAP. The rise of PAP between 8.30

and 9.05 a.m. is caused by a partial obstruction of the Swan-Ganz catheter and not valid.

Discussion

Changes in HR during spontaneous increases of ICP in patients with severe head injury have been reported by other investigators before (2, 4, 6). The increases of HR in association with ICP rises confirm these observations (Fig. 2). However, it may be sometimes difficult to discover such relationship (Fig. 1), especially when only isolated measurements of ICP are performed. By continuous monitoring of ICP with other vital parameters these interrelations are more easily detected and sudden changes of HR may indicate ICP changes, implying the need of therapy to reduce ICP.

A further advantage of continuous ICP measurement lies in the better management of mechanical ventilation with respect to its influence on ICP. High tidal volumes are often required in patients with multiple injuries beause of the increased pulmonary shunt and dead space (7). On the other hand, the increased mean intrathoracic pressure leads to an elevation of ICP (Fig. 3) which may be hazardous to patients with severe head injury.

The interrelations between the cardiovascular system and ICP are demonstrated in Fig. 4. Probably induced by catecholamine release (5) the ICP rise is associated with increase of PAP. The hemodynamic measurement performed at 9.20 a.m. reveals an enhanced stress on the cardiorespiratory system. CI, LVSWI and Qa/Qt are increased compared with the data assessed after treatment at 10.30 a.m.

Conclusions

A continuous assessment of ICP with other vital parameters may be of great value for the intensive care of patients with severe head injury. Interrelations between ICP and cardiorespiratory system become more evident. Alterations of cardiovascular patterns are realized in time permitting an instant treatment of an expected elevation of ICP before the ICP has reached its peak. Damage to the brain could be prevented better by this procedure. It further allows one to control the efficacy of such treatment.

References

1. Brock, M., Dietz, H.: Intracranial pressure I. Berlin, Heidelberg, New York: Springer 1972
2. Cooper, R.L., Hulme, A.: Changes of the EEG, intracranial pressure and other variables during sleep in patients with intracranial lesions. Electroenceph. Clin. Neurophysiol. 27, 12-22 (1969)
3. Hase, U.: Intrakranielle Drucksteigerung. (Meßmethoden, Pathophysiologie, Therapie). Neurochirurgia 21, 145-156 (1978)
4. Kjällquist, A., Lundberg, N., Ponten, U.: Respiratory and cardiovascular changes during rapid spontaneous variations of ventricular fluid pressure in patients with intracranial hypertension. Acta Neurol. Scand. 40, 291-317 (1964)

5. Nishimura, M.C., Hoff, J.T.: Sequential hemodynamic changes in experimental neurogenic pulmonary edema. In: Intracranial pressure IV. Brock, M., Dietz, H. (eds.), pp. 333-336. Berlin, Heidelberg, New York: Springer 1980
6. Tindall, G.T., McGraw, C.P., Vanderveer, R.W., Iwata, K.: Cardiorespiratory changes associated with plateau waves in patients with head injury. In: Intracranial pressure I. Brock, M., Dietz, H. (eds.), pp. 227-231. Berlin, Heidelberg, New York: Springer 1972
7. Wolff, G.: Die künstliche Beatmung auf Intensivstationen. 2. Aufl. Berlin, Heidelberg, New York: Springer 1977

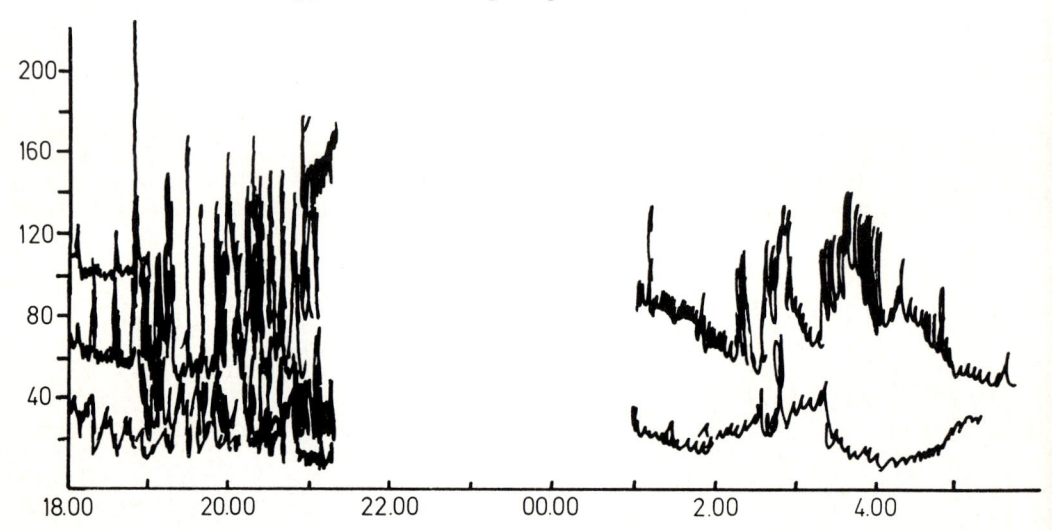

Fig. 1. Computer generated chart of the 19-year old patient. The left half seems to be an accumulation of artefacts

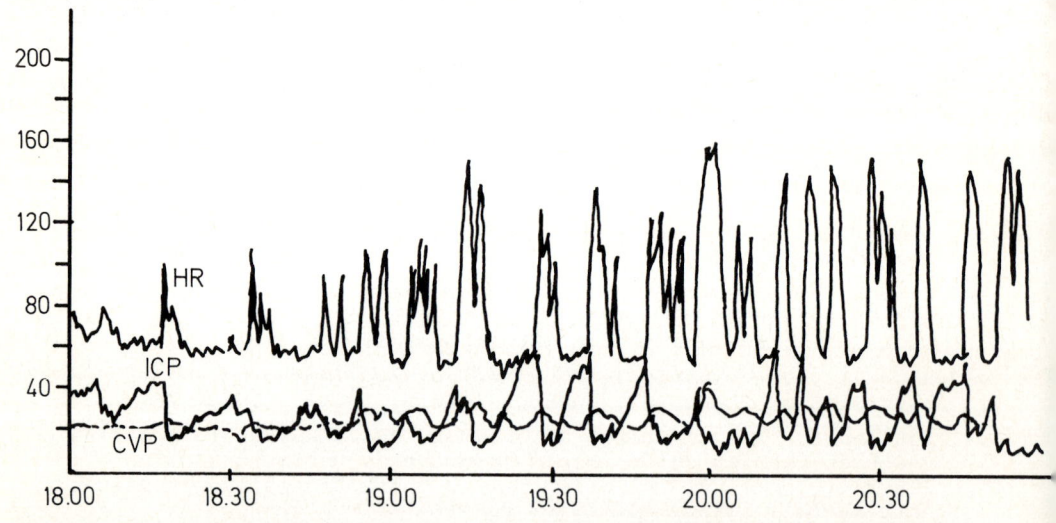

Fig. 2. The left half of Fig. 1, this time extended on the time axis. The upper curve represents the HR, the middle one the ICP. There is a specific relationship of the elevation of ICP to the peaks of HR

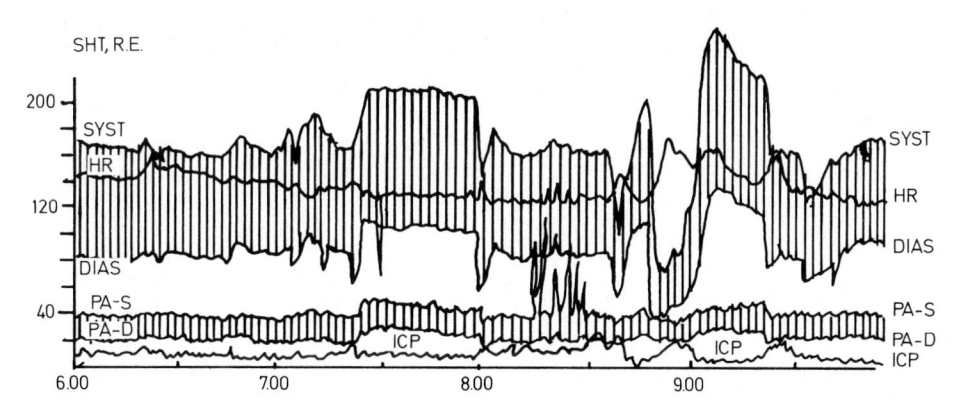

Fig. 3. Computer generated chart of the 16-years old patient. It displays the systemic BP (SYST, DIAS), HR, PAP (PA-S, PA-D), CVP and ICP. The arrows indicate the moments when tidal volume of mechanical ventilation has been increased

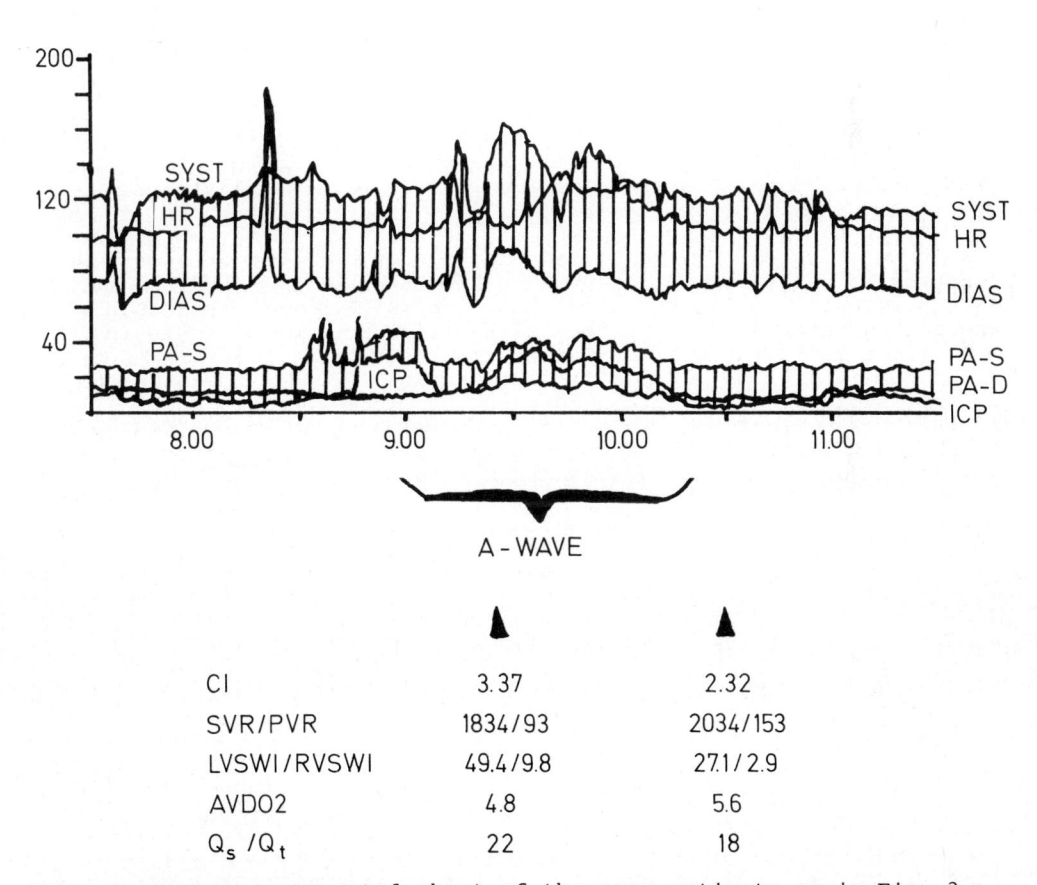

CI	3.37	2.32
SVR/PVR	1834/93	2034/153
LVSWI/RVSWI	49.4/9.8	27.1/2.9
AVDO2	4.8	5.6
Q_s/Q_t	22	18

Fig. 4. Computer generated chart of the same patients as in Fig. 3. The hemodynamic measurement during the plateau wave of ICP at 9.20 a.m. reveals an increased stress on the cardiovascular system

Possibilities and Results by Using the Rhinosurgical Approach in Cases of Anterior Cranial Fossa Injuries

W. ELIES

In cases of blunt and open frontal head injuries maxillo-facial and/ or paranasal sinus wall fractures are often found. The rupture of the dura, lying behind the posterior wall of the frontal sinus or covering the floor of the anterior cranial fossa, is not uncommon. Rhinorrhoea - the typical clinical finding and the diagnostic sign of a cerebrospinal fluid leakage as well as early meningitis are found in only two thirds of the patients (1-4, 7-9). The other patients can get late meningitis over even dramatic complications from the paranasal air sinuses years or decades after injury. If one reviews the literature, the incidence of dural tears in cases of frontal head injuries differs greatly. There are percentages given between 1.6% and 75% (1-4, 7-9). Also the rate of recurrence of cerebrospinal fluid fistulas differs between 0.5% and 20% (2, 3, 8, 9). For the closure of dural ruptures, the reconstruction of the frontal bone and particularly of the floor of the anterior cranial fossa operative techniques are known (1-4, 6, 8, 9). The first aim of the surgeon is the watertight closure of the dura. If it is impossible autologeous fascia or lyophilised homologeous dura can be used. The fixation of grafts can be assured by fibrin glue. For the reconstruction of frontal bone defects are bone grafts or bone cement in use. The reconstruction of the floor of the anterior cranial fossa is more difficult but possible. Surgical methods using bone grafts or arteficial materials (ceramics) are described (3, 4, 6, 9). Because of the involved paranasal sinuses and therefore impaired mucosal discharge complications (mucocele, pyocele) have to be avoided by a frontoethmoidectomy. The aim of the surgeon also is to achieve optimal drainage from the paranasal air sinuses to the nose.

For the surgery of frontobasal dura ruptures two approaches are known: the transfrontal neurosurgical and the rhinosurgical way through the frontal and ethmoidal air sinuses. Because of the lower operative discomfort, the greater exposure of the anterior cranial fossa and the achievement of the sinus drainage we prefer the rhinosurgical approach for the treatment of frontobasal cerebrospinal fluid fistulas.

During the last three years we operated on 110 patients suffering from a frontal head injury. Surgery was done during the first four weeks after trauma in 74 cases. The other 36 patients were operated on up to 29 years after the injury. An important problem is the reconstruction of the posterior wall of the frontal sinus. 35 cases showed defects of the posterior wall after trauma or fronto-temporal craniotomy. In 17 of these cases a meningocele was seen and in 10 the meningocele had blocked the fronto-nasal duct. The result was a muco- or pyocele. Depending on this finding the posterior wall of the frontal sinus has to be reconstructed. In 29 cases we have carried out a wire osteosynthesis of the anterior or posterior wall of the frontal sinus. Complications were not seen. Without adequate primary treatment of the air sinuses muco- and pyoceles are not infrequent complications. There were 6 during the first year and 21 between the second and 28th year. In 4 cases we found at the operative revision artificial glue (Histoacryl) present the frontal sinus. Macroscopically the lateral recess of the sinus or the frontonasal duct were obliterated. Microscopically severe inflammation and fibrotic tissue were found (Fig. 1). In 70 cases a dura rupture was seen and in other 25 patients bone defects of the anterior cranial fossa could be demonstrated. In comparison to only 51 cases having either rhinorrhoea or early meningitis there is the indication for the operative exploration in every doubtful case.

The rhinosurgical approach allows also the decompression of the optic nerve. Because the bony canal of the optic nerve is the upper-lateral border of the sphenoid sinus it is easy to drill away his medial-inferior bony wall by using a diamond drill. We have done this in 15 patients suffering from a posttraumatic blindness. The function of the optic nerve recovered in 8 cases.

In 23 cases of our patients a large defect of the anterior cranial fossa was found and 15 of them showed a meningocele into the ethmoidal air cells. In these cases we have carried out the reconstruction by the use of heterologous bone grafts. Artificial materials can also be used. After repair of the dura the bone graft has to be individually formed for the patient and is then pushed parallel to the anterior skull base into the sphenoid sinus. The anterior end of the graft is situated on the ethmoidal recess of the maxillary sinus. The empty space between the graft and the skull base can be filled up by a free muscle graft. During the last three years we have carried out 25 of such reconstructions. 22 were unilateral and 3 bilateral. Two complications were seen: a mucocele of the frontal sinus and a dislocation of a bone graft. Histological examinations of graft specimen 3 and 9 months after insertion showed connective tissue formation but no inflammation (Fig. 2).

Our experiences show the advantages of the rhinosurgical approach over the frontal one. There is the possibility for an adequate repair of dural ruptures. Additionally the reconstruction of the anterior skull base and the posterior wall of the frontal sinus, the decompression of the optic nerve and the achievement of an optimal sinus drainage is to carry out at the same operative procedure.

References

1. Boenninghaus, H.G.: Rhinochirurgische Aufgaben bei der Chirurgie des an die Schädelbasis angrenzenden Gesichtsschädels. Arch. Ohr.-Nas.-Kehlk.-Heilk. 207, 1-228 (1974)
2. Boenninghaus, H.G.: Die Behandlung der Schädelbasisbrüche. Stuttgart: Thieme 1960
3. Dietz, H.: Die frontobasale Schädelverletzung. Berlin, Heidelberg, New York: Springer 1970
4. Elies, W.: Rhinoneurochirurgische Aspekte der Nebenhöhlen- und Rhinobasistraumatologie. Arch. Ohr.-Nas.-Kehlk.-Heilk. 223, 455-457 (1979)
5. Fukado, Y.: Results in 350 cases of surgical decompression of the optic nerve. Transact. Ophthal. Soc. NZ 25, 96-99 (1973
6. Jahnke, K.: Zur Rekonstruktion der Frontobasis mit Keramikwerkstoffen. Laryng. Rhinol. 59, 111-115 (1980)

7. Kley, W.: Die Unfallchirurgie der Schädelbasis und der pneumatischen Räume. Arch. klin. exp. Ohr.-Nas.-Kehlk.-Heilk. 191, 1 (1968)
8. Langnickel, R.: Die Bedeutung der operativen Versorgung von Verletzungen der vorderen Schädelgrube durch den Oto-Rhino-Laryngologen. Akt. Traumatol. 5, 221-231 (1975)
9. Probst, Ch.: Frontobasale Verletzungen. Bern: Huber 1971

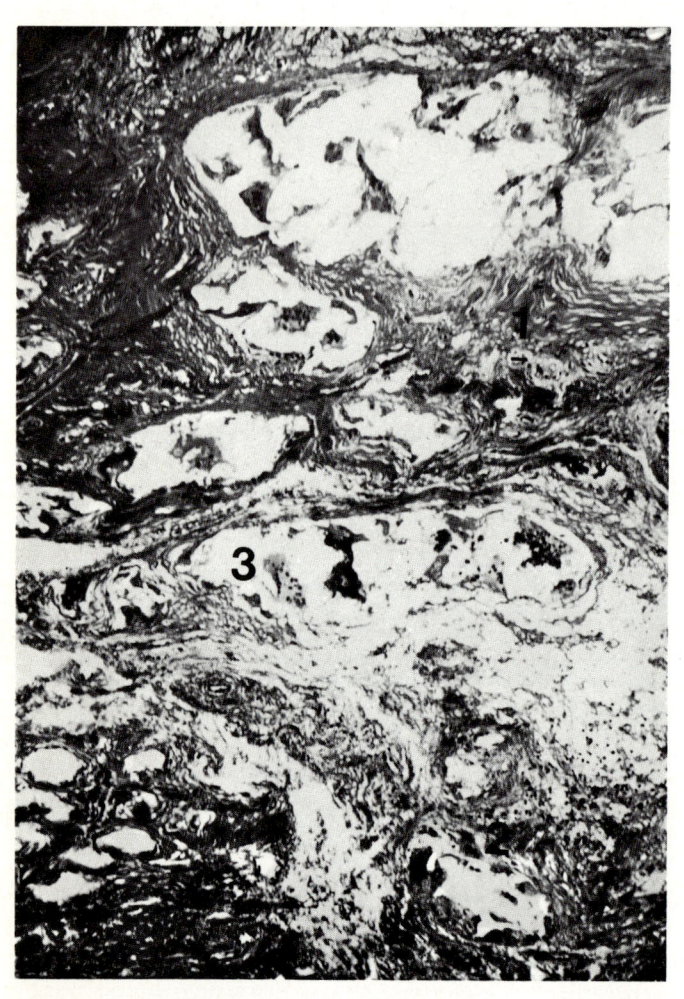

Fig. 1. Mucosa of the frontal sinus 3 years after the use of artificial glue. Connective tissue (1), round cells (2), giant cells (3). HE; 110 x

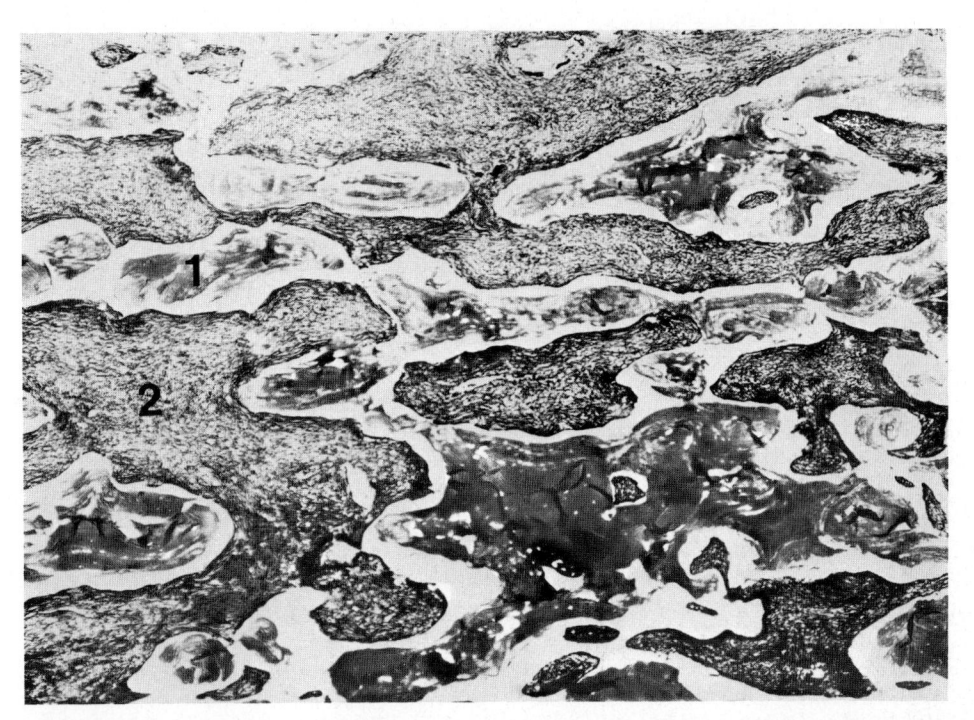

Fig. 2. Histological aspect of a heterologous bone graft 3 weeks after implantation. Heterologous bone (1), connective tissue (2). HE; 62.5 x

Experiences with Microvascular Decompression in the Cerebellopontine Angle in Trigeminal Neuralgia

A. KÜHNER and H. PENZHOLZ

Introduction

Vascular compression of the trigeminal nerve as possible cause of tic douloureux was already discussed by DANDY (4) and somewhat later by GARDNER (6). Single cases of vascular compression in trigeminal neuralgia were reported in the literature (2, 12, 13, 16). This vascular compression theory failed to gain acceptance at the time but the introduction of microsurgery allowed better demonstration of these pathological changes. In 1967 JANETTA (8) advocated microvascular decompression (MDV) as treatment of choice in trigeminal neuralgia. Since that time 14 years have passed and excellent longterm results have been published (9, 10) but still this method encounters a widespread scepticism evoking last but not least the destiny of TAARNHOJ's operation. SWEET himself reported in 1975 (18) that he cut the trigeminal nerve root in a patient despite a clear-cut arterial compression. Only few neurosurgeons, especially in the U.S. (1, 7-11, 14, 17, 19-22) and in Australia (15, 20) adopted this procedure. In the European literature there is only one report concerning this technique (5).

Being of the opinion that no surgical method should be rejected unless it has been proven to be ineffective or too dangerous we started in 1977 with microvascular decompression operations.

Patients

Since 1977 45 consecutive patients have been treated by MVD. Besides 35 cases of typical tic our series includes 6 cases of secondary atypical neuralgias (initially typical neuralgia associated with permanent pain due to previous destructive procedures) and 4 cases of primary atypical facial pain. The ages of these patients ranged from 19 to 82 (!) years and averaged 58 years. Follow-up was obtained in all patients by means of questionnaire or direct examination.

Technique

Our first patients have been operated in the sitting position. Considering air embolism being too great a risk all further patients were operated in the lateral position. The patient's head is fixed in the pin-headrest turned 30 degrees to the ipsilateral side and well flexed. The upper part of the body is slightly elevated. In this position there is no risk of air embolism and gravity retracts the cerebellum. A vertical incision about 8 cm long is made 2 cm beside the mastoid process. A 3 x 3 cm craniectomy is performed in the superolateral part of the posterior fossa and enlarged laterally to the margin of the transverse and sigmoid sinuses. The opened mastoid air cells are waxed. The dura is incised just beneath the sinus extending downwards. The petrosal vein is divided after bipolar coagulation and the arachnoid around the trigeminal nerve is opened. This and all further steps are carried out using the microscope. After aspiration of CSF the cerebellar hemisphere recedes and the Leyla retractor is placed over the superolateral corner of the hemisphere. This high approach facilitates exposure of the trigeminal nerve root. In fact the retractor is only necessary for the exposure of the root entry zone. The trigeminal nerve is carefully inspected, special attention has to be paid to the root entry zone and the lateral surface of the pons. If an artery, considered to compress the nerve, is found, it is gently separated by cutting its arachnoid attachments from the nerve and the surface of the pons. The artery is then mobilized and a small Teflon or muscle pledget is placed between nerve and blood vessel. Compressing veins are coagulated and divided.

Operative Findings

Typical Neuralgia. 36 operations were performed in 35 patients (Table 1). In 18 cases (51%) the superior cerebellar artery (SCA) compressed the nerve which shows an indentation adn a deformation of it's usually straight course (Fig. 1). In 4 cases (11%) a vein gave rise to an unequivocal compression and in 2 others a vein and the SCA compressed the nerve. Usually the vascular compression took place in the "axilla" of the nerve root but in some cases (Fig. 1) it was more laterally. In one case a small angioma compressing the nerve was found. This AVM was localized in the space between the trigeminal nerve and the tentorium and could not be demonstrated on angiography. Arterial or venous contacts without any indentation or deformation of the nerve were found in 7 cases. A tumor was found twice (1 meningioma, 1 cholesteatoma) and in one patient there was only a thickened arachnoid.

Secondary Atypical Neuralgia. 7 operations were executed in 6 patients (Zable 1). In 5 of these originally typical neuralgias we found a clear-cut compression by the SCA, in another a compressing vein perforating and splitting the fascicles in the root entry zone. In the resting case there was a contact with the SCA.

Table 1. Operative findings in 45 cases of trigeminal pain

	Typical tic n = 35	Secondary atypical pain n = 6	Primary atypical pain n = 4
Arterial compression	18	4	2
Venous compression	4	1	1
Arterial and venous compression	2	–	–
Angioma	1	–	–
Tumor	2	–	–
Total compression	27	5	3
%	77 78	83	75
Vascular contact	7	1	1
Arachnoiditis	1	–	–

Primary Atypical Neuralgia. 4 operations were carried out in 4 patients. In 2 of them there was evidence of arterial compression by the SCA and in 1 a vein was thought to compress the nerve. In the 4th patient an arterial contact was found.

Results

After MVD 28 (30%) of 35 patients with typical tic were pain-free at discharge (Table 2). Some of them presented nevertheless some twinges of tic pain in the early postoperative period. 7 patients (20%) were improved, persistent mild tic pain was well controlled by low dosed Carbamazepine (Tegretol). It is of interest to state that 5 of the latter had no compressive lesions (Table 2). In presence of vascular compression 92% of this group were relieved and 8% were improved.

In the group of secondary atypical neuralgias all patients were completely relieved from tic whereas the permanent and/or burning pain persisted.

In the primary atypical group 3 patients had complete relief and one was improved at discharge.

It should be mentioned that despite careful dissection of the trigeminal nerve 17 of 45 patients had some transient sensory loss in the face. This has to be taken into consideration in the evaluation of early results.

Follow-up of our patients ranges from 2 months to 3 1/2 years, averaging 15 months. In this period we observed 4 relapses (12%) in patients with typical tic (Table 2) which all occurred within seven months.

With regard to the operative findings relapses occurred only once (4%) in the presence of a clear-cut vascular compression whereas in the contact group 2 patients out of 7 (29%) had pain recurrence within 6 months and underwent thermorhizotomy.

Table 2. Results of MVD in 35 patients with typical trigeminal neuralgia

Lesion	N	Relief	Improved[a]	Failure	Relapse
Arterial compression	18	16	2	0	1
Venous compression	4	4	0	0	0
Arterial and venous compression	2	2	0	0	0
Angioma	1	1	0	0	0
Total vascular contact	25	23	2	0	1
%	71	66	6	0	4
Vascular contact	7	2	5	0	2
Arachnoiditis	1	1	-	-	1
Tumor	2	2	-	-	0
Total	35	28	7	0	4
%	100	80	20	0	12

Follow-up of all 27 patients with typical tic douloureux due to a compressive lesion is summarized in Table 3. 11 patients are free from tic for more than 1, 6 for more than 2 and 3 of them for more than 3 years. Only one patient had a relapse of mild tic after MVD, controlled by Tegretol. The overall recurrence rate in our series of MVD for typical trigeminal neuralgia is 12%.

Complications

Most of the complications observed concerened cranial nerves and cerebellum (Table 4). There was no mortality. Vertigo was the most frequent complication (22%) followed by diplopia due to trochlear nerve dysfunction (16%) and impairment of ipsilateral hearing (13%). Ataxia occurred in 9% and 2 patients had a facial paresis (4%). All these complications fortunately were transient except decreased ipsilateral hearing persisting more than 6 months in 3 patients. Despite careful and gentle dissection and decompression facial numbness was seen in the early postoperative period in 17 patients (38%). In most cases it disappeared within some weeks but 3 patients reported persisting facial numbness for more than 6 months. This was said to be insignificant and not disturbing. In no case dysesthesia or anesthesia dolorosa occurred.

Our major complication was a spontaneous right frontal intracerebral hematoma which recovered spontaneously. There was no meningitis in spite of CSF leaks from the wound in 3 cases.

Table 3. Follow-up of 27 patients with typical neuralgia due to compressive lesions

Type of compression		≤ 3 months	6 - 12 months	12 - 24 months	24 - 39 months
Vascular	Relief	23	17	11	6
n = 25	Improved	2	1	0	0
	Relapse	0	1	0	0
Tumor	Relief	2	1		
n = 2	Relapse	0	0		
Total	27	27	20	11	6

Table 4. Complications of MVD in 45 cases

Type of complication	n	%	>6 months
Diplopia (N. IV)	7	16	0
Numbness (N.V)	17	38	3
Facial palsy	2	4	0
Hearing impairment	6	13	3
Vertigo	10	22	0
Ataxia	4	9	0
CSF leak	3	7	0
Hematoma (frontal)	1	2	spontaneous recovered
Mortality	0	0	

Discussion

Our personal experience confirms previous reports of operative findings and results of MVD in trigeminal neuralgia. An unequivocal vascular compression was found in 71% of our patients with typical tic douloureux and thus compares favorably with the rate of 72.5% reported by HAINES (7). In all of our cases the offending artery was the SCA, a compression by the AICA as reported by others (1, 7-9) was not observed in our series. The analysis of 252 published cases reveals a frequency of arterial compression of 64%. Venous compressions are less frequent as shown by the analysis of 204 reported cases with 19% of venous compressions. In our series we observed venous compressions in 11%; HAINES (7) reported 12.5%. It is interesting to state that 5 of our 6 patients with secondary atypical neuralgia presented a clear-cut vascular compression too. Besides vascular compressions we had 2 tumors and 1 angioma in our series. Similar observations were reported (1, 9).

Complete relief of tic pain at discharge was seen in 80% of our series the other patients were improved with substantial reduction in the intensity of pain and easily controlled on small doses of Carbamazepine. In the literature 200 of 219 patients (91%) of a compiled series were reported to be pain-free at discharge.

It is interesting to state that all our patients with secondary atypical pain are reported to be free of tic pain after MVD. This experience reinforces our conviction of the pathogenetic significance of vascular compressions.

The long term recurrence rate in our series is 12% and compares favorably with other reports (1, 19, 22). For a (compiled) series of 200 published cases 13 recurrences (7%) within the first year were reported. In a smaller (compiled) series of 95 patients 11 (12%) had relapses within 2 years. JANETTA (10) reported 11% of relapses within the first 6 months just as in our series. Some authors had no recurrences within the first year (5, 11, 15, 17, 20).

When dealing with results and relapses of MVD in tic pain it is of interest to correlate operative findings and results. In presence of clear-cut vascular cross-compressions we had better results (92% relief) and less relapses (4%) than in those cases where only a vascular contact was found (29% relief and relapses respectively). Similar experiences are reported (19), whereas the pathogenetic role of vascular compression is admitted by all authors. In our experience the role of vascular contacts is difficult to emphasize. Our relatively poor results might be due to inadequate decompression but it has also to be discussed if vascular contacts really may cause trigeminal neuralgia. Others (19) are convinced that vascular contacts are not responsible for tic pain and advocate partial root section in these cases.

Performed by a skilled microneurosurgeon MVD has low morbidity and no mortality. In our series and those of others (1, 11, 20, 22) totalizing 140 cases there was no mortality. In JANETTA's (10) series of 450 patients 4 (0.9%) died from intracranial complications, but there was no mortality in his last 200 cases (10). One of DUPLAY's (5) 16 patients died from myocardial infarction in the early postoperative period (we had a similar case after thermorhizotomy).

A complication not mentioned in the literature was frequent in our series: 10 patients had disturbing vertigo within the first week.

Diplopia and acoustic nerve dysfunction were typical complications and are also reported by others (1, 5, 10, 20-22). These dysfunctions are generally transient, but 3 of our patients reported permanent impairment of hearing. In JANETTA's (10) series this occurred in 0.9%. Transient facial paresis is rare but was present in 2 of our patients, similar cases are reported in the literature (1, 5). Cerebellar dysfunction occurred in 4 of our patients and in 2 of APFELBAUM's (1) series. All these transient cranial nerve dysfunctions are probably due to traction damage. We observed no meningitis and no wound infection. A particular complication was reported by WILSON (22): in 2 of his patients a CSF rhinorrhea via the mastoid air cells occurred.

There is no doubt that this procedure is safe and has low morbidity if some guide lines are respected: this operation should be left to neurosurgeons properly trained in microsurgical techniques. Correct positioning of the patient is very important. We prefer like others (20, 22) the lateral decubitus position although others (1, 8, 11, 17) favor the sitting position. The absence of risk of air embolism is in our opinion an advantage of the former. On the other hand the cerebellar hemisphere recedes better laterally in the lateral position minimizing thus the risk of pressure damage of the cerebellum. The root entry zone can only be correctly visualized if the head is turned about 30 degrees to the ipsilateral side. Craniectomy has to be carried up to the transverse sinus and laterally to the margin of the sigmoid sinus.

What can we tell a patient to whom we offer MVD? In our experience there is a 27% chance of finding the responsible lesion and an 80% chance of pain relief. Compressive lesions are to be expected in about 77% with pain relief in 93%. The recurrence rate in this group is 4%.

Conclusion

The posterior fossa microvascular decompression seems to be an ideal method for relief of trigeminal neuralgia without the indesirable side-effect of permanent facial numbness, paresthesias or anesthesia dolorosa which are a disagreable and sometimes disabling feature of destructive methods. This is especially true when compressive lesions are found, since we had better results and less relapses in this group. The pathogenetic role of vascular contacts is, in our opinion, obscure and warrants continuing trial and discussion.

The follow-up of our series is too short to allow the procedure to be considered curative, but our experience confirms previous reports in all aspects. The absence of mortality and the low morbidity authorizes us to offer this operation to all patients in good general condition, especially to younger ones.

References

1. Apfelbaum, R.I.: A comparison of percutaneous radiofrequency trigeminal neurolysis and microvascular decompression of the trigeminal nerve for the treatment of tic douloureux. Neurosurg. 1, 16-21 (1977)
2. Broager, B.: Transtentorial trigeminotomy at the pons - three cases of arterial root compression. Acta Neurol. Scand. 44, 257 (1968)

3. Constans, J.P. et al.: Anèvrysme géant du tronc basilaire révelé par une névralgie faciale essentielle. Neuro-Chirurgie 22, 493-502 (1976)
4. Dandy, W.E.: Concerning the cause of trigeminal neuralgia. Am. J. Surg. 24, 447-455 (1934)
5. Duplay, J. et al.: Contribution à la chirurgie non mutilante de la névralgie faciale essentielle. Neuro-Chirurgie 20, 593-598 (1974)
6. Gardner, W.S., Miklos, M.V.: Response of trigeminal neuralgia to decompression of sensory root. JAMA 170, 1773-1776 (1959)
7. Haines, S.J., Janetta, P.J., Zorub, D.S.: Microvascular relations of the trigeminal nerve. J. Neurosurg. 52, 381-386 (1980)
8. Janetta, P.J.: Arterial compression of the trigeminal nerve at the pons in patients with trigeminal neuralgia. J. Neurosurg. 26, 159-162 (1967)
9. Janetta, P.J.: Observations on trigeminal neuralgia, hemifacial spasm, acoustic nerve dysfunction and glossopharyngeal neuralgia. Neurochirurgia 20, 145-154 (1977)
10. Janetta, P.J.: Treatment of trigeminal neuralgia. Viewpoint. Neurosurgery 4, 93-94 (1979)
11. Kelly, D.L.: Posterior fossa neurovascular decompression for tic douloureux and hemifacial spasm. N. Carol. Med. J. 38, 534-536 (1977)
12. Kempe, L.G., Smith, D.R.: Trigeminal neuralgia, facial spasm, intermedius and glossopharyngeal neuralgia with persistent carotid basilar anastomosis. J. Neurosurg. 31, 445-451 (1969)
13. Kuhlendahl, H.: Versuch einer Begründung der Pathologie der Neuralgie. Habilitationsschrift, Düsseldorf (1953)
14. Nugent, G.R.: Discussion of Apfelbaum's paper. Neurosurgery 1, 21 (1977)
15. Petty, P.G., Southby, R.: Vascular decompression of the lower cranial nerves: observations using the microscope with particular reference to trigeminal neuralgia. Aust. N. Z. J. Surg. 47, 314 (1977)
16. Provost, J., Hardy, J.: Microchirurgie tu trijumeau. Anatomie fonctionelle. Neuro-Chirurgie 16, 459-470 (1970)
17. Rhoton, A.L.: Microsurgical neurovascular decompression for trigeminal neuralgia and hemifacial spasm. J. Florida MA 65, 425-428 (1978)
18. Sweet, W.H.: Percutaneous differential thermal trigeminal rhizotomy for the management of facial pain. Adv. Neurosurg. 3, 274-286 (1975)
19. Tarlov, E.: Percutaneous and open microsurgical techniques for relief of refractory tic douloureux. Surg. Clin. N. Am. 60, 593-630 (1980)
20. Weidmann, M.J.: Trigeminal neuralgia. Surgical treatment by microvascular decompression of the trigeminal nerve root. Med. J. Aust. 2, 628-630 (1979)
21. Wilkins, R.H.: Discussion of Apfelbaum's paper. Neurosurgery 1, 21 (1977)
22. Wilson, C.B. et al.: Microsurgical vascular decompression for trigeminal neuralgia and hemifacial spasm. West. J. Med. 132, 481-484 (1980)

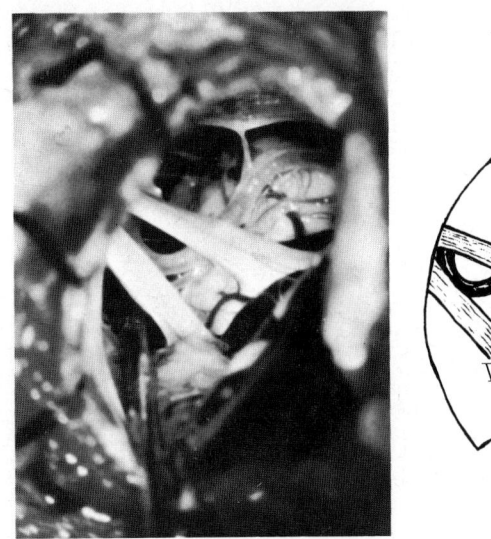

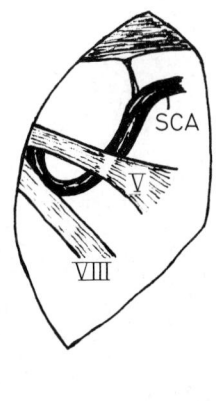

Fig. 1. Compression of the trigeminal nerve by the SCA *(left)*.
Same case, schematic drawing *(right)*

Spondylitis – A Complication Following Lumbar Disc Operations
M. Klinger

From 1962 till 1977 a total of 1289 lumbar disc operations were performed at the Neurochirurgische Universitätsklinik Erlangen. In 9 of these patients spondylitis was found to occur, so that an incidence of 0.7% may be calculated. In comparison to the data in the literature where the incidence ranges from 0.2% - 4.0%, this incidence of 0.7% is quite low. Particularly interesting is the fact that spondylitis did not occur in the first 9 years of this 15-year-period, this complication has been diagnosed repeatedly since 1972.

Spondylitis is an inflammatory lesion originating in the intervertebral space and leading to an erosion of the surface of the lumbar vertebra. A displacement of the vertebral bodies in relationship to each other, leading to spondylolisthesis, is often observed. In view of the slow metabolism in this region, the process of healing is very protracted. Healing of this lesion leads to block formation of the two vertebral bodies.

The characteristic symptom is the occurrence of postoperative pain in the lumbar spine. Every movement, even the slightest, causes almost intolerable pain. Because this clinical entity is rather rare, it is often not thought of and the hospital personnel often do not believe the intensity of the patient's pain. For this reason, our first patient with this clinical syndrome was initially thought to be a hypochondriac.

Examination always reveals a decreased mobility in the lumbar spine and massive muscular spasm. Furthermore, the affected lumbar segments are extremely sensitive to pressure. There is no change in the neurological status. In 5 of our 9 patients, the increase in lumbar pain occurred right after the operation, in the other four patients the deterioration became apparent 2 - 5 weeks later. The majority of the patients had fever with temperatures from 38°C to 39.5°C.

Although the number of leucocytes was never raised in the postoperative phase, there was always a massive rise in the erythrocyte sedimentation rate (ESR). This rise in the ESR is a relatively early parameter which occurs within the first two weeks after operation. In all our cases the ESR in the second hour was always 100 or over (Table 1).

The final diagnosis can be made only with the help of X-rays. However, these changes cannot be seen until the third week at the earliest and usually only after a period of 6 weeks. The time relationship between the clinical picture indicating the onset of pain and the radiological changes is seen in Fig. 1.

Table 1. Clinical findings in cases of spondylitis

Case	Fever	Raised ESR	Positive X-ray	Delayed healing of wound	Cystitis
1	+	+	+		+
2	+	+	+		+
3	+	+	+		
4		+	+		
5		+	+	+	+
6		+	+		
7	+	+	+		
8	+	+	+	+	+
9		+	+		
	5	9	9	2	5

The typical radiological changes can be seen in the case of a 48-year-old woman, who was operated for a lumbar disc compressing the fifth lumbar nerve root. First the bony contour at the ventral border of the affected intervertebral disc became indistinct (Fig. 2). Then the bony structure of the adjacent vertebral body is eroded in its ventral part. As a rule the upper vertebral body is affected first, but both of the adjacent vertebral bodies may show signs of inflammation simultaneously (Fig. 3). Later the two vertebral bodies are shifted in relation to each other, resulting in a spondylolisthesis. When the acute inflammatory phase is over, the outer border of the inflammation is seen as a sclerotic line in the vertebral body. Finally there is bony scar formation in the intervertebral disc and the two vertebral bodies form a single bony block (Fig. 4).

Treatment consists of absolute bed rest in a plaster cast for the duration of the entire process. The state of the infection may be monitored by the ESR rates which are estimated at weekly intervals. An antibiotic with good penetration into bone, such as Cillimycin is given as a rule, although the bacterial etiology of the inflammation is not proven in the majority of cases, the exception being one case of spinal empyema.

Of special interest is the question of predisposing factors. A review of the clinical data of our nine patients revealed an already raised ESR in the preoperative stage. Furthermore cystitis was found to be present in 4 patients at the time of operation (see Table 1) and in two of these delayed wound healing occurred in the postoperative phase. Thus the presence of an infection at a different site in the body seems to predispose to postoperative spondylitis.

Possibly older patients have a higher chance of having spondylitis as seven of our nine patients were over the age of 40.

These clinical observations again raise the question if there is a correlation between a preoperative infection such as a cystitis and postoperative spondylitis especially in patients over the age of 40.

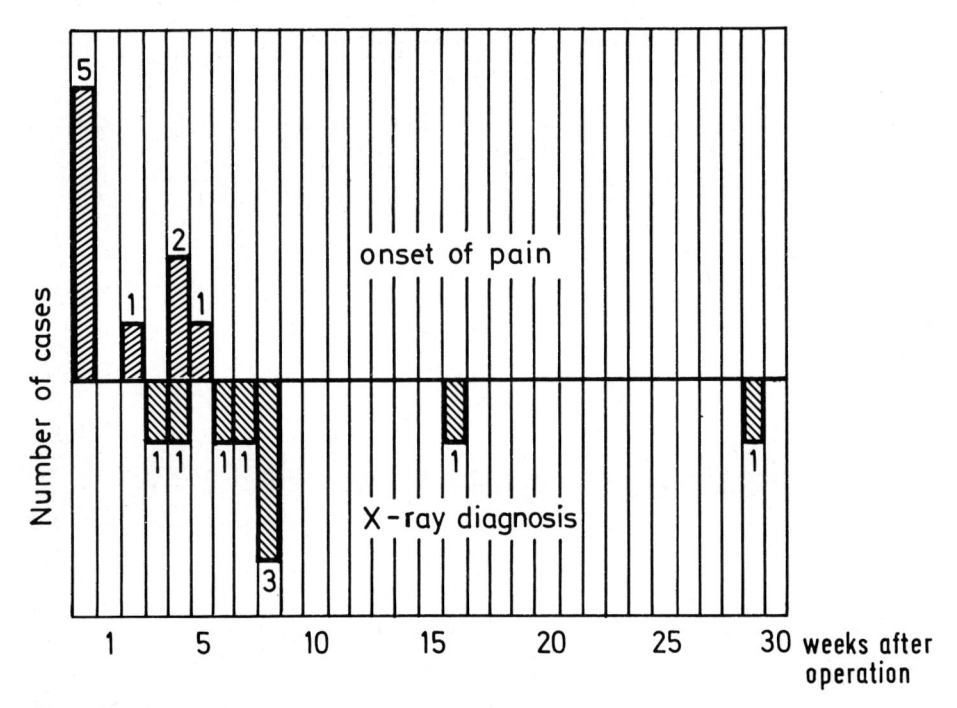

Fig. 1. Relationship of clinical to radiological symptomatology

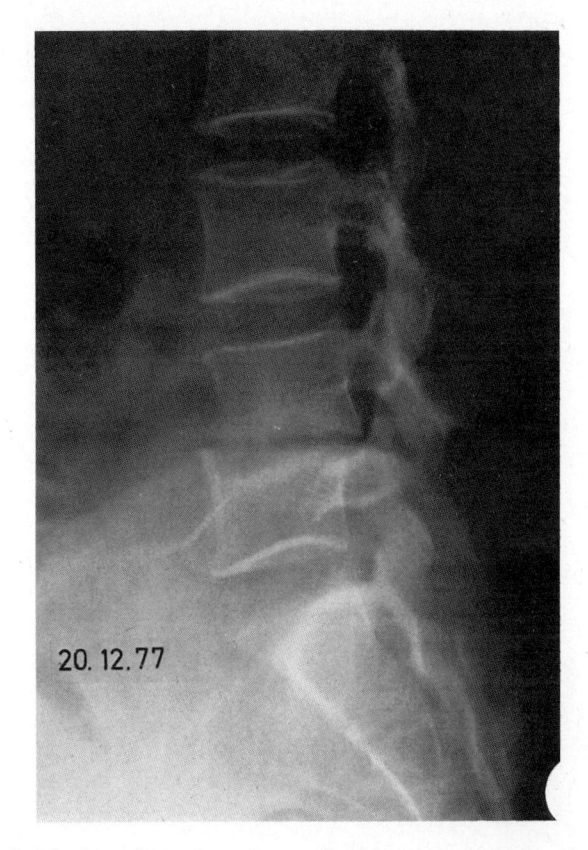

Fig. 2. Initial signs of spondylitis with erosion of the upper ventral portion of the fifth lumbar vertebrae below the lumbar disc which had been operated on 6 weeks before

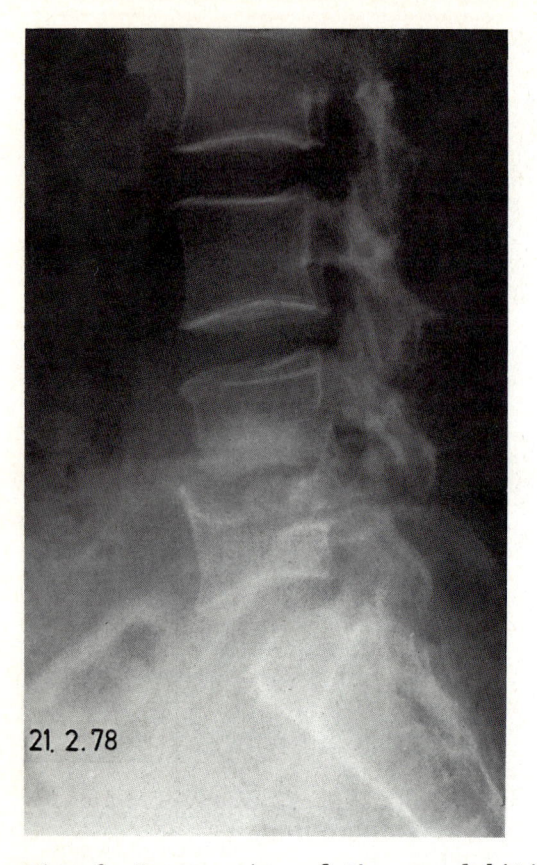

Fig. 3. Progression of the spondylitis (12.2.1978) with erosion of the fifth lumbar vertebrae below the operated intervertebral disc (Courtesy of Dr.Persch, Gunzenhausen)

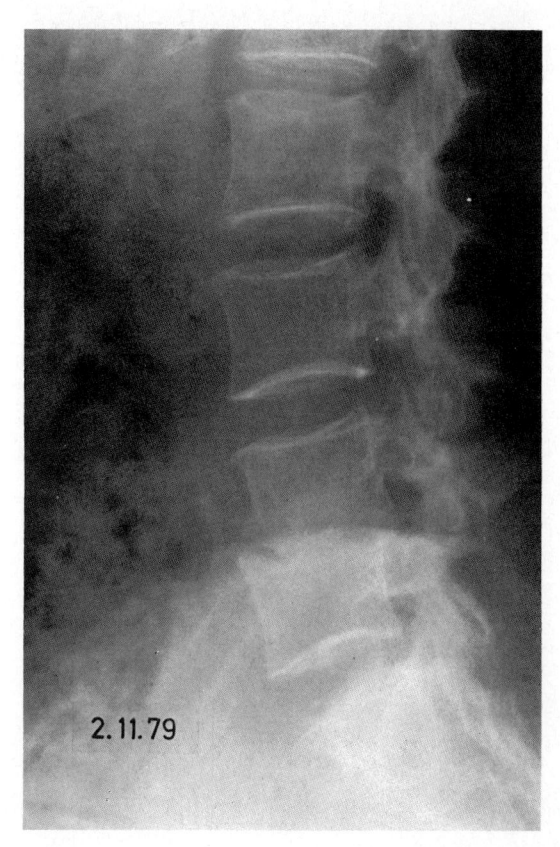

Fig. 4. Two years later (2.11.1979) the inflammation has subsided and the two vertebral bodies heal together into a single bony block (Courtesy of Dr.Persch, Gunzenhausen)

Subject Index

accident, traffic 275
accumulation, intracranial 149
accuracy, diagnostic 34
acidosis, metabolic 238
ADP 230
aeroembolism check, Doppler
 sonographic 52
alloplastic material 280
alterations, perifocal glial 27
AMP 230
anastomosis 145,340,344
-, microvascular 340
anesthesia dolorosa 391
aneurysm 208
- of anterior communicating artery
 135
- of basilar artery 136
-, carotid, diagnostic evidence
 44
-, cerebral, diagnosis and postoperative observation 132-138
-, demonstration by CT 133
-, localization 132
- of middle cerebral artery 133
- of supraclinoid carotid artery
 133
angioma 387
angiogram, preoperative 133
angiography 121,183,200,333,334
antibiotics 214,395
anticoagulants 293
apex, petrous 44,46
appallic syndrom 222-228
approach, basal 56
-, interhemispheric 58,63
-, lateral 55
-, medial 56
-, operative 80
-,-, rostral brain stem 57-63
-, pterional 57,59
-, subtemporal 58,59
-, transcallosal 59

-, unilateral 55
arachnoiditis 388
arteriovenous angioma 120,129
artery, superior cerebellar 387
arthritis, rheumatoid 288
astrocytoma 3,5
- of brain, seizures 5
atacia 389
atelextasis 266
atherosclerosis 340
ATP 230,238
atrophy, cortical 160

barbiturate 259-265
base ring 17
--, stereotactic 20,22
biopsy of the brain 25-32
-, stereotactic 27
bleeding, intracerebral 148
-, traumatic intracerebral, extent
 of brain damage 113
-,--, mortality rate 113
-,--, state of consciousness 113
-,--, surgery 112-116
-,--,- contraindicated 113
-,--,- indicated 113
blindness 383
blood-brain barrier 138,189,191,
 208
blood volume cerebral 266
body, vertebral 395
bone, cement 324
-, chip 279
-, graft 279, 24,383
brain abscess 214-221
-,-, diagnosis 73-79
-,-, puncture 73,74
-,-, surgery 74
-,-, treatment 73-79
-,-,-, aspiration 76
-,-,-, conservative 74

brain death 201
--, neuroendocrinological aspects 200-202
- edema 209,214-221,278,302,316, 350,357
--, cell volume 254-258
- stem lesion 47-51
--, rostral, operative approaches 57-63
--, spontaneous 47-51
- tumors, deep-seated 64-72
burn, cerebral edema after 236-243
burning, experimental 237
B-waves, correlation with PVI 166
- and periventricular lucency 164-172
bypass, extra-intracranial 333-339,340

calcification 34
carbamazepine 390
cardiac output 378
catecholamine 236,239
catheter, ventricular 176
-,-, revisions 177
cauda equina 275,281
cell, glial 254
central cord destruction 302
cerclage 324
cerebellum 391
cerebral blood flow 189,190, 216,259,333-339
- metabolic rate 190
cerebroside 208
cerebrospinal fluid 245,387
--, circulation 368
--, reduced absorption 160
cerebrovascular disease, classification 140
--, indication and timing of operation 139,140
--, operative treatment 169-146
- resistance 230
cerebroside 208
cervical spine 279,287,299,305-311, 322
chloride 256
cholesteatoma 387
-, primary 43
cholesterol 208
chordoma 287
chromatography 209

circulatory arrest 259
cisternography, CT 41
-, metrizamide 36
clearance, Kr^{85} 206
clivus 287,289
clot 344
coagulation 293
collapse of spongiosa 283
collection, subdural 186
column, vertebral 275,281
compliance, intracranial 367
complications, recognition of postoperative 147
compression 308,316
computerized tomography 1-186
consolidation, bone 280
construction of tumor on X-ray and scalp 16
content fluid 237
contusion, space-occupying 112
coordinate 20
-, base ring 17
-, CT 17
-, stereotactic 19
cortex, adrenal 249
-, brain, oxygen supply during hypocapnie 229-235
cortisol 248,249
cranio-cervical dysplasia 287
Crutchfield extension 312
CSF drainage, follow-up studies 147-155
-, Leskell 350
-, ventriculoperitoneal 348
CT, functional indication 17,20
-, non-functional indication 17,20
- parameters of brain tumors 33
- scan, coronal scout view 22
--, false negative 8
--,- positive 9
--, misinterpretation 27
- stereotaxy 19
cushion, intimal 341
cyst 38
- arachnoidal 36
-, intracranial 36-41
-, retrosellar 40
-, suprasellar 39
cystitis 395

damage of root 281
decompression in trigeminal neuralgia 386-393

-, overrapid 177
dehydration 177
dementia 164
dexamethasone 248,357
diagnosis, preoperative, brain tumor 33-35
-, radiological 183-186
diaphanoscopy 344-347
dinucleotide 214
diplopia 389,391
disc, herniated 299
-, intervertebral 250,277,281, 306,395
-, lumbar 394-399
dislocation 275,278,305
-, fracture 281,312-314,316,324
disturbance of consciousness 169
-, gait 164,165,169
duct, frontonasal 383

edema of the brain 209,214-221, 278,302,316,350,357
--, cell volume 254,258
-, cerebral 244,248
-,- following burns, sodium, potassium, magnesium and zinc 236-243
-, cytotoxic 254
-, fluid 215
-, intimal 341
-, vasogenic 254
EIAB 141
elasticity 368
electrolyte concentration 238
embolism 222,386
-, pulmonary 316
empyema of the interhemispheric fissure 78
-, spinal 385
-, subdural, diagnosis 73-79
-,-, effusion 75
-,-, puncture 74,75
-,-, surgery 75
-,-, treatment 73-79
encephalitic reaction 77
encephalitis 77
endarterectomy, carotid 139,141
endothelium 344
energy, oxidative 256
enhancement, metrizamide 36,37
enzyme, hydrolytic 260,262
ependymoma 350
epinephrine 222

fixation, dorsal 306,323
fluid collection, subdural 186
fossa, anterior cranial 382-385
-, middle cranial, base 43
-,--, schematic representation 45
-, rhomboid 348
Fourier transformation 372
fracture 108
-, compression 281,299,312-314, 324
-, fragment 281
-, hangman 305
-, mobile 305
-, skull 112
free radical 262
frontonasal duct 383
fundoscopic examination 176
fusion, cervical, transoral 287-292

gangrene, cerebral 75
gantry, CT 21
gas gangrene, cerebral 75
gibbus 308
Glasgow-Coma Scale 101,105
glioblastoma 3,4,254
-, perifocal edema 5
- statistics 4
gliosis 350
glucocorticoids 214
glucose 189,214-221
glycosyl-ceramide 210
glucuronidase, β- 260
glue, fibrin 382
glutamic acid 254
glycolipid 208
glycolysis 215
gradient, ion 254
graft, bone 279,324,383

Harrington method 281-286
headache in meningioma 5
heart function 222
hemangioma, cavernous 117,125,130
hemangioendothelioma, malignant 120
hematoma 279
-, absorption 87
-, bilateral subdural 99
-, cerebellar 84
-, chronic subdural, CT-follow-up 95-110

hematoma, chronic, preoperative
   CT 98
-, CT 129
-, deep-lying 115
-, epidural 91,293
-, extradural 101-107
-,-, chronic 101
-,- with delayed course, surgical
   treatment 108-111
-,-, mortality 103,105
-,-, surgically treated 110
-, giant 112,116
-, intracerebral 91,389
-, multiple 112,115
-, radicular 277
-, solitary 114
-, spinal epidural 293-298
-, spontaneous intracerebral,
   atypical 85
-,--, classification of neurological status 86
-,--, CT-era 85
-,--, mortality 84,85,87
-,--,- and age 89
-,--, operative mortality 86,87,
   90-92,102,103
-,--, pre-CT-era 85
-,--, prognosis 86
-,--, results of operative treatment 86
-,--, treatment 84-89
-,--, typical 85
-, subdural 91,367
-, supratentorial 84
-, traumatic intracerebral 113
-,--, frequency of diagnostic
   methods 93
-,-,--, influence of the CT scan
   103
-,--, postoperative outcome 90
-,--, prognosis 90-94
-,--, survival rate 90
hematomyelia 300
hemoglobin 229
hemorrhage 275,278
-, diapedetic 302
-, fatal intracerebral, cryptic
   nature 117
-, intracerebral 149
-, massive brain stem 50
-, neonatal intracranial 174
-, spontaneous intracranial, due
   to aneurysms 132
-, subdural 210

histamine 236
hormone, adenocorticotrophic 248
-, follicle-stimulating 248,250
-, growth 248,249
-, human prolactin 201,202
-, luteinizing 201,202,248,249
-, releasing 201,202
hydrocephalus 367
-, communicating 173
-,-, idiopathic 174
-,-, post-meningitis 174,180
-, intermittent pressure 164
-, intermittently normotensive
   164
-, internus 348
-, malresorptive 133,209
- with myelomeningocele 173,174
-, normal course, etiology 157,
   160
-,- pressure, B-waves and periventricular lucency 164-172
-,--, clinical and CT follow-up
   156-163
-,--, clinical improvement 157,
   160
-,--,- outcome 156-163
-,--, correlation between clinical
   response and ventricular size
   159,160,162,163
-,--,- with CT 156-163
-,--, CT follow-up studies 159
-,--, etiological factor 159
-,--, following trauma 159
-,--, idiopathic 157-165
-,--, importance of periventricular lucency 165
-,--, posttraumatic 163
-,--, preoperative test 165
-,--, ventricular size 156-163
-, obstructive 173
-,-, idiopathic 174
-, occlusive 153
-, overshunting 149
-, posthemorrhagic 138
-, post-meningitis 181
-, postoperative complications
   149
-, undershunting 149
hypalgesia 299
hypercapnia 190
hyperextension 299
hyperglycemia 238
hyperventilation 229,230
hypesthesia 299

hypocapnia 229-235
-, arterial 190
-, oxygen supply in brain cortex 229-235
hypotension 203-207
-, systemic 206,207
hypoxemia, arterial 191
hypoxia 259
hypoxydosis 222

impedance, cerebral 254
impression, basilar 287
incontinence, urinary 164,165
index, cardiac 378
-, Huckman 156
-, pressure-volume 166
-, stroke work 378
infarct, cerebral 139
infarction, brain stem 47,48
infection 148,367
injection, bolus 368,372
injury, anoxic 257
-, brain 262
-,-, neuroendocrinological aspects 200-202
-, head 102,378,379
-,-, dexamethasone and radioimmuno-assay 244-247
-, open 277
-,-, sphingolipids 208-213
-, severe brain 202
-, spinal 277,278,299-304
insulin 238
intimal cushion 341
ion activity, extracellular 205
-, sodium 256
ischemia 259,333
-, cerebral 254

joint, interpedicular 282

kyphosis 281,314

lactate 215,229
laminectomy 279,282,308,312,323
-, decompression 277
lesion, avascular 120
-, calcified 121
-, experimental cold 259-265
-, hypodense 139

ligamentum flavum 299
lipoprotein 260
lucency, periventricular 176
luxation 278,308
lysosome 260

magnesium 236-243
malformation, angiomatous 117
-, cerebrovascular, CT 119
-,-, clinical findings 118
-,-, pathology 119
-, cryptic cerebrovascular 117-131
-,--, usefulness and limitation of CT 117
-, Dandy-Walker 37
-, vascular 293
-, venous 293
marking external 11
mastoid 386
medulla oblongata 316
medulloblastoma 348
meningioma 3,387
-, diagnostic evidence 44
-, headache 5
- statistics 5
meningitis 210,382
mental disorder 165,169
metabolism oxidative 189-199
metastases, cerebral 80
-, intracranial 80-83
6-methylprednisolone 357-366
metrizamide CT 36-41
-- cisternography 36,37
- enhancement 36
microcephaly 177
microelectrode 204
microvascular decompression 386-393
monitoring, intracranial pressure 177
mucocele 382
myelin 208
myelitis, acute 293
myelography 276

narrow spinal canal 302
necrosis, hemorrhagic 302,316
neomycin sulfate 75
nerve, trigeminal 386,387
neuralgia, atypical 386,388
-, trigeminal, microvascular decompression in cerebellopontine angle 386-393

neurinoma, diagnostic evidence   44
neuroblastoma   254
neurolysis   283
neurotraumatology   112
norepinephrine   222

obliquity, alemannic   13
occlusion, carotid artery   146
odontoid   287,288,305,306
oligodendroglioma   3
-, seizures   5
osmolarity   256
osteosynthesis   306
overdrainage   147,173
overmanipulation, iatrogenic   177
oxygen consumption   254,378
- debt   257
- uptake   230
oxygenation   230
-, hyperbaric   75,141

pain   390,394
-, facial   386
paraparesis   275
paraplegia   275,277,278,294,308
paresis, facial   389
pentobarbital   260
perfusion, cerebral   204,333
-, ventriculo-cisternal   257
perifocal edema, glioblastoma   5
periventricular lucency   176
permeability, membrane   256,257
-, vessel   236
pH, extracellular   206
phosphocreatine   230
phospholipid   262
pons   387
posterior fossa, CT localization
   52-56
--, operative approach   52-56
potassium   236,243
- activity, extracellular   207
pressure, carbon dioxide   229
-, cerebral perfusion   189
-, epidural   368
-, intracranial   259,266,348,367-
   377,378-381
-,-, measurement   165
-,-, monitoring   1-7
- negative   177
- recording, continuous   166
prolactin, human   202

prolapse, disc   248,278,306
prolonged reversible ischemic
   neurological, deficit   139
pseudarthrosis   277,305
pseudospecificity of CT   27
pseudo-tumor, inflammatory   9
prostaglandin   236
pulse amplitude   371,372
- pressure, ratio   166
- rate   266
pump, sodium-potassium   238
puncture, lumbar   293,368
-, stereotactic   19
PVL, preoperative   171
pyocele   382
pyruvate   215,229,230

radicular syndrome   277,323
radiculopathy, traumatic   313
radioimmunoassay   200
reference point   12
--, brain tumor projection   13
--, head   13
--, skull, X-ray   11
rehabilitation   275,277
reposition, surgical   305
resistance, cerebrovascular   230
resorption rate   86
retention, urinary   299
retrobulbar lesion   9
rhinorrhea   382,383,391
rhythm, circadian   224
-,- of catecholamines, cortisol
   and prolactin in apallic syndrome   222-228
ring, stereotactic   20,22
root damage   281
-, lumbar nerve   395
-, spinal nerve   302
rupture, dural   383

scalp, construction of tumor   16
scanning, coronal   81
scaphocephaly   177
sclerosis, multiple   210
scoliosis   281
seizures, astrocytomas of brain   5
-, oligodendroglioma   5
-, psychomotor   5
shunt, pulmonary   378
- response   165
-, time interval between insertion
   and complications   152

shunting, cerebrospinal fluid 164, 170
sinus, frontal 382
-, paranasal air 382
-, sagittal 229
-, sigmoid 391
sitting position 52
slit ventricle 173-182
sodium 236-243,257
- nitroprusside 203,206,207
sonography, Doppler 333
space, dead 266-271
-, epidural 378
-, extracellular 254
-, intervertebral 394
spasm, muscular 394
sphingolipids, head injury 208-213
sphingomyelin 208
spinal cord 275,276,281
spine, cervical 279,287,299,305-311,322
-, lumbar 279,394
spondylarthritis 302
spondylitis 394-399
spondylodesis 282,306
spondylolisthesis 394,395
spondylosis 302
spongiosa 282
spots, café-au-lait 120
stabilization 278
-, dorsal 305
-, ventral 324
staphylococcus aureus 214
steal 334
stenosis, aqueduct 174
stereotactic device, CT scanner gantry 21
stereotaxy 17-24
-, advantages of 20
-, functional 18
-,- indications 19
-, non-functional indications 19
stress 250
-, surgical 248
stroke 333
-, completed 139,141
stump, vessel 340
subluxation 275,312-314,323
sulfatide 208
surgery stereotactic 17-24
survival, time 259
swelling 256
-, brain 107,245

-, cell 257
symptoms, onset 3
syringiomyelia 371
system, hypothalamic-pituitary 201,202

target point 20
tear, dural 382
test, pressure-volume 367
testosterone 248,249
tetraparesis 288,289
tetraplegia 299
thermorhizotomy 388
thrombus 344,345
thyrotropin 201
tic douloureux 389
transducer 372
transient ischemic attack 139
transillumination 344
transoral fusion of cervical vertebrae 287-292
transverse lesion 323
--, cord 323
trauma, cervical 315-321
-, head 103
trepanation, basal 53
-, lateral suboccipital 52
-, medial suboccipital 53
-, pterional 61
-, unilateral suboccipital 53
trigeminal neuralgia, microvascular decompression 386-393
trimetaphan camsylate 203,206,207
tumor, brain 8,11-16
-,-, CT parameter 33
-,-, deep-seated, operation 64-72
-,-, diagnosis 34
-,-, earlier diagnosis 3-6
-,-, preoperative diagnosis 33-35
-,-, projection, reference points 13
-,- stem 66
-,-, suspected 7-10
-, cerebellopontine 348
-, cerebral 244
-, construction on X-ray and scalp 16
-, deep-seated 14,66,68
-, gliomatous, diagnosis 29
- localization 11
--, transfer from X-ray to scalp 12

tumor of middle cranial fossa,
   diagnosis   42-46
-, occipital   14
-, parietal   14
- parts, ring-shaped   34
-, retrobulbar   7-10
-, ring-shaped   34
-, temporal   14

unconcsciousness, prolonged   91
underdrainage   147
uptake, oxygen   230
urinary retention   299

valves, contrast medium study
   177
valvulography   176
vascular brain stem   47
---, etiology   48
---, mortality   48
vascularity   34
vasodilatation   230
vasoregulation   372
vein, petrosal   387
ventilation, mechanical   378,379
vertebra   394

vertigo   390
ventriculocisternostomy   348
ventriculogram   183
ventriculography   186
ventriculostomy   41

water content   215

X-ray, computational transfer
   of CT findings   12
-, construction of tumor   16
-, CT findings   11
-, reconstruction of CT layers
   11
-,- on deep-seated tumors   14
-,- on occipital tumors   14
-,- on parietal tumors   14
-,- on temporal tumors   14
-, skull, reference point   11
-, transfer   11
-,- of CT layers   12
-,- of tumor localization to
   scalp   12

zinc   236-243

Modern Neurosurgery

Editor: M. Brock

1982. Approx. 158 figures, 95 tables.
Approx. 500 pages
ISBN 3-540-10972-2

Contents: Technical Developments. – Head Injuries. Intensive Care. – Chemotherapy of Brain Tumours. – Surgery of the Pituitary Region. – Surgery of Ventricular Tomours. – Spinal Cord. – Reconstructive Vascular Surgery. – Vasospasm. – Aneurysm Surgery. – Functional Neurosurgery. – Subject Index.

Modern Neurosurgery is a new Springer-Verlag series whose volumes appear at four-year intervals.

The editor of Modern Neurosurgery is the Editor of Congress Publications of the World Federation of Neurosurgical Societies (WFNS). Each volume contains about 50 papers selected from the several hundred submitted to the corresponding WFNS Congress.

The aim of **Modern Neurosurgery** is to provide a precise and broad overview of the state of art of Neurosurgery as viewed by international authorities.

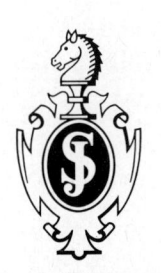

Springer-Verlag
Berlin
Heidelberg
New York

Advances in Neuro-surgery

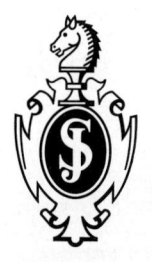

Springer-Verlag
Berlin
Heidelberg
New York

Volume 9

Brain Abscess and Meningitis Subarachnoid Hemorrhage: Timing Problems

Editors: W. Schiefer, M. Klinger, M. Brock
1981. 219 figures, 134 tables. XIX, 519 pages
ISBN 3-540-10539-5

Contents: Brain Abscess and Meningitis. – Subarachnoid Hemorrhage: Timing Problems. – Free Topics. – Subject Index.

Special aspects of two clinically important syndromes are covered in this volume. The first – brain abscesses and meningitis – is a growing problem due to the continuously changing spectrum of causative organisms and their rapid development of resistance to antibiotics. The bacteriology, clinical symptomology and treatment results of brain abscesses are presented here, with special reference to recent research on antibiotic penetration of the blood-brain barrier. The diagnostic use of computer tomography is also covered.

The second major topic – the course of treatment to be followed at the time of subarachnoid hemorrhage and thereafter – is presented in contributions reflecting the present level of experience with this difficult problem. Various aspects of the timing involved are discussed by prominent neurosurgeons. Featured in their discussion are reports on positive results obtained from antifibrinolytic therapy.

Volume 8

Surgery of Cervical Myelopathy Infantile Hydrocephalus: Long-Term Results

Editors: W. Grote, M. Brock, H.-E. Clar, M. Klinger, H.E. Nau
1980. 178 figures in 215 separate illustrations, 138 tables.
XVII, 456 pages
ISBN 3-540-09949-2

Contents: Cercvical Myelopathy. – Hydrocephalus in Childhood. – Free Topics. – Subject Index.

Volume 7

Neurosvascular Surgery Specialized Neurosurgical Techniques

Editors: F. Marguth, M. Brock, E. Kazner, M. Klinger, P. Schmiedek
1979. 202 figures in 249 separate illustrations, 85 tables.
XXII, 394 pages
ISBN 3-540-09675-2

Contents: Neurovascular Surgery. – Specialized Neurosurgical Techniques. – Free Topics. – Subject Index.